UNDERSTANDING PACIFIC PEOPLES HEALTH AND WELLBEING CHALLENGES IN AOTEAROA NEW ZEALAND

Sir Collin Tukuitonga,
Li'amanaia Roannie Ng Shiu and
Malaeulu Seuta'afili Patrick Thomsen (Eds)

UNDERSTANDING PACIFIC PEOPLES HEALTH AND WELLBEING CHALLENGES IN AOTEAROA NEW ZEALAND

Pacific Islander Studies

Collection Editors

Moeata Keil & Patrick Thomsen

First published in 2026 by Lived Places Publishing

British Library Cataloguing in Publication Data
A CIP record for this book is available from the British Library.

ISBN: 9781918026276 (pbk)
ISBN: 9781918026290 (ePDF)
ISBN: 9781918026283 (ePUB)

Cover design by Fiachra McCarthy
Book design by Rachel Trolove of Twin Trail Design
Typeset by Newgen Publishing, UK

Lived Places Publishing
P.O. Box 1845
47 Echo Avenue
Miller Place, NY 11764

www.livedplacespublishing.com

In loving memory of Tunumafono Fa'amoetauloa Avaula Colenso Fa'amoe MNZM (1972–2025). A giant in the disability community: Pacific leader and advocate who will always be remembered for a lifetime of courage, compassion and change making.

Ia manuia lava lau malaga.

Contents

Foreword

Pacific peoples have some of the worst health statistics in Aotearoa-New Zealand and despite several dedicated government policies and strategies over the years, they continue to show poor health outcomes. Ethnic inequities are pervasive and persistent with no sign of improvement largely as a result of the broader determinants of health. Risk factors such as obesity, unhealthy diets, and smoking disproportionately affect Pacific people. Adverse socioeconomic circumstances such as low income and cold, damp, and over-crowded houses are responsible for much of the health inequities seen in the country (Ministry of Health, 2020). High and rising prevalence of non-communicable diseases (NCDs) such as diabetes and heart disease reflect the impact of the commercial determinants of health on Pacific people. Undue consumption of highly processed foods and sugar-sweetened beverages is a major factor driving NCDs in Pacific people (Parnell et al., 2011). Prevention and control of NCDs including reducing the prevalence of childhood obesity is a key priority for Pacific people (Ministry of Health, 2020). It is not simply a matter of individuals making better choices but governments, civil society organisations, and the private sector making a collective effort to address the socioeconomic and commercial determinants of health in Aotearoa-New Zealand.

We have highlighted a number of critical issues affecting Pacific people in Aotearoa-New Zealand in this the first reference publication addressing the health of Pacific peoples in the country. These include a focus on children and young people, mental health and wellbeing, disabled people, and particular health concerns of Pacific Rainbow+ communities. The hope is that researchers and students of Pacific health will contribute to the generation of knowledge about various communities that make up the broader Pacific population group in Aotearoa-New Zealand.

A significant proportion of Pacific children and young people grow up in challenging social and economic environments. There is some evidence that longer term poverty has a more severe negative effect on children's outcomes than shorter term experiences of poverty. Childhood poverty negatively influences adult employment, education, income, health, and cognitive outcomes (Ministry of Social Development, 2018). The Pacific Islands Families (PIF) study has provided detailed health and development information on Pacific children in Aotearoa-New Zealand. It is an important source of information about Pacific children and young people. The study is embarking on information collection from the birth cohort as they approach 22 years. Additional information about Pacific children and young people can be obtained from the Growing Up in New Zealand (GUiNZ) Study (Growing Up in New Zealand, 2023). Further reducing the number of Pacific children living in poverty is an urgent priority for Aotearoa-New Zealand.

Increasing awareness of the importance of mental health and wellbeing is an important part of health improvement in Aotearoa-New Zealand. Additional updated information on the specific mental health needs of Pacific peoples is needed especially in relation to access and use of mental health services. Furthermore, there is an urgent need for better services for people with disabilities, addictions, and those of the Rainbow+ communities.

Improving the health and wellbeing of Pacific peoples is an urgent public policy for Aotearoa-New Zealand. A continuation of the same strategies and health plans will not deliver better health outcomes. Opportunities exist in the health reforms and the Pae Ora Legislation but plans need to be adequately resourced. Information in this reference text will help Pacific researchers and communities to monitor and report on the progress being made.

References

Ministry of Health. (2020). *Ola Manuia: Pacific Health and Wellbeing Action Plan 2020–2025*. https://www.health.govt.nz/system/files/documents/publications/ola_manuia-phwap-22june.pdf

Ministry of Social Development. (2018). *Rapid Evidence Review: The Impact of Poverty on Life Course Outcomes for Children, and the Likely Effect of Increasing the Adequacy of Welfare Benefits*. https://www.msd.govt.nz/documents/about-msd-and-our-work/publications-resources/information-releases/weag-report-release/rapid-evidence-review-the-impact-of-poverty-on-life-course-outcomes-for-children-and-the-likely-effect-of-increasing-the-adequacy-of-welfare-benef.pdf

Parnell, W., Wilson, N., Thomson, C., Mackay, S. and Stefanogiannis, N. (2011). *A Focus on Nutrition: Key Findings of the 2008/09 New Zealand Adult Nutrition Survey*. Ministry of Health.

Growing Up in New Zealand. (2023). *Home*. https://www.growingup.co.nz/

Contributors

Book Editors

Li'amanaia Dr Roannie Ng Shiu (Sāmoa) is Manager of the Pacific Academy of Sciences in Samoa, Co-Director of Te Poutoko Ora a Kiwa at Waipapa Taumata Rau, the University of Auckland and Adjunct Associate Professor of Science at the National University of Samoa. She is a public health, human geography and climate health expert. Her research focuses on equity and advancing the wellbeing of Pacific peoples globally.

Malaeulu Seuta'afili Associate Professor Patrick Thomsen (Sāmoa) is the newly appointed (March 2026) Associate Dean Pacific at the University of Otago Wellington's School of Medicine within the Department of Primary Healthcare and General Practice. Previously he was a Senior Research Fellow in Pacific Health and a Senior Lecturer in Global Studies at *Waipapa Taumata Rau*, the University of Auckland.

Professor Sir Collin Tukuitonga (Niue) is the Associate Dean Pacific in the Faculty of Medical and Health Sciences at Waipapa Taumata Rau, The University of Auckland. He is a leading public health physician and advocate for reducing health inequalities for Māori and Pacific people, was knighted in 2022 for his service and leadership in Pacific health. Sir Collin has been the Director of Public Health for New Zealand, the Head of Surveillance and

Prevention of NCDs at the World Health Organisation and the Director-General of the Pacific Community (SPC).

Chapter Authors

Phylesha Brown-Acton MNZM (Niue) is a proud fakafifine woman, advocate and community organiser, having served Pacific communities for over 20 years. As founder of F'INE Pasifika Aotearoa Trust, she has been at the forefront of advocating and serving Pacific Rainbow+ communities in various regional and global forums, including at the United Nations. As a researcher, her work focuses on empowering Pacific Rainbow+ communities and individuals to improve wellbeing outcomes for themselves and their families.

Tunumafono Faamoetauola Avaula Colenso Faamoe MNZM (Sāmoa - 1972–2025) was the founder and National Executive Officer of the Tōfā Mamao Collective, a grassroots movement advocating for the rights and inclusion of Pacific Disabled People in Aotearoa-New Zealand. Remembered as a giant in the Pacific Disability Movement, Tunumafono was highly respected in wider Pacific communities and as a key figure in South Auckland local government and community development.

Associate Professor David Taufui Mikato Fa'avae (Tonga) is a renowned scholar of Pacific/Pasifika education. Currently based at the University of Auckland, alongside Pacific masculinities, Associate Professor Fa'avae's work covers indigenous studies and sociology of education and is considered a contemporary leader in the utilisation of methodologies like talanoa-vā and Pacific philosophies.

Dr Edmond Fehoko (Tonga) was born and raised in New Zealand. Completing his studies with a BA (Criminology and Social Sciences), MA (Hons) and PhD (Public Health) at Auckland University of Technology, Dr Fehoko is currently a senior lecturer with the Department of Human Nutrition and Associate Dean Pacific with the Division of Sciences at the University of Otago.

Dr Siale Foliaki MNZM (Tonga) is a leading Pacific psychiatrist with over 20 years of experience dedicated to improving Pacific mental health in Aotearoa-New Zealand. Dr Foliaki was awarded the New Zealand Order of Merit in 2023 for his services to Pacific mental health. He is also the Board Director for Vaka Tautua, who provide mental health and disability support for older Pacific people in Auckland, Wellington, Canterbury and Otago.

Dr Corina Grey (Sāmoa, Pākehā) is the first Pacific Woman Director of Public Health for New Zealand's Ministry of Health. As a physician and epidemiologist, Dr Grey has over two decades of experience working in the health sector and public sector agencies. Her work has consistently focused on addressing health inequalities/inequities and improving outcomes, particularly for Pacific and Māori communities.

Dr John Huakau (Tonga, England) is the Principal Advisor at the Pasifika Medical Association Group and an Honorary Lecturer at the University of Auckland. John's academic background is in statistics, epidemiology, and public health. John has over 11 years of experience with Whānau Ora and Commissioning for Outcomes.

Dr Leon Iusitini (Sāmoa, Cook Islands, Pākehā) is a researcher at the Auckland University of Technology. He has been a member of the Pacific Islands Families Study research team since 2006.

His research interests are in the wellbeing of Pacific populations in New Zealand, especially Pacific child development.

Dr Sam Manuela (Cook Islands) is a Senior Lecturer in Psychology at The University of Auckland. His research focuses on Pacific peoples' wellbeing, ethnic identity, and mental health. He has additional interests in psychometrics, ethnicity data, and data sovereignty across Aotearoa New Zealand and the Pacific region.

Professor Vili Nosa (Niue) is a professor of public health in the Department of Pacific Health as part of the School of Population Health within the Faculty of Medical Health Sciences at Waipapa Taumata Rau – University of Auckland and an Adjunct Professor in Public Health, School of Public Health at the University of Queensland, Brisbane, Australia. His research focuses on Pacific health issues in Aotearoa-New Zealand and the Pacific region, with specialisations in Pacific addictions research such as alcohol, tobacco, illicit drugs and substance abuse.

Dr Karaponi Okesene-Gafa (Niue, Samoa, Cook Islands) is a prominent obstetrician, gynaecologist, and the Head of Pacific Health at Waipapa Taumata Rau, the University of Auckland. She is a passionate advocate for Pacific women's health, focussing her research on addressing high BMI in pregnancy and improving outcomes for multi-ethnic populations. Her work also involves developing pathways for Pacific doctors and raising awareness about conditions such as endometrial cancer.

Dame Teuila Percival (Sāmoa) is a consultant paediatrician at KidzFirst Children's Hospital, South Auckland, and an associate professor in the Department of Paediatrics at the University of

Auckland. Dr Percival was made a Dame (DNZM) in the King's Birthday Honours in 2023 and awarded the Queen's Service Order (QSO) in 2010 for service to the Pacific Community and children.

Asetoa Sam Pilisi (Niue, Sāmoa) is a PhD candidate at the University of Auckland's School of Population Health, exploring wellbeing, self-care, and burnout among Pacific peoples. Alongside his doctoral research, Asetoa oversees Pacific health workforce development, from preparing secondary students for health pathways to strengthening clinical, service, and research capacity across Aotearoa and the Pacific.

Debbie Sorensen ONZM (Tonga) serves as the CEO of the Pasifika Medical Association Group and an Honorary Professional Teaching Fellow at Waipapa Taumata Rau, the University of Auckland. Debbie has led the development of the Pasifika Medical Association Group over the past 15 years, transforming it into the largest Non-Governmental Pacific organisation in the Pacific region.

Dr Brittany Stanley-Wishart (Samoa, Cook Islands, Lebanon, Scotland, Ireland) is currently completing her psychiatry fellowship and serves on the board for Malologa Ltd and YWCA Greater Wellington. She blends Western training with Indigenous knowledge to support more holistic, collaborative, and meaningful mental health care for the community.

Professor El-Shadan Tautolo (Sāmoa, Cook Islands) has ties to Fa'asito'o Uta and Tanugamanono in Samoa and Tongareva in the Cook Islands. He is a professor in the Centre for Pacific Health and Development Research at the Auckland University of Technology. Professor Tautolo has also been the Director of the

Pacific Islands Families Study since 2014. He is passionate about the health of Pacific families and continually strives to use his research to support the needs of Pacific communities.

Sione Tu'itahi (Tonga) is an educator, writer, and public health leader whose work spans planetary health, health determinants, human rights, and Indigenous knowledge. He is Executive Director of the Health Promotion Forum of New Zealand, former President of IUHPE, and a World Health Organization technical adviser on planetary health promotion and Indigenous knowledge.

Allyssa Verner-Pula is a doctoral candidate at Waiapa Taumata Rau, The University of Auckland, in Pacific Studies. She was the research associate on the Manalagi Project and completed her Master's degree in Pacific Studies. She is also an award-winning podcaster and blogger focusing on elevating Pacific young peoples' experiences and voices.

Pastor Dr Paul Muamai Vui Siope, **Malaeulu Leatuavao Rebekah Rimoni**, **Fuimaono Puasina Salanoa**, **Nuualii Tupaimatuna**, **Luse Hellen Folau**, **Leah Sosofa Leata Purea**, and **Fetaui Iosefo** are members of the 'Aiga Komiti Sa and Tapasā Mo Aiga (TMA), working collectively in community wellbeing, counselling, and Indigenous healing within the Samoan diaspora.

Setting the scene: Pacific health research in Aotearoa-New Zealand

Sir Collin Tukuitonga; Roannie Ng Shiu

Chapter summary

This chapter presents a historical and contemporary analysis of the dynamics of Pacific peoples in Aotearoa New Zealand in relation to its significance to health research. Tracing Pacific peoples' journey from early migrations to Aotearoa New Zealand, and the systemic inequalities which has created health disparities for Pacific peoples, this chapter draws attention to the significant socioeconomic challenges that have created adverse effects on health and wellbeing for our communities. The chapter emphasises the importance of addressing these issues through a public health lens, focusing on social determinants of health. It highlights the resilience of Pacific communities, particularly during the COVID-19 pandemic, and underscores the necessity of culturally competent healthcare solutions. By exploring population and health trends among Pacific peoples, the chapter aims to provide an understanding of the multifaceted issues affecting our communities and calls for targeted action to remedy historical injustices while promoting health equity in New Zealand, which is why this book matters for Pacific peoples and Aotearoa New Zealand today.

Introduction

Aotearoa New Zealand has had strong historic links with the Pacific region since at least 1901 when the Cook Islands and Niue became colonial territories of New Zealand. Tokelau later joined the New Zealand realm in 1925 which enabled Tokelauans citizenship and rights of residence like Cook Islanders and Niueans. After the Second World War, there was rapid growth in the Pacific population in Aotearoa. This growth and movement of Pacific migrants to New Zealand was welcomed and encouraged by the New Zealand government given the post-war labour shortages. Initial labour programmes were focussed on bringing young Pacific men to work as agricultural and forest workers while young Pacific women were employed as domestic workers. New Zealand experienced a manufacturing boom in the late 1960s and early 1970s. This boom coupled with a labour shortage led to another wave of migration from the Pacific.

However, New Zealand soon faced an economic downturn with increasing unemployment and Pacific people were no longer welcomed. A new, tumultuous relationship between Pacific people and New Zealand began, highlighted by the Dawn Raids of 1974–1976. The New Zealand police were given powers and rights to enter people's homes and to stop and ask anyone on the street for documents to prove they were in New Zealand legally in order to identify those who had overstayed their visa permit. The irony of this directive is that Pacific people were exclusively targeted despite the majority of overstayers coming from Europe or North America. As part of this new government directive, New Zealand police raided homes with known Pacific families at dawn for searches giving rise to the term Dawn Raids. Since the Dawn Raids and what has been described by Dr Melani Anae (2020) as 'the most blatantly racist attack on Pacific peoples by the New Zealand government in New Zealand's history,' this history of racial discrimination has had permeating effects on the health and wellbeing of Pacific people in Aotearoa.

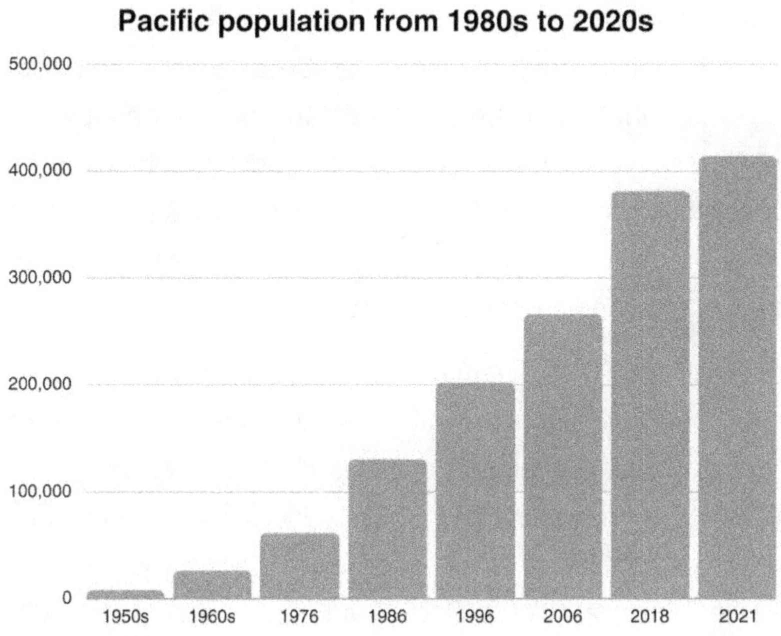

Today, Pacific people in Aotearoa New Zealand, represent a diverse and vibrant population group of about 17 well-established Pacific ethnicities that contribute to the country's social and multicultural fabric. The impact that Pacific people have had on Auckland culturally, economically, and socially has meant that Auckland is often described as the world's largest Polynesian city. While Pacific people have made positive contributions to Aotearoa New Zealand, persistent inequalities and the lack of investment in the health and wellbeing of Pacific families have had a range of impacts. Addressing health inequalities in Pacific communities and understanding the issues that impact on the health and wellbeing of Pacific families is important for the future of the country.

Taking a public health view and social determinants of health (SDH) approach to addressing Pacific health issues allow us to better understand, and nuance, the determinants that impact on the health and wellbeing of Pacific peoples in Aotearoa New Zealand. SDH are the non-medical factors that influence health outcomes which describe the conditions in 'which people are born, grow, work, live and age and the wider set of forces and systems shaping the conditions of daily life' (Solar & Irwin, 2010). Addressing health inequities in Pacific communities contributes to a more just and equitable society.

Focusing on SDH and framing health as a social phenomenon enables us to think critically about what is needed to create a more equitable social environment for Pacific communities. Realising health equity, that is, the absence of unfair and avoidable or remediable differences in health among social groups requires significant resourcing to address historic health disparities and inequities for Pacific communities in New Zealand who have experienced higher rates of long-term illnesses and infectious diseases and lower life expectancies. Addressing these inequities is crucial to achieving health outcomes that are fair and just for all populations in Aotearoa-New Zealand.

In August 2021 when this anthology of Pacific health in Aotearoa New Zealand was initially proposed, Aotearoa New Zealand and Auckland specifically went through significant COVID-19 lockdowns. Many of the authors and contributors to this edition were at the forefront of New Zealand's pandemic response. Pacific communities were disproportionately affected by the pandemic as several COVID-19 outbreaks occurred in Pacific communities. The silver lining of the COVID-19 outbreaks and the subsequent vaccination drives demonstrated the resilience of Pacific communities and the effectiveness of Pacific leadership in addressing Pacific health problems. The challenge now remains on how the learnings from the pandemic and Pacific leadership in Pacific health issues continues to help address current health challenges.

Population trends and patterns

The Pacific population represents 9% of the total population (an estimated 459,200) (Stats NZ, 2023). The seven largest Pacific groups in Aotearoa are Samoan, Tongan, Cook Island, Niuean, Fijian, Tokelauan, and Tuvaluan (Stats NZ, 2023). As a well-established ethnic group more than 60% of the population was born in Aotearoa New Zealand and of those born overseas, more than 60% have lived in Aotearoa for more than 10 years (Ministry for Pacific Peoples, 2021). Pacific populations continue to have relatively high birth rates which contributes to strong population growth and relatively high net migration which tends to be associated with younger age groups leading to a projected population growth of 1.9% over the next 10 years. These trends contrast with Europeans who are ageing faster and growing slower compared to other ethnic groups (Brundson, 2023).

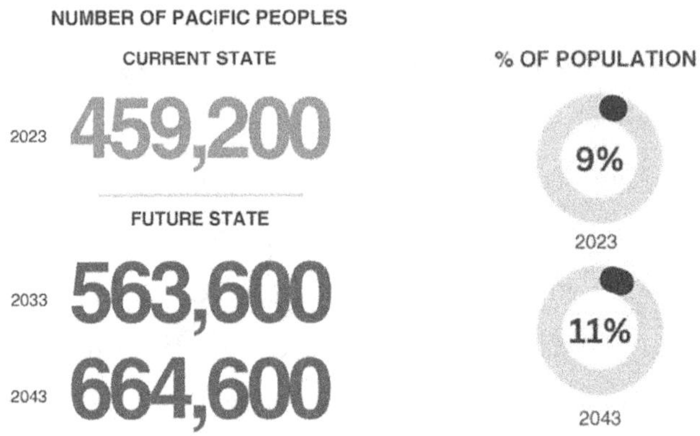

The majority of Pacific communities live in Auckland; the number of Pacific people living in rural areas is likely to increase from its current state of 7.2%.

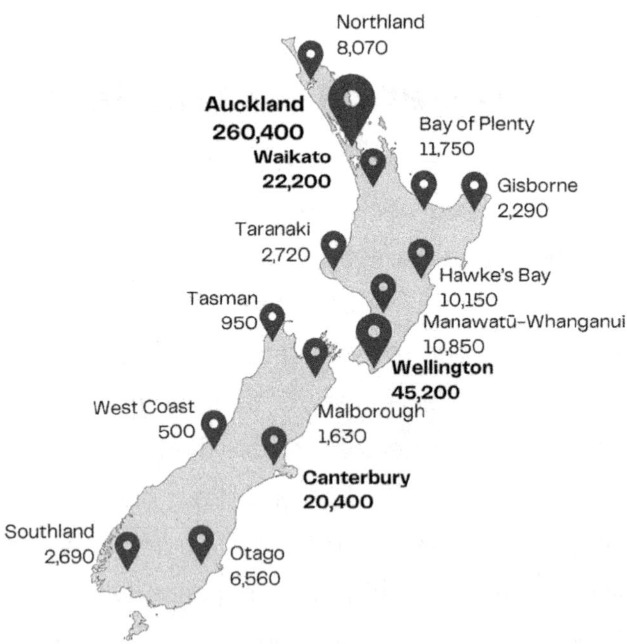
Northland
8,070
Auckland
260,400
Waikato
22,200
Bay of Plenty
11,750
Gisborne
2,290
Taranaki
2,720
Hawke's Bay
10,150
Manawatū-Whanganui
10,850
Wellington
45,200
Tasman
950
West Coast
500
Malborough
1,630
Canterbury
20,400
Southland
2,690
Otago
6,560

Almost half of the Pacific population identify as Samoan (49%) with the number of Pacific people identifying with more than one ethnic group increasing as 50% of Pacific children aged 0–14 years identify with more than one ethnic group. A key contemporary demographic feature of Aotearoa New Zealand is the number of people who identify as both Māori and Pacific, currently at 58,000, 50% of whom are younger than 15 years old (Ministry of Health, 2023).

The Pacific population has a much younger age structure than the country's total population. Approximately 33% of Pacific peoples in Aotearoa are younger than 15 years old and 50% are younger than 25 years old. In an ageing population, the Pacific working-age population is projected to increase from almost 300,000 in 2023 to 420,000 by 2043, which is an important demographic feature for Aotearoa-New Zealand as a whole (Stats NZ, 2023).

These trends point towards a growing, youthful, and ethnically diverse population. While the majority of Pacific people will continue to reside in urban cities, there will be an increase of Pacific people living in rural areas who also identify as Māori. This will have important implications for the future health and wellbeing of Aotearoa New Zealand, as a whole. Unaddressed health issues within the Pacific population can have economic consequences, including increased healthcare costs and lost productivity. Therefore, investing in the health of Pacific children and young people today is an investment in the future health and wellbeing of New Zealand.

Socioeconomic trends

A key feature of SDH is understanding the social and economic conditions in which people live in. These include income and social protection, education and literacy, unemployment and job insecurity, working life conditions, and food security. The following table provides an overview of key socioeconomic indicators compared to Europeans.

	PACIFIC PEOPLES	EUROPEANS
Median personal annual income	$24,300	$34,500
Unemployment rate (June 2022)	5.4%	2.9%
School leaver with NCEA 2 or above	76.2%	81.1%
Individual home ownership	21%	58%
Severe housing deprivation (per 10,000)	245.5	41.2
Dwellings lack basic amenities (disabled)	17.3%	5.6%
Dwellings lack basic amenities (not disabled)	9.7%	3.1%
% children living in material hardship	25.6%	7.6%

These comparisons demonstrate the social and economic gaps between Pacific communities and their European counterparts. To put into context what some of these comparisons mean in real terms, we can look to current figures on gender and ethnic pay gaps where the biggest pay gap in Aotearoa New Zealand is between European men and Pacific women at 25%. At this rate it will take about 110 years respectively to reach pay equity (Human Rights Commission, 2021).

The median personal annual income reflects the over-representation of Pacific people in low skilled occupations (53%) such as labour hire and packing type activities compared to 22% in highly-skilled occupations. Education achievement can provide some explanation. In 2021, Pacific achievement in school with NCEA 2 or above at 76% is comparable to 79% for all ethnicities. The gains made at school, however, have yet to be translated into tertiary education with 23% of Pacific people holding a Level 4 or higher qualification compared to 35% for the overall population (Brundson, 2023).

Pacific cultures often emphasise the importance of family and community and this is reflected in Pacific peoples preferred way of living. Pacific families are more likely to live in rented, large intergenerational homes. Intergenerational homes and large households can enable Pacific language retention and promote general family wellbeing. However, these homes are often insufficient in size, have poor insulation and are more likely to have issues with mould leading to overall poorer physical and mental health for Pacific families (Stats NZ, 2023). Affordable, safe, and warm housing is important for health and wellbeing. Recognising and integrating multigenerational and collective ways of living is also an important consideration for healthcare policy and practice that can positively impact the overall health and wellbeing of Pacific families and communities.

Home ownership is an important factor in securing intergenerational wealth, financial stability, and economic mobility. Pacific peoples experienced a net and percentage decrease in home ownership since the 1980s, where in 1986 half of Pacific peoples lived in owner-occupied dwellings, which fell to just over one-third in 2018 (Stats NZ, 2023). The fact that Pacific peoples are less likely to own their homes today than their parents and grandparents' generations, speaks to further challenges in realising optimal health outcomes for Pacific communities that are tied to structural issues in wider society. In fact, Pacific peoples experience severe housing deprivation at greater rate than the total population. With homelessness prevalence at 578 per 10,000 people compared with 217 people per 10,000 people for the total population (Stats NZ, 2023).

Health trends

Pacific peoples together with Māori have the poorest health outcomes in Aotearoa New Zealand. Information on health outcome trends for Pacific peoples is limited and available projections may be unreliable due to quality of underlying data. Research has shown that there are substantial health disparities for Pacific peoples leading to a gap in life expectancy at birth between Pacific men (75.4 years) and women (79 years) compared to European men (81 years) and women (84.5 years). This gap is largely explained by premature deaths that could have been prevented with early health interventions, improved socioeconomic conditions, and better access to medicine and health care.

	LIFE EXPECTANCY - PACIFIC	LIFE EXPECTANCY - EUROPEAN
MEN	75.4 YEARS	81.0 YEARS
WOMEN	79.0 YEARS	84.5 YEARS

Health inequities for Pacific peoples are experienced throughout their life course. Improved maternal health care will help to stem some of these trends, particularly by ensuring that every Pacific mother has access to a lead maternity carer within their first trimester. This will help to decrease the infant death rate for Pacific babies at 7.1 per 1,000 live births, the highest for all ethnic groups in New Zealand (MOH, 2023).

Rheumatic fever, a disease that is almost nonexistent in most high-income countries, remains stubbornly high for Pacific children, having lasting lifelong effects as they become adults (MOH, 2023). Dame Teuila Percival's chapter on Pacific children and young people will provide important insights into the state of Pacific child health in Aotearoa-New Zealand.

Pacific adults experience long term chronic illnesses at a higher rate and earlier age compared to the total population. Pacific adults are more than likely to experience multimorbidity, that is the presence of two or more chronic conditions. For example, 35% of Pacific peoples aged 65 years have multimorbidity compared with 15% of Europeans. The vast majority of these commonly-diagnosed conditions include cancers, heart disease, and renal diseases (Gurney et al., 2020).

One of the most concerning health issues for Pacific women in Aotearoa, is living with the consequences of obesity. The obesity epidemic has continued to increase globally, in Aotearoa and in the Pacific, worsening the health outcomes of Pacific women throughout their life course. Obesity not only affects the life of women, but also of their families and communities. Te Whatu Ora, Counties Manukau in South Auckland where the highest proportion of Pacific people reside, Pacific women with overweight and obesity who birthed in their facility were 17.2% and 72.1%, respectively. The parallel rise in diabetes in pregnancy as a consequence is also concerning (Counties Manukau Health, 2020).

To address the high prevalence of cancers for Pacific women requires improved access to diagnostic health care (Meredith, Sarfati et al., 2012). Highest proportion of Pacific women with endometrial cancer were in obesity class III (BMI ≥ 40kg/m^2) with most having risk factors for diabetes, impaired glucose tolerance (IGT), hypertension, hyperlipidemia, and nulliparity.

As a youthful, diverse, and growing population, understanding Pacific people's experiences of mental illness within New Zealand (including risk and protective factors), is one of the first steps to developing solutions that can lead to more equitable mental health outcomes for future generations of Pacific people. Despite the higher overall prevalence of mental disorders, the rate of Pacific people receiving mental health treatment has previously been identified as 35% lower than the rate for the total New Zealand population (Ministry of Health, 2005). Providing culturally competent and integrated healthcare services is essential to meeting the unique needs of Pacific communities. While there has been more research and resourcing into mental health for Pacific people improving access to culturally safe mental health services remains a priority.

Research and data needs for a healthy and informed future

Research and data on the health of Pacific peoples is a challenge with substantial gaps in data quality and availability. However, this anthology provides a starting point to provide an overview of key health issues for Pacific people in Aotearoa New Zealand, written by Pacific health scholars that moves beyond merely statistics and descriptions but provides a nuanced understanding of Pacific peoples' health and wellbeing. Subsequent editions in the future will begin to capture better data and research initiatives that focus on Pacific health issues to inform evidence-based policies and describe data innovations that allow for the monitoring of the effectiveness of interventions and the overall state of Pacific health. Addressing the complex issues surrounding access to healthcare for Pacific people in New Zealand requires a comprehensive, collaborative, and culturally competent approach involving government agencies, healthcare providers, community organizations, and the Pacific community itself.

References

Brundson, N. (2023). Insights into New Zealand's Pacific people. *Infometrics*. https://economics.infometrics.co.nz/article/2023-11-insights-into-new-zealands-pacific-people

Counties Manukau Health. (2020). *Women's Health and Newborn, Annual Report: 2019 - 2020*. https://www.countiesmanukau.health.nz/assets/About-CMH/Reports-and-planning/Maternity/2020_CMH_maternity_Annual_Report.pdf

Gurney, J., Stanley, J. and Sarfati, D. (2020). The inequity of morbidity: Disparities in the prevalence of morbidity between ethnic groups in New Zealand. *Journal of Comorbidity*, 10, 2235042X20971168.

Human Rights Commission. (2021). Inquiry into the Pacific Pay Gap. Human Rights Commission. https://tikatangata.org.nz/our-work/inquiry-into-the-pacific-pay-gap

Ministry of Health. (2005). *Te Orau Ora: Pacific Mental Health Profile. Wellington: Ministry of Health.* https://www.moh.govt.nz/notebook/nbbooks.nsf/0/9f56f480f030606acc2570180070fc77/$FILE/pacificmentalhealthprofile.pdf

Ministry of Health. (2023). *Te Mana Ola: The Pacific Health Strategy.* Ministry of Health. https://www.health.govt.nz/publication/te-mana-ola-pacific-health-strategy

Melani Anae, The Platform: The Radical Legacy of the Polynesian Panthers, Bridget Williams Books, Wellington, 2020

Meredith, I., Sarfati, D., Ikeda, T., & Blakely, T. (2012). Cancer in Pacific people in New Zealand. *Cancer Causes & Control*, *23*(7), 1173–1184. https://doi.org/10.1007/s10552-012-9986-x

Ministry for Pacific Peoples 2021 Pacific wellbeing strategy. Wellington: Ministry for Pacific Peoples.

Solar, O. and Irwin, A. A Conceptual Framework for Action on the Social Determinants of Health. WHO Social Determinants of Health Discussion Paper 2 (Policy and Practice), 2010.

Stats NZ, Pacific housing: people, place, and wellbeing, 2023

Pacific identity and wellbeing

Sam Manuela

Chapter summary

This chapter explores the dynamic nature of Pacific ethnic identities/ethnicity and wellbeing, emphasising the pivotal role of relationships and connections in shaping the multifaceted identities of diverse Pacific communities. This chapter argues that the vā, an indigenous Pacific socio-spatial concept, is fundamental to understanding Pacific identities and wellbeing, acting as a framework that underscores the significance of relationships. In doing so, the chapter posits that measurements of Pacific identities and wellbeing require drawing on a combination of Pacific and psychological theories and methods. The positive correlation between components of Pacific ethnic identity being protective of wellbeing is highlighted, with an emphasis on unravelling the mechanisms at play for effective intervention strategies.

Introduction

There is a vast diversity of Pacific nations represented in Aotearoa, with differing and shared histories, including differences in place of birth, and an increasing number of multi-ethnic peoples – particularly in younger age groups (Stats NZ, 2005). Recognising this diversity means recognising that there is no single way Pacific peoples may view and understand their ethnic identity. Ethnic identity and wellbeing are multifaceted constructs. Psychological research has historically leaned towards a more parsimonious definition and understanding of the two. However, recent theorising has adopted more cultural nuance and recognition of the social, political, and contextual influences on the ways ethnic identity and wellbeing can be understood and experienced. In contrast, Pacific research on identities and wellbeing are centred on the cultural knowledge systems embedded within Pacific worldviews. These provide deeper and more meaningful explanations on how Pacific peoples can experience a sense of who they are and what it means to live well. This chapter will integrate psychological and Pacific literature, theories, and research on ethnic identity and wellbeing, offering another perspective on the relationship between these two constructs and how they add to health research in Aotearoa New Zealand.

Clarity between ethnicity and ethnic identity

The associations between ethnicity and health outcomes are becoming increasingly complex, particularly with how ethnicity is categorised for identifying with multiple ethnic groups (Yao et al., 2025). Understanding the relationships between ethnicity and health provides crucial information about the social and systemic issues contributing to health disparities. However, care must be taken to ensure that findings do not present ethnic minorities in a deficit manner, nor present ethnicity itself as a variable responsible for health disparities. Furthermore, care must be taken to ensure that ethnicity is not conflated with ethnic identity. Ethnicity is viewed in social sciences as a social construct. It is defined by Stats NZ (2005) as the ethnic group or groups that people identify with or feel they belong to, a measure of cultural affiliation, and is self-perceived. While this definition shares some similarities with ethnic identity, ethnicity and ethnic identity are measured differently. Ethnicity is usually measured as a response to a question where people can indicate the ethnic group/s they identify with. This provides categorical data about which ethnic group (or groups – see Yao et al., 2025 for a discussion on multi-ethnic data analyses). Categorical ethnicity does not provide information about the extent to which someone's ethnicity holds meaning to their sense of self, beyond self-affiliation. Conflating ethnicity and ethnic identity risks attributing health inequities to cultural or psychological differences when there may be no empirical justification for doing so – otherwise known as the cultural attribution fallacy (Matsumoto & Jones, 2009). Ethnic identity provides more detail about how a sense of self can influence their experiences within systems, further influencing their health and wellbeing (Haslam et al., 2009).

Psychological perspectives on ethnic identity and wellbeing

There are parallels between Pacific and psychological theories of identity. While psychology has advanced what is currently known about the relationships between identity and wellbeing, Eurocentric biases in psychological theories and methods limit their applicability to understanding Pacific identities and wellbeing (Henrich et al., 2010). Despite this, there are parallels that can be drawn between psychological and Pacific perspectives.

Ethnic identity

Psychology describes ethnic identity as a multifaceted construct comprising feelings, thoughts, and attitudes towards being a member of an ethnic group (Yip, 2018). Ethnic identity includes self-identification with an ethnic group, attitudes towards group membership, a sense of belonging, behaviours (Phinney, 1990), and perceptions about how central ethnicity is to one's identity (Sellers et al., 1998). Broader concepts of ethnic-racial identity include aspects of content (such as attitudes, beliefs, and relationships) and *processes* (how people explore, form, and maintain their ethnic identities (Umaña-Taylor et al., 2014). Ethnic identity development is proposed as consisting of both exploration of what one's ethnicity means to them, and a commitment to that identity (Phinney & Ong, 2007), recognising how this occurs within social, cultural, historical, and political contexts, often against a backdrop of discrimination for ethnic minorities (Yip, 2018).

A key distinction in understanding identity, and thus ethnic identity, is understanding different self-construals (Cross et al., 2011). There are three types of self-construal:

1. *Independent self-construal*: Understanding the self as distinct from others, emphasising personal abilities, traits, and preferences. There is an assumption that individual goals are emphasised over group goals.
2. *Interdependent self-construal*: Understanding the self as connected to others, emphasising group roles, and group goals over individual goals.

3. *Relational self-construal*: Understanding the self in terms of close, dyadic relationships.

An individual's self-construal may be a combination of independent, interdependent, and relational, however socialisation within different cultural contexts may put greater emphasis on one. For example, a stronger emphasis on relationships within Pacific cultural contexts may mean Pacific peoples are more socialised in understanding their selves in terms of the relationships that they have with others.

Ethnic identity differs from ethnicity in that it is multi-factorial and dimensional, providing more information about the extent to which one's ethnicity is a centrally defining aspect of their self. Measures of ethnic identity are useful in this regard as they provide information on individual variability. The most common measure is the Multigroup Ethnic Identity Measure (Phinney, 1992; Phinney & Ong, 2007) which can provide information about how salient someone's ethnic group affiliation is to their life. Recognising variability in how people understand their ethnic identity and the extent to which it is a salient part of their life is associated with health and wellbeing outcomes. For instance, positive ethnic identity is associated with wellbeing (Espinosa et al., 2018; Smith & Silva, 2011), providing evidence for the contributions that strong ethnic identity can have for positive health outcomes.

Wellbeing

Prevailing psychological definitions present wellbeing as a subjective experience that includes emotional responses, satisfaction within different domains of life, and global judgements of life satisfaction (Diener et al., 1999). Thus, wellbeing has two broad affective and cognitive components. The affective component refers to the positive and negative emotions, moods, and feelings associated with our everyday experiences. The cognitive component refers to how people think about their lives and what leads them to evaluate it positively. For instance, life satisfaction may be understood as a person's assessment of whether there is a discrepancy between their current situation and their ideal situation. Wellbeing has also been defined as a balance between having psychological, social, and physical resources to meet psychological, social, and physical challenges (Dodge et al., 2012). Bridging these two definitions, wellbeing can be understood as a combination of satisfaction with different domains of life, together with the feelings and emotions that go with them, and being able to face the challenges that can affect them.

Measurements of wellbeing provide information about individual variability in the ways that people appraise their life. Such measures include the Satisfaction with Life Scale (Diener et al., 1985) which asks people to rate on a more global level how satisfied they are with their life as a whole, and the Personal Wellbeing Index (Cummins et al., 2003), which asks people to rate how satisfied they are with different domains of their life including: standard of living, health, achievements in life, personal relationships, safety, sense of community, and future security.

Psychology presents ethnic identity and wellbeing as separate but positively related constructs. Understanding the mechanisms of the positive relationship between ethnic identity and wellbeing indicates those who have a secure understanding of what their ethnicity means to them have a psychological resource that can help counter negative experiences and thus protect their wellbeing. Understanding the mechanism of this relationship is important, and Pacific perspectives of ethnic identity offer valuable theoretical insights into how the two are connected.

Pacific identities and wellbeing

Pacific identities can refer to ethnic-specific identities (e.g., a Cook Island ethnic identity) or a broader 'Pacific' identity reflecting the shared experiences and common histories that transcend the uniqueness and nuances of ethnic-specific identities within the Aotearoa context. The 'Pacific' label and other derivatives (e.g., Pasifika) are contested terms with origins in the early Pacific migration to Aotearoa. Despite this, the broader Pacific category provides a wider group which people can identify with simultaneously (or separately) with ethnic-specific Pacific identities. There is also a growing proportion of people with multiple ethnic backgrounds, including Pacific ethnicities (e.g., Tongan and Māori, Niuean and European). Layered on this is the mobility of Pacific peoples, recognising that identities can develop across multiple locations with different social influences within them. For instance, how ethnic identity develops in the Cook Islands may differ from Aotearoa. This is commonly categorised as 'Island-born' and 'New Zealand-born', recognising different socialising experiences that can influence how Pacific peoples view the world around them.

Pacific cultures emphasise interdependence and relationships – leaning strongly into a holistic worldview that includes physical, mental, emotional, spiritual, cultural, social, and environmental domains (See Figure 1). A useful concept for understanding

Pacific worldviews is vā. Albert Wendt articulates vā as a space that relates, that creates meaning, and how these meanings can change with context (Wendt, 1996). As Ka'ili (2005) posits, vā emphasises a space between rather than emptiness (Ka'ili, 2005). Mila-Schaaf bridges multiple understandings of vā to describe how relationships within social spaces shape identity; thus, Pacific identities are continuously shaped within the contexts of multiple relationships (Mila-Schaaf, 2006).

It is within the vā that connections and relationships are identified, formed, negotiated, maintained, and nurtured. A relational self-construal is the closest comparison from psychological perspectives where a sense of self is defined by the relationships to others in a given context. However, a relational self-construal is limited as the focus is on dyadic relationships, ignoring the wider sense of connections that people may experience with multiple peoples, past and present. Vā positions relatedness as culturally situated. The meanings and relationships depend on whom the vā is shared with, underpinned by respective cultural values for each Pacific group. For instance, Tongan culture recognises a father's oldest sister as holding a high status within a family at formal and informal social occasions. Roles and expectations are learned through socialisation within Tongan families and cultural events. Emphasis is put on maintaining relationships – tauhi vā. Learning and understanding the intricacies of these relationships within Tongan cultural concepts informs what it means to be Tongan – a Tongan ethnic identity.

The emphasis on relationality extends into a multitude of familial and wider social relationships for many Pacific peoples. For instance, the vā between a parent and children will have different meanings between the vā between a manager and employees, or a teacher and students. These relationships may change over time, but the vā remains as the constant space in which those relationships are negotiated and create meaning for the self. This presents Pacific identities as fluid and dynamic, with core elements remaining consistent over time, but our connections to them changing as our contexts change.

Components of Pacific identities

While vā provides a unique cultural lens to understand identity, there are similarities between Pacific and psychological perspectives that extend further than relational aspects of identity and self-hood. These include the ethnic labels we use, positive affect, attitudes, and beliefs around what our ethnicity means to us. Further to this, Pacific perspectives of identity lean more into a holistic conceptualisation with an emphasis on the groups we affiliate with, and the relationships that we have with those around us. Pacific identity perspectives include spirituality which can be derived through religious orientations, or more spiritually-based connections with others and lands. This recognises that Pacific identities also encompass connections and a sense of belonging to places, lands, and environments. Related to spirituality, religiosity has been identified as a link between broader domains of Pacific identities and wellbeing (Manuela & Sibley, 2014). Aspects of spirituality and environments are often missing from Western psychological perspectives of ethnic identity.

Measurements of Pacific identities and wellbeing requires drawing on a combination of Pacific and psychological theories and methods. The Pacific Identity and Wellbeing Scale (Manuela &

Sibley, 2013; Manuela & Sibley, 2015) identifies six domains common across Pacific and psychological perspectives of identity and wellbeing (see Table 1), and also provides a way to assess the dimensionality of each of these domains. This means that although there may be common aspects across Pacific identity and wellbeing research, there is no uniform way Pacific peoples experience or understand their identity and wellbeing. A measure designed for Pacific peoples allows researchers to understand individual variability in the extent to which Pacific peoples view their ethnicity as a part of their identity. This recognises that just as there is no single 'Pacific' community, there is also no single way of 'being' Pacific or what Pacific identity can mean for a Pacific person.

Research with the Pacific Identity and Wellbeing Scale has shown how specific components of Pacific ethnic identity are protective of wellbeing. Experiences of ethnic discrimination can negatively affect Pacific peoples physical and mental health (Kapeli et al., 2020; Pascoe & Smart Richman, 2009). Discrimination is an identity related stressor, despite ethnic identity being positively related to wellbeing. However, the impact of discrimination on wellbeing depends on *how* Pacific peoples identify with their ethnicity. Manuela (2021) showed that for Pacific peoples that reported low scores on Group Membership Evaluation (see Table 1), experiences of discrimination had a more detrimental effect on satisfaction with family, life, and health. However, for those that reported high scores on Group Membership Evaluation, there was no significant association between discrimination and the same satisfaction domains. This pattern of findings suggests that high ethnic identity acts as a buffer against the harmful effects of discrimination for Pacific peoples.

Wellbeing

Drawing on vā provides another way to conceptualise Pacific wellbeing. Vā can also refer to the space between people and objects, or people and places, and thus provides a socio-spatial understanding of the relationships between people and their environment. From this, Pacific wellbeing can be understood as a layered array of relationships that occur across multiple domains

Table 1: Factors and definitions of the Pacific Identity and Wellbeing Scale (Manuela and Sibley, 2013; 2015).

Factor	Definition
Perceived Familial Wellbeing	Satisfaction with different aspects of one's family life.
Perceived Societal Wellbeing	Satisfaction with different aspects of New Zealand society, including government and local community.
Group Membership Evaluation	Subjective evaluations of a perceived connections to the broader Pacific category, and positive affect.
Pacific Connectedness and Belonging	A sense of belonging and connections with Pacific others.
Religious Centrality and Embeddedness	The extent to which one feels religion is intertwined with their identity.
Cultural Efficacy	The extent to which one feels they are able to participate within Pacific cultural contexts.

of life. These are illustrated by the numerous Pacific models of health.

The Fonofale model (Pultou-Endemann, 2021) uses the architecture of a fale to symbolise various domains important to the holistic health and wellbeing of Pacific peoples. The foundation of the fale representing family – the foundation of Pacific social structures and providing overall support for the structure. The roof representing culture – such as values, beliefs, language. Four pou (posts) each representing physical, spiritual, mental, and other sociodemographic domains. Surrounding the fale is a cocoon representing time, context, and the environment. Te Vaka Atafaga (Kupa, 2009) presents an outrigger canoe as a metaphor for Tokelau health and wellbeing. Elements of the vaka reflect various domains including te mafaufau (mental), te tino o te tagata (physical), kaiga (family), talitonuga (belief systems), inati (social systems), and puipuiga o te tino o te tagata (environment). A Tongan framework of health is Fonua ola (Tu'itahi, 2015) that uses an ecological model to represent different domains of 'ataki (environment), koloa (economic), sino (physical), 'atamani (mental), anga fakafonua (cultural) and laumalie (spiritual), and how these need to be understood across multiple levels including taautaha (individual), famili (family), kolo (local), fonua (national), and mamani (global).

There are more models than what are mentioned above, each imbued with the cultural nuance of their respective ethnic specific cultural worldviews. While there are subtle differences across the models, there are broad similarities that exist. Pacific models of health emphasise holism, drawing attention to physical, mental, spiritual, familial, social, cultural, and environmental domains

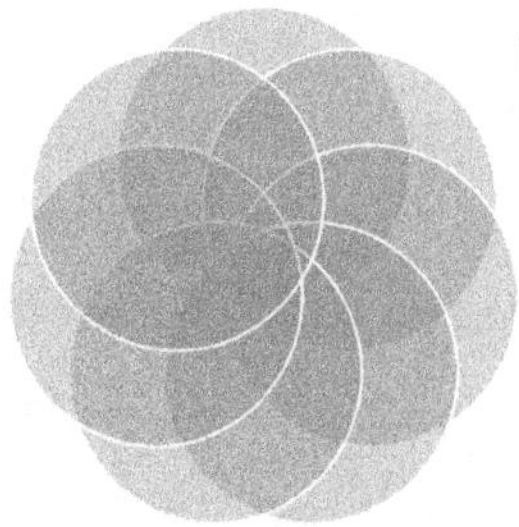

Figure 1: *Common domains across Pacific models of health and wellbeing.*

of life, and their interwoven nature (See Figure 1). Though Pacific models offer conceptual understandings, there are similarities and critical differences to psychological measures of wellbeing. For example, the previously mentioned PWI presents satisfaction across seven different domains of life. There are some similarities between Pacific and psychological perspectives (such as relationships and health), however psychological perspectives do not include domains important for Pacific peoples, such as spirituality, environment, and a specific focus on families (the PWI presents satisfaction with spirituality/religion as an optional item). Any broad approach to Pacific wellbeing should be holistic and recognise the interwoven nature of each domain, together with nuance in how these domains may be understood or experienced.

Pacific wellbeing can be understood as balance across each domain, recognising the reciprocal influence each can have on each other. For instance, overall wellbeing would largely reflect positive appraisals across each domain. However, overall positive wellbeing is not necessarily dependent on each domain being strong. People will experience hardships, difficulties, and negative experiences that could negatively impact on their wellbeing. However, strength in other domains can provide support to help counteract difficulties in another domain. For example, someone experiencing emotional difficulties (mental domain) can be supported by family members (familial), and their church communities if they are religious (spiritual). In this way, although a person may have difficulty in one area of their life, their wellbeing can be supported by strengths in other areas of their lives. However, it must be considered that some domains may carry more weight or be more salient in a person's life. This means that wellbeing is a subjective experience that also depends on idiosyncratic values in conjunction with shared Pacific values.

Another way that wellbeing can be understood is by understanding the vā between people and places *within* each domain. Negative impacts on wellbeing can be understood as transgressions of the relationships, or damage to the vā where violation of sacred spaces can manifest as emotional distress. For example, a fight between a brother and sister will mean the vā between them has been disturbed (crossing familial and cultural domains). Another example is the effects of climate change threatening the relationship and sense of belonging one has to their land (crossing environmental, social, and spiritual domains). It is normal to experience fluctuations in relationships people have with each other, and the relationships we have with the spaces we occupy. Understanding the nature and quality of the relationships in the vā is critical to understanding wellbeing. Should a relationship be strained, repairing and nurturing the vā can restore the relationship. Thus, tauhi vā or teu le va (care for or nurture the relationship) are culturally-situated practices that can both maintain wellbeing and restore it. Bringing this all together, a way of understanding wellbeing that is centred on Pacific worldviews is the harmony across and within broad domains of life, and the totality of the quality of the relationships within each domain (Ka'ili, 2005; Tu'itahi, 2015).

It is through vā that the similarities and differences between Pacific and Western psychological concepts of identity and wellbeing are illuminated. Both highlight identity and wellbeing as multifaceted. Psychological perspectives lend explanations to relational self-concepts that speak to the self being defined in terms of relationships with others, which aligns well with Pacific perspectives of the relational self. However, this is still largely predicated on Western values that emphasise more individual over collective relationships. Pacific perspectives provide a culturally meaningful and situated explanation of identity through vā, which provides a more nuanced understanding of the layered relationships that exist between different peoples. Furthermore, positive affect derived from the nurturing or healing of these relationships reflect wellbeing. From a Western perspective, this means identity and wellbeing are separate but related, while from Pacific perspectives, identity and wellbeing are relational aspects of an integrated whole – identity and wellbeing are both understood through vā.

Conclusion

Pacific identities and wellbeing within Aotearoa can be understood as the thoughts, feelings, and emotions associated with one's Pacific ethnicity. They are multi-faceted – a combination of physical, cultural, spiritual familial, mental, and environmental domains. Key to Pacific identities and wellbeing are relationships, best understood as connections that are experienced and nurtured in the vā – socio-spatial spaces that connect. A sense of self is developed in terms of the relationships Pacific peoples have with other people and their surrounding environments. A sense of wellbeing is developed in terms of the nature and quality of those relationships. Wellbeing also encompasses a combination of affect (positive feelings) and evaluations (such as satisfaction) within each domain. Thus, Pacific wellbeing can be understood as the overall nature, quality, and subjective evaluation of one's life within and between life domains.

Combining aspects of psychology that align well with Pacific knowledges, Pacific identities, and wellbeing are presented as a layered array of relationships that are formed, maintained, and nurtured in the vā. The self is understood in terms of relationships with others, and the nature of those relationships across multiple domains of life contribute to wellbeing. In this sense, Pacific identities and wellbeing are intricately tied and inseparable, where self and wellbeing are the totality and quality of the spaces in which people are connected to others.

References

Boven, N., Exeter, D., Sporle, A. and Shackleton, N. (2020). The implications of different ethnicity categorisation methods for understanding outcomes and developing policy in New Zealand. *Kōtuitui: New Zealand Journal of Social Sciences Online*, 15(1), 123–139. https://doi.org/10.1080/1177083X.2019.1657912

Cross, S. E., Hardin, E. E. and Gercek-Swing, B. (2011). The what, how, why, and where of self-construal. *Personality and Social*

Psychology Review, 15(2), 142–179. https://doi.org/10.1177/1088868310373752

Cummins, R. A., Eckersley, R., Pallant, J., Van Vugt, J. and Misajon, R. (2003). Developing a national index of subjective wellbeing: The Australian Unity Wellbeing Index. *Social Indicators Research,* 64(2), 159–190. https://doi.org/10.1023/A:1024704320683

Diener, E. D., Emmons, R. A., Larsen, R. J. and Griffin, S. (1985). The satisfaction with life scale. *Journal of Personality Assessment,* 49(1), 71–75. https://doi.org/10.1207/s15327752jpa4901_13

Diener, E. D., Suh, E. M., Lucas, R. E. and Smith, H. L. (1999). Subjective well-being: Three decades of progress. *Psychological Bulletin,* 125(2), 276–302. https://doi.org/10.1037/0033-2909.125.2.276

Dodge, R., Daly, A. P., Huyton, J. and Sanders, L. D. (2012). The challenge of defining wellbeing. *International Journal of Wellbeing,* 2(3), 222–235. http://doi.org/10.5502/ijw.v2i3.4

Espinosa, A., Tikhonov, A., Ellman, L. M., Kern, D. M., Lui, F. and Anglin, D. (2018). Ethnic identity and perceived stress among ethnically diverse immigrants. *Journal of Immigrant and Minority Health,* 20(1), 155–163. https://doi.org/10.1007/s10903-016-0494-z

Haslam, S. A., Jetten, J., Postmes, T. and Haslam, C. (2009). Social identity, health and well-being: An emerging agenda for applied psychology. *Applied Psychology,* 58(1), 1–23. https://doi.org/10.1111/j.1464-0597.2008.00379.x

Henrich, J., Heine, S. J. and Norenzayan, A. (2010). The weirdest people in the world? *Behavioral and Brain Sciences,* 33(2–3), 61–83. https://doi.org/10.1017/S0140525X0999152X

Ka'ili, T. O. (2005). Tauhi vā: Nurturing Tongan sociospatial ties in Maui and beyond. *The Contemporary Pacific,* 17(1), 83–114. http://doi.org/10.1353/cp.2005.0017

Kapeli, S. A., Manuela, S., & Sibley, C. G. (2020). Perceived discrimination is associated with poorer health and well-being outcomes among Pacific peoples in New Zealand. *Journal of Community & Applied Social Psychology,* 30(2), 132–150. https://doi.org/10.1002/casp.2433

Kupa, K. (2009). Te Vaka Atafaga: A Tokelau assessment model for supporting holistic mental health practice with Tokelau people in Aotearoa-New Zealand. *Pacific Health Dialog,* 15(1), 156–163.

Manuela, S. (2021). Ethnic identity buffers the effect of discrimination on family, life, and health satisfaction for pacific peoples in New Zealand. *Pacific Health Dialog,* 21(7), 390–398.

Manuela, S. and Sibley, C. G. (2013). The Pacific Identity and Wellbeing Scale (PIWBS): A culturally-appropriate self-report measure for Pacific peoples in New Zealand. *Social Indicators Research,* 112(1), 83–103. https://doi.org/10.1007/s11205-012-0041-9

Manuela, S. and Sibley, C. G. (2014). Exploring the hierarchical structure of Pacific identity and wellbeing. *Social Indicators Research,* 118(3), 969–985. https://doi.org/10.1007/s11205-013-0472-y

Manuela, S. and Sibley, C. G. (2015). The Pacific Identity and Wellbeing Scale-Revised (PIWBS-R). *Cultural Diversity and Ethnic Minority Psychology,* 21(1), 146–155. https://doi.org/10.1037/a0037536

Matsumoto, D. and Jones, C. A. L. (2009). Ethical Issues in Cross-Cultural Psychology. In: D. M. Mertens and P. E. Ginsberg, eds., *The Handbook of Social Research Ethics*. 1st ed. SAGE Publications, Inc, 323–336. https://doi.org/10.4135/9781483348971.n21

Mila-Schaaf, K. (2006). Va-centred social work: Possibilities for a Pacific approach to social work practice. *Social Work Review,* 18(1), 8–13.

Pascoe, E. A. and Smart Richman, L. (2009). Perceived discrimination and health: A meta-analytic review. *Psychological Bulletin,* 135(4), 531–554. https://doi.org/10.1037/a0016059

Phinney, J. S. (1990). Ethnic identity in adolescents and adults: Review of research. *Psychological Bulletin,* 108(3), 499–514. https://doi.org/10.1037/0033-2909.108.3.499

Phinney, J. S. (1992). The multigroup ethnic identity measure: A new scale for use with diverse groups. *Journal of Adolescent Research,* 7(2), 156–176. https://doi.org/10.1177/07435548 9272003

Phinney, J. S. and Ong, A. D. (2007). Conceptualization and measurement of ethnic identity: Current status and future directions. *Journal of Counseling Psychology,* 54(3), 271–281. https://doi.org/ 10.1037/0022-0167.54.3.271

Pultou-Endemann, F. K. (2021). *Fonofale Model: Pacific Health & Wellbeing.* https://www.mpp.govt.nz/assets/Resources/Fonofale-presentation-to-Pacific-Wellbeing-Talanoa-May-2021.pdf

Sellers, R. M., Smith, M. A., Shelton, J. N., Rowley, S. A., & Chavous, T. M. (1998). Multidimensional model of racial identity: A reconceptualization of African American racial identity. Personality and social psychology review, 2(1), 18–39. https://doi.org/10.1207/ s15327957pspr0201_2

Smith, T. B. and Silva, L. (2011). Ethnic identity and personal well-being of people of color: A meta-analysis. *Journal of Counseling Psychology,* 58(1), 42–60. https://doi.org/10.1037/a0021528

Stats NZ. (2005). *Statistical Standard for Ethnicity.* https://www.stats.govt.nz/methods-and-standards/standards-and-classifi cations/

Tu'itahi, S. (2015, August 19). Why Pasifika Health Models? Do They Work? (From Fonua to Fonua Ola). [PowerPoint slides]. Health Promotion Forum of New Zealand. https://hpfnz.org.nz/ assets/Uploads/From-Fonua-to-Fonua-Ola.pdf

Umaña-Taylor, A. J., Quintana, S. M., Lee, R. M., Cross Jr, W. E., Rivas-Drake, D., Schwartz, S. J., Syed, M., Yip, T., Seaton, E. and Ethnic and Racial Identity in the 21st Century Study Group. (2014). Ethnic and racial identity during adolescence and into young adulthood: An integrated conceptualization. *Child Development*, 85(1), 21–39. https://doi.org/10.1111/cdev.12196

Wendt, A. (1996). Tatauing the Post-Colonial Body. *New Zealand Electronic Poetry Centre*. http://www.nzepc.auckland.ac.nz/authors/wendt/tatauing.asp

Yao, E. S., Meissel, K., Atatoa Carr, P., Bullen, P., Peiris-John, R., Manuela, S., & Clark, T. C. (2025). Unpacking tick-boxes: considerations and recommendations for collecting, analysing, and interpreting ethnicity data. *Journal of the Royal Society of New Zealand*, *55*(6), 1432–1451. 1–20. https://doi.org/10.1080/03036758.2025.2467275

Yip, T. (2018). Ethnic/racial identity—A double-edged sword? Associations with discrimination and psychological outcomes. *Current Directions in Psychological Science*, 27(3), 170–175. https://doi.org/10.1177/0963721417739348

The health of children and young people

Dame Teuila Percival

Chapter summary

This chapter sheds light on the profound health challenges faced by Pacific children, underscoring pervasive inequities that stem from structural issues such as poverty and poor housing. Pacific children encounter preventable serious morbidity, particularly respiratory and infectious diseases, further accentuating health disparities. Notably, chronic conditions such as rheumatic heart disease and bronchiectasis, contribute to the overall health burden. The chapter expresses deep concern over the existing inequities in healthcare for Pacific children, including high incidences of family violence, emphasising the pivotal role positive health and wellbeing plays in childhood as a critical foundation for adult life

Introduction

Health is a state of physical, mental, social, and emotional well-being and not merely the absence of disease (World Health Organization, 1946). Health for children and young people also includes optimizing development and the capacity to realize potential (National Research Council and Institute of Medicine, 2004).

Childhood is a unique phase of human development which is critical for laying the foundations of good health in our Pacific community. It is a time in life when there are normal changes in an individual's growth, physiology, cognitive, and emotional social development with associated health needs encompassing these expected age-related changes.

Positive trajectories toward health and wellbeing in adult life are established in the very early years of life. Young children's physical health and development provide the foundation for later health, educational, and social outcomes, including cardiovascular disease, obesity, smoking, and depression (Heckman et al., 2014.

The period between childhood and adult life is similarly a time of change and development with associated health and development needs. How this transition from childhood to adult life is defined and recognised differs between cultures and is variably referred to as adolescence, youth, or young people. Adolescence is a term used for teenagers aged 10–19 years and young people with an upper age range of 24 years.

Regardless of the lower or upper age limits, the defining feature of young people or adolescents is increasing autonomy and independence of the individual with less reliance on the parents and caregivers seen in childhood. Adolescence too, is a critical phase in human development of the individual and group which influences adult health and socio-economic success (Patton, 2016). The life course trajectory of health and wellbeing is largely set by young adulthood (Patton, 2016; Sawyer et al., 2012) and the health inequities seen in adolescents account for many of the later adult disparities including cancer, diabetes, and cardiovascular disease.

Children and young people make up over half of the Pacific population in New Zealand. In the 2013 census 35.7% of Pacific were children aged 0–14 years and 54.9% of Pacific people were under the age of 25 years (Stats NZ, 2014). Despite decades of reports calling for change, Pacific children and young people continue to face significant health and social disparities (Health Quality & Safety Commission, 2021; Ministry of Health, 2008). Pacific children experience higher rates of hospitalisation, respiratory illness, and infectious disease. They have higher rates of obesity. They experience disparities in health promotion resourcing, preventative health care, and inequitable access to effective management of chronic conditions (Health Quality & Safety Commission, 2021). Given the importance of this population group for setting the bedrock of adult health and wellbeing, this is a major concern for the Pacific communities of New Zealand.

Determinants of children and young people's health

Housing quality, overcrowding, household income, and unemployment are important determinants of morbidity and mortality for children (Child and Youth Mortality Review Committee, 2021; Ingham et al., 2019; Jaine et al., 2008). It is worth noting some unique child health determinants. Children of course live in families, environments, and communities that provide them with the opportunity to be healthy and reach their fullest potential. Maternal education is one of the strongest predictors of child health, independent of socioeconomic status (Gakidou et al., 2010; Pamuk et al., 2011). The health of caregivers is an obvious determinant of children's health. Infants born to diabetic mothers have increased risk of growth, neurodevelopmental, and other congenital abnormalities (Ornoy, 2005; Perna et al., 2015). Postpartum and maternal depression is a recognised risk factor for socio-emotional and cognitive development in children (Canadian Paediatric Society, 2004; Meaney, 2018; Stein et al., 2008).

Positive determinants and mitigations of poor child health outcomes are also noteworthy. Higher socioeconomic status can mitigate the negative effects of postnatal depression (Stein et al., 2008). The presence of grandparents in families can reduce externalising aggressive behaviour problems in at risk children (Sheridan et al., 2011) and increasing family social capital can reduce delinquent behaviour in adolescents (Hoffmann et al., 2020). In Aotearoa, strong alignment with Pacific culture can also be associated with better infant and maternal risk factors (Borrows et al., 2011).

Pacific child and adolescent deaths

Inequities in children and young people's survival is impacted by the effectiveness of the health system as well as social determinants such as household income and living conditions.

New Zealand child deaths have been decreasing through the decades, however there continues to be persistent inequity without narrowing of the gap between mortality rates for Pacific children aged 0–15 years and non-Pacific Non-Māori (NPNM; Duncanson et al., 2020).

Deaths of Pacific children and young people in New Zealand are analysed and reported regularly by the Child and Youth Mortality Review Committee. Its most recent report (Child and Youth Mortality Review Committee, 2021) details continuing disparities in the mortality rate of Pacific children and young people.

Between the years 2015 and 2019, the risk of death for Pacific infants (aged 28 days – < 1 year of age) was over three times that of NPNM (rate ratio 3.82, 95 per cent CI 2.98–4.89). Sudden Unexpected Death in Infancy (SUDI) remains the most common cause of death for this infant age group and Pacific continue to have a higher rate of SUDI deaths (Rate ratio 8.57, 95 per cent CI 5.74–12.79) than NPNM. The second most common cause of death in infants beyond the neonatal period is medical conditions and Pacific infant deaths for medical conditions are twice that of NPNM (Child and Youth Mortality Review Committee, 2021).

In older children (1–9 years) the leading causes of death for Pacific children are medical conditions, most commonly respiratory illness followed by infections and neoplasms. Injury deaths, including transport related and drowning are also an important cause of death for preschool and school aged Pacific children (Child and Youth Mortality Review Committee, 2021).

In the younger Pacific adolescent age group (10–14 years) medical conditions and respiratory illness continue to be the leading cause of deaths. In older adolescents (15–19 years) medical conditions remain important but now with equal numbers of suicide deaths, followed closely by injury related deaths. The disparity in mortality is also seen in Pacific young people dying at twice the rate of NPNM for medical conditions for 15–19 year-olds (rate ratio 2.05, 95 per cent CI 1.34–3.12) and 20–24 year-olds (rate ratio 2.55, 95 per cent CI 1.81–3.59) (Child and Youth Mortality Review Committee, 2021).

Case Study: Pacific SUDI

Sudden unexpected death in infancy (SUDI) is the leading cause of death for New Zealand infants aged from 28 to 364 days. It most commonly occurs in otherwise healthy infants as a result of suffocation in bed or sudden infant death syndrome. Pacific infants continue to experience SUDI rates almost four times as high as European/other infants (Duncanson et al., 2020). Protection against this avoidable tragic death is possible through supporting families with infant safe sleep behaviours, access to health services and resources, adequate housing, household heating, effective smoking cessation, and enabling safe places for infants to sleep. This requires coordinated culturally competent Antenatal, Well Child and Primary Health Care service with an understanding of Pacific communities and commitment to supporting Pacific families with SUDI prevention.

Neonates: Preparing for life

The neonatal period covers the first 28 days of life. Prematurity and low birth weight can be associated with acute health issues such as hypoglycaemia and respiratory distress but also longer term morbidity with increased rates of hospitalisation in the first year of life and neurodevelopmental delay (Allen, 2002; Darlow et al., 1997; Wilson-Costello, 2007).

Preterm births are babies born before 37 weeks gestation. The preterm birth rate for Pacific babies in New Zealand is now 8.8% of live births, which is higher than that of other ethnic groups (Health New Zealand, Te Whatu Ora, 2022). The rate of Pacific low birth weight babies at term is low compared with other ethnic groups (Health New Zealand, Te Whatu Ora, 2022; Simpson et al., 2017). Rates of congenital anomalies noted at birth are not dissimilar to other New Zealand babies (Simpson et al., 2017).

The healthcare journey and outcome for Pacific babies born with prematurity or critical congenital abnormalities is perhaps an area for focus though. Pacific and Māori babies born at 23–26 weeks gestation are less likely to be resuscitated than their NPNM counterparts (Perinatal Mortality Review Committee, 2021). Pacific and Māori babies diagnosed with Hypoplastic Left Heart syndrome are more likely to have an outcome of late fetal death, stillbirth, palliative care, or infant death compared with NZ European babies despite similar complexity of heart defects. Why there is inequitable treatment and outcomes with extreme prematurity resuscitation and critical congenital conditions is not explained but conceivably discussions with families about viability and treatment options requires cultural competence of clinician teams and health systems (Perinatal Mortality Review Committee, 2021; Pio et al., 2020; Soszyn et al., 2019).

Pacific adolescents and young people

Adolescents tend to be overlooked in population health and clinical care, one reason why they have had fewer health gains compared with other age groups (Patton et al., 2016). This is a critical age when the foundations of adult health, chronic disease, and wellness are set. It is a time with new and different health problems related to behaviour, emotional control, and the onset of sexual activity.

Pacific have high levels of typical adolescent health problems, including infectious diseases, obesity, Type 2 diabetes, injury, poor access to sexual and reproductive health, and mental distress and depression (Ministry of Health, 2008; Simpson et al., 2017).

Pacific teenage pregnancy rates (defined as women giving birth aged 15–19 years) are lower than Māori but higher than that of European (Simpson et al., 2017). Teenage motherhood has been associated with poorer educational and economic outcomes (Boden et al., 2008). Outcomes need not however be negative and can be positive both for baby and teenage parent with appropriate support of family, wrap around services, and the community (The Families Commission, 2011).

Injuries are a major health problem accounting for one-quarter of New Zealand adolescent hospital bed days and three-quarters of deaths. Pacific rates of trauma related hospitalisation are similar to other New Zealanders except for pedestrian traffic injuries and assaults where Pacific are over represented (Ameratunga et al., 1999).

Rates of obesity in Pacific children and adolescents are disproportionately high with well described associations of poor dietary and physical activity behaviours (Chiavaroli et al., 2019; Rush et al., 2013). Alcohol consumption is an additional association to consider in obese Pacific young people (Moors, 2016).

There are increasing rates of Type 2 diabetes in Pacific adolescents (Sjardon et al., 2018). Pacific young adults with Type 2 diabetes also have very high risk of early complications with 44% having micro albuminuria at diagnosis and 56% having retinopathy at a median of 6 years post diagnosis (Beig et al., 2017).

Pacific secondary school students living with chronic illness or disability report generally positive family and school environments, but a high prevalence of food and housing insecurity and poor access to healthcare with notable discrimination by healthcare providers (Roy et al., 2020). Whereas culturally competent chronic disease management and health promotion are key, there is also a need to specifically consider young people's needs and views.

Illness and disease

The burden of serious childhood illnesses is high in Pacific children with highest preventable hospitalisation rates, including lower respiratory tract infections, invasive bacterial infections, and acute rheumatic fever (ARF; Craig et al., 2008; Duncanson et al., 2019). Chronic life limiting conditions as a result of repeated acute respiratory and infectious illness such as bronchiectasis and rheumatic heart disease (RHD) are also higher in Pacific children and young people compared with Māori and European/others (Twiss et al., 2005).

Respiratory conditions

Respiratory conditions are a major cause of Pacific child and youth morbidity (Asthma and Respiratory Foundation of New Zealand, 2015; Craig et al., 2008; Duncanson et al., 2019; Grant et al., 2001). These conditions which include acute upper and lower respiratory infections, bronchiolitis, pneumonia, asthma, and wheeze make up over a third of child admissions to hospital (Duncanson et al., 2019; Trenholme et al., 2012).

Pacific children have consistently experienced high hospitalisation rates for asthma and wheeze, higher than Māori and over three times that of European/other children (Duncanson et al., 2019; Gilles et al., 2013). Despite having high prevalence of asthma symptoms and more severe asthma requiring hospitalisation, Pacific children are less likely to receive effective care in the community, in particular escalation of treatment to include inhaled corticosteroids and long-acting β2-agonists (Gilles et al., 2013). Lower respiratory infection which includes bronchiolitis and pneumonia have highest hospitalisation rates in Pacific children (Grant et al., 2001). Pacific children are likely to experience repeated hospitalisation (Trenholme et al., 2012) and more severe disease and complications including empyema (Burton et al., 2015; Mahon et al., 2016; Wright et al., 2011).

Bronchiectasis is a chronic respiratory disease thought to be caused by a cycle of lung infection and inflammation producing permanent lung damage, chronic illness, disability, and potentially premature death. It has declined in other developed countries. In New Zealand, bronchiectasis is an ongoing concern particularly in Pacific and Māori children who have over 80 per cent of cases. The incidence for under 15 year olds is highest in Pacific at 17.8/100,000 compared with 4.8/100,000 for Māori and 1.5/100,000 for European (Twiss et al., 2005).

Risk factors for respiratory conditions like pneumonia and asthma include poverty, poor housing, crowded households, frequent, and severe lower respiratory infections in childhood, exposure to tobacco smoke (Ingham et al., 2019; Tin Tin et al., 2016; World Health Organization, 2018).

As well as preventative strategies, given the high rates and severity of respiratory illness in Pacific children including chronic sequelae, there is a need to focus on ensuring equitable and effective healthcare and resources.

Infectious diseases

Infections are common in childhood but become concerning when they are serious, requiring hospitalisation, or there is the development of chronic illness and/or disability. Pacific child hospitalisation rates for infectious diseases are over twice that of European children (Hobbs et al., 2016).

Serious skin infections include cellulitis, skin abscesses, lymphadenitis, and other. Pacific children and young people are hospitalised with serious skin infections at twice the rate of Māori and almost four times the rate of European children. Of concern is that these rates are not declining and may be increasing particularly in the 5–14 year old age group (Oben et al., 2019; Simpson et al., 2017).

Post-streptococcal glomerulonephritis (PSGN) is an immune mediated illness that can follow streptococcal skin infection. It is the commonest cause of severe acute glomerulonephritis in New Zealand children, with the majority (85%) of the patients being either Pacific or Māori (Wong et al., 2009). Significant short-term complications include hypertension, hypertensive encephalopathy, renal failure, and congestive heart failure. Long-term renal morbidity is uncommon but also a concern for this largely preventable disease (Wong et al., 2013).

ARF is preventable multisystem inflammatory disease that develops in about 3% of children and young people with untreated Group A streptococcal sore throat infection (Ministry of Health, 2012; Webb et al., 2015). The severe complication of ARF is RHD which can lead to cardiac failure, disability, and premature death. Rates of ARF are highest in Pacific children and young people. There has been a concerted effort to prevent rheumatic fever with community programmes such as school sore throat clinics, with some reduction in Māori rates. However, Pacific rates have not decreased (Institute of Environmental Science and Research, 2018; Ministry of Health, 2021) which raises the need for tailoring and developing programmes to fit better with Pacific families and communities.

Meningococcal disease is a serious invasive bacterial infection manifesting as septicaemia or meningitis or both. The case fatality rate of 10% in developed countries (Stephens, 2007). There have been two major epidemics in New Zealand, in the 1970's and again between 1991 and 2008. The current background rate is 1–3 cases per 100,000 (Sexton et al., 2004). In 2018 there were 120 cases reported in and 139 in 2019 with a steady rise from 45 cases in 2014 (Institute of Environmental Science and Research, 2019b). All ages can be affected but disease is most common in under 1 year old infants. Ethnic disparities are marked both in non-epidemic and epidemic outbreaks with disproportionately highest rates in Pacific followed by Māori (Institute of Environmental Science and Research, 2019b). Currently there is no funded Meningococcal vaccine in our universal New Zealand schedule. Household crowding, poverty, and access to early treatment as with other infectious diseases are important modifiable risk factors. Meningococcal vaccines are not universally funded in New Zealand but are available for purchase or free for individuals with high-risk medical conditions.

Case study: Measles 2019 epidemic in Auckland and Samoa

The 2019 New Zealand Measles outbreak had 2,174 reported cases. Over 80% were in Auckland, predominantly South Auckland (Institute of Environmental Science and Research, 2019a). The burden of infection was highest in very young infants followed by adolescents and young adults. Pacific and Māori were disproportionately affected and 75% of all hospitalisations were Pacific or Māori (Turner, 2019). The outbreak peaked in September and then slowly tapered off through the subsequent 4 months. The outbreak was fueled by historically poor immunisation rates with under immunised young people and vulnerable as yet unvaccinated infants.

Just a 3-hour plane ride away, in Samoa, the first measles case was reported on 30 September 2019 and the first death on 16th October. With historically low Measles vaccination (MMR) coverage and the national vaccination programme suspended in July 2018 due to two infant deaths, the national MMR coverage was probably 30% at best in 2019 (Boodoosingh et al., 2020) when Measles spread from Auckland. This was the "perfect storm" for an epidemic. What followed was a National State of emergency, 5,707 reported Measles cases, 1,860 hospitalisations, and 83 Measles deaths. 87% of deaths were in under 5 year old children (Craig et al., 2020). Samoa, with a National hospital bed capacity of 190 moved to over 200 Measles inpatients a day, 12 ventilated children, and 10 high dependency beds. The country responded setting up Measles dedicated emergency departments and hospital and welcomed overseas medical team support. On 5th and 6th of December, the Government shut the country down for a mass door to door Measles vaccination programme. The curfew was lifted on 7th of December when the government estimated they had reached 90% MMR coverage.

New Zealand and Samoa are linked with frequent two-way travel and both had low MMR coverage, insufficient to protect vulnerable infants who suffer by far most of the disease burden and deaths.

Optimising development and potential

Development and behaviour

Children's early development – their first learning experiences and the bonds they form with family deeply affect their future physical, cognitive, emotional, and social development. Optimising the early years of our children's lives is the best investment to ensure positive learning and educational success.

The Pacific Islands Families Study (PIFS) is a longitudinal study following 1398 Pacific children from birth. When the cohort was screened for developmental problems as 2 year olds, most children (65%) had no developmental delay, with 35% having some form of delay, the most common being cognitive or language (Paterson et al., 2011). PIFS also looked at behaviour problems in their cohort and found 14.2% of 2 year olds had behavioural problems in the clinical range (Paterson et al., 2007). Notably there was variation in the group with externalising behaviour associated with discipline and internalising behaviour symptoms associated with cultural orientation, number of years in New Zealand and maternal education.

Ear health and adequate hearing are critical to language development and learning (Moore et al., 2020). The PIFS found that over 25% of 2 year olds had Otitis Media with effusion, commonly known as Glue Ear (Paterson et al., 2006) and at 11 years of age significant problems with previously unknown hearing loss and auditory processing difficulties (Purdy et al., 2019). Pacific children aged 0–4 years old are more likely to be admitted to hospital with acute otitis media than European children. In contrast Pacific have lower rates of elective admission for ventilation tubes and less outpatient Ear Nose & Throat (ENT) first appointments than European children (McCallum, 2015). This disparity in treatment was not as marked in older children.

New Zealand's Universal Well-Child-Tamariki-Ora programme (WCTO) including the Before-School-Check at Age 4 years is designed to identify developmental concerns enabling early intervention and family support.

There is mounting concern that the WCTO programme does not meet the needs of Pacific families through its transactional methodology and use of mainstream developmental/behaviour screening tools (Ministry of Health, 2021). Māori and Pacific are less likely to complete Well Child and B4School checks (Gibb et al., 2019). There is also variation in programme application and inconsistent referral to health and specialist services of children who meet appropriate criteria (Richards et al., 2019).

Family violence and child abuse

Every year, 10 New Zealand children die as a direct result of child abuse (Duncanson et al., 2009; UNICEF, 2003). Underlying this is the additional morbidity of child maltreatment with inflicted injuries, neglect, and emotional abuse. Whereas there is a larger discussion on the underlying community, family, and societal issues that produce an environment where children are hurt, the first step is to acknowledge and recognise that child abuse occurs.

Pacific children have higher rates of hospitalisation for child maltreatment including assaults and neglect than European but lower than Māori children (Craig et al., 2008). Oranga Tamariki received 56,900 reports of concern in the 12 months to June 2021 with 35,100 of these progressing for Care & Protection investigation. Pacific made up just over 10% cases needing investigation. In addition Pacific make up 6% of children needing statutory level intervention who are classified as in the custody of the CEO, Ministry for Children (Oranga Tamariki, Ministry for Children, 2021).

Family Violence is common in New Zealand, including among Pacific families (Paterson, 2007). Exposure to family violence can cause ongoing child morbidity and in New Zealand Pacific children it has been associated with increased GP visits in exposed children (Schulter et al., 2009). Physical discipline of Pacific children is fairly common with over 80% of fathers reporting smacking and 14.2% reporting hitting their 2-year olds with an object (Schulter et al., 2011).

From a health and Pacific community view, the importance of identifying both child abuse and family violence is the associated physical, mental health, and social morbidity (Ferguson et al., 1997; Schulter et al., 2011) and the need for a Pacific lens on the social determinants that lead to child maltreatment and similarly Pacific leadership for services that support children and families.

Health promotion and healthcare

Poor access to effective and culturally appropriate primary and community health care for Pacific has been well documented (Foliaki et al., 2020; Ryan et al., 2019; Southwick et al., 2012). Pacific children and young people also experience less effective healthcare in the community (Gilles et al., 2013; Pio et al., 2020; Teevale et al., 2013) and secondary care (Cloete et al., 2019; McCallum, 2015).

WCTO core nurse contacts should occur at scheduled ages for growth and developmental screening, identification of issues, and timely intervention. There has been a widening of the WCTO equity for Pacific with less enrolments at birth and less scheduled core contacts (Ministry of Health, 2020). Health promotion and family support should be provided in a culturally appropriate, effective way through the continuum of Lead Maternity Carer, Well Child Nurse Dental Health, and Primary Care. Measures of Pacific child health show marked disparity however, just 43% of Pacific babies live in smoke free homes at 6 weeks of age and only 48% are breastfed at 3 months of age (Ministry of Health, 2020). As with WCTO, children are entitled to free universal dental health services until they leave secondary school. Pacific children have highest rates of dental decay and yet their enrolment, clinic attendance, and receipt of preventative treatment such as fluoride tooth varnish in pre-schoolers is less than other children (Auckland District Health Board, 2021).

Conclusion

Pacific children and young people face continuing health inequity. Illnesses associated with poverty and poor housing are most prevalent in our Pacific children. Our children experience preventable serious morbidity with respiratory and infectious diseases and the chronic conditions of rheumatic heart disease and bronchiectasis uncommon in other developed countries. The continuing inequity in healthcare for Pacific children, in different contexts, with different conditions from resuscitating extreme preterm babies to management of chronic illness in young people is concerning. The health and wellbeing of Pacific children and young people lays the critical foundation for adult life and our Pacific community. Whereas addressing the upstream determinants of health are critical, the solutions to poverty and housing affordability are distant. Healthcare is surely more tangible and the sector should be able to address racism, cultural competence, and Pacific specific effectiveness and health outcomes.

References

Auckland District Health Board. (2021). *Oral Health in the Auckland Region. Report for Community and Public Health Committee (CPHAC) – Commissioning for Equity.*

Allen, M. C. (2002). Preterm outcomes research: A critical component of neonatal intensive care. *Mental Retardation and Developmental Disabilities Research Reviews,* 8(4), 221–233. https://doi.org/10.1002/mrdd.10044

Ameratunga, S. N., Alexander, C. S., Smith, G. S., Lennon, D. R. and Norton, R. N. (1999). Trauma-related hospitalizations among urban adolescents in New Zealand: priorities for prevention. *The Journal of Adolescent Health, 25*(1), 75–83. https://doi.org/10.1016/s1054-139x(98)00088-3

Asthma and Respiratory Foundation of New Zealand. (2015). *Te Hā Ora (The Breath of Life): National Respiratory Strategy.* The Asthma Foundation. https://www.asthmafoundation.org.nz/assets/images/National-Respiratory-Strategy-online-version.pdf

Beig, J., Khandkar, M., and Cundy, T. (2017). Type 2 diabetes in young adults in Central Auckland: demography and complications. *Internal Medicine Journal, 48*(1), 67–73. https://doi.org/10.1111/imj.13623

Boden, J. M., Fergusson, D. M., and Horwood, J. L. (2008). Early motherhood and subsequent life outcomes. *Journal of Child Psychology and Psychiatry, 49*(2) 151–60. http://doi.org/10.1111/j.1469- 7610.2007.01830.x

Boodoosingh, R., Ama'ama, S., and Schoeffe, P. (2020). A perfect Story: The Social and Institutional Contexts of Samoa's 2019–2020 Measles Epidemic and Lessons learned for the Covid-19

Pandemic. *Journal of Samoan Studies, 10*, 5–24. http://doi.org/10.47922/KSBD7726

Borrows, J., Williams, M., Schulter, P., Peterson, J., and Helu, S. (2011). Pacific Islands Families Study: The Association of Infant Health Risk Indicators and Acculturation of Pacific Island Mothers Living in New Zealand. *Journal of Cross-Cultural Psychology, 42*(5), 699–724. https://doi.org/10.1177/0022022110362750

Burton, C., Walls, T., Price, N., Glasgow, T., Walker, C., Beasley, S., and Best, E. (2015). Paediatric empyema in New Zealand: a tale of two cities. *The New Zealand Medical Journal, 128* (1415), 25–33.

Bernard-Bonnin, A. C., Canadian Paediatric Society, and Mental Health and Developmental Disabilities Committee. (2004). Maternal depression and child development. *Paediatrics & Child Health, 9*(8), 575–583. http://doi.org/10.1093/pch/9.8.575

Chiavaroli V., Gibbins J. D., Cutfield W. S., & Derraik J. G. B. (2019). Childhood obesity in New Zealand. *World Journal of Pediatrics, 15*(4), 322–331. http://doi.org/10.1007/s12519-019-00261-3

Child and Youth Mortality Review Committee | Te Ropu Arotake Auau o te Hunga Tamaki Taiohi. (2021). *15th data report: 2015–19.* Health Quality & Safety Commission. www.hqsc.govt.nz/our-programmes/mrc/cymrc

Craig A., Heywood A., & Worth H. (2020) Measles epidemic in Samoa and other Pacific Islands. *The Lancet. Infectious Diseases, 20*(3), 273–275. https://doi.org/10.1016/S1473-3099(20)30053-0

Craig E., Anderson P., Taufa S., Jackson C., & Han DY. (2008). *The Health of Pacific Children and Young People in New Zealand.* New Zealand Child and Youth Epidemiology Service. https://www.otago.ac.nz/nzcyes/otago086561.pdf

Darlow B. A., Horwood L. J., Mogridge N., & Clemett R. S. (1997). Prospective study of New Zealand very low birthweight infants: Outcome at 7 to 8 years. *Journal of Paediatrics and Child Health, 33*, 47–51. http://doi/10.1111/j.1440-1754.1997.tb00990.x

Dunconson M., Smith D., & Davies E. (2009). *Death and serious injury from assault of children under 5 years in Aotearoa-New Zealand: A review of international literature and recent findings.* Office of the Children's Commissioner. https://www.occ.org.nz/assets/Uploads/Reports/Child-abuse-and-neglect/Death-and-serious-injury.pdf

Duncanson, M., Richardson, G., Wicken, A., van Asten, H., & Adams, J. (2020). *Child Poverty Monitor 2020: Technical Report (Child Poverty Monitor Series).* New Zealand Child and Youth Epidemiology Service. http://hdl.handle.net/10523/10585

Duncanson, M., Oben, G., Adams, J., Richardson, G., Wicken, A., & Pierson, M. (2019). *Health and wellbeing of under-15 year olds in Aotearoa 2018.* New Zealand Child and Youth Epidemiology Service. http://hdl.handle.net/10523/9641

Ferguson D. M., & Lynskey M. T. (1997). Physical punishment/maltreatment during childhood and adjustment in young adulthood. *Child Abuse & Neglect, 21*(7), 617–630. https://doi.org/10.1016/s0145-2134(97)00021-5

Foliaki, S., Pulu, V., Denison, H., Weatherall, M., & Douwes, J. (2020). Pacific meets west in addressing palliative care for Pacific populations in Aotearoa/New Zealand: a qualitative study. *BMC Palliative Care, 19*(1), 1–12. https://doi.org/10.1186/s12904-020-00604-2

Gakidou, E., Cowling, K., Lozano, R., & Murray, C. J. (2010). Increased educational attainment and its effect on child mortality in 175 countries between 1970 and 2009: a systematic analysis. *The Lancet*, 376(9745), 959–974. https://doi.org/10.1016/S0140-6736(10)61257-3

Gibb S., Milne B., Shakleton N., Taylor B., & Audas R. (2019). How universal are universal preschool health checks? An observational study using routine data from New Zealand's B4 School Check. *BMJ Open*, *9*(4), e025535. https://doi.org/10.1136/bmjopen-2018-025535

Gilles T, Tomlin A, Dovey S.M., & Tilyard M. (2013). Ethnic disparities in asthma treatment and outcomes in children under 15 years in New Zealand; analysis of national databases. *Primary Care Respiratory Journal: Journal of the General Practice Airways Group, 22*(3),312–318. https://doi.org/10.4104/pcrj.2013.00068

Grant, C. C., Pati, A., Tan, D., Vogel, S., Aickin, R., & Scragg, R. (2001). Ethnic comparisons of disease severity in children hospitalized with pneumonia in New Zealand. *Journal of Paediatrics and Child Health, 37*(1), 32–37. https://doi.org/10.1046/j.1440-1754.2001.00583.x

Health New Zealand | Te Whatu Ora. (2022). *Report on Maternity web tool: Preterm birth rates by ethnicity (2022).* Health New Zealand. Retrieved December 5, 2025, from https://www.tewhatuora.govt.nz/for-health-professionals/data-and-statistics/maternity/report-on-maternity-web-tool

Health Quality & Safety Commission. (2021). *Bula Sautu – A window on quality 2021: Pacific health in the year of COVID-19.* Health Quality & Safety Commission. https://www.hqsc.govt.nz/assets/Health-Quality-Evaluation/PR/BulaSautu_WEB.pdf

Heckman, J., Humphries, J. E., Veramendi, G., & Urzua, S. (2014). Education, Health and Wages (No. w19971; p. w19971). *National Bureau of Economic Research.* https://doi.org/10.3386/w19971

Hobbs, M., Morton, S., Atatoa Carr, P., Ritchie, S. R., Thomas, M. J., Saraf, R., Chelimo, C., Harnden, A., Camargo, C. A., & Grant, C. C. (2016). Ethnic disparities in infectious disease hospitalisations in the first year of life in New Zealand. Journal of Paediatrics and Child Health, 53(3), 223–231. https://doi.org/10.1111/jpc.13377

Hoffmann, J. P., Thorpe, J. D., & Dufur, M. J. (2020). Family Social Capital and Delinquent Behavior in the United Kingdom. *Social Sciences, 9*(10). http://doi.org/10.3390/socsci9100178

Ingham, T., Keall, M., Jones, B., Aldridge, D. R. T., Dowell, A. C., Davies, C., Crane, J., Draper, J. B., Bailey, L. O., Viggers, H., Stanley, T. V., Leadbitter, P., Latimer, M., & Howden-Chapman, P. (2019).

Damp mouldy housing and early childhood hospital admissions for acute respiratory infection: a case control study. *Thorax, 74*(9), 849–857. https://doi.org/10.1136/thoraxjnl-2018-212979

Institute of Environmental Science and Research (ESR). (2019a). *Measles Weekly report. Week 51:14–20 Dec 2019.* https://surv.esr.cri.nz/PDF_surveillance/MeaslesRpt/2019/WeeklyMeasles23122019.pdf

Institute of Environmental Science and Research (ESR). (2019b). *Invasive Meningococcal Disease report: 2019.* https://surv.esr.cri.nz/PDF_surveillance/MeningococcalDisease/2019/MeningococcalDisease_Q4_2019.pdf

Institute of Environmental Science and Research (ESR). (2018). *Biannual Rheumatic fever report Jan-Dec 2018.* https://surv.esr.cri.nz/PDF_surveillance/RheumaticFever/Rheumaticfeverbi-annualreportJan-Dec2018.pdf

Jaine R, Baker M, Venugopal K. (2008). Epidemiology of acute rheumatic fever in New Zealand 1996–2005. *Journal of Paediatrics and Child Health. 44*(10), 564–571. https://doi.org/10.1111/j.1440-1754.2008.01384.x

Mahon C, Walker W, Drage A, Best E. (2016). Incidence, aetiology and outcome of pleural empyema and parapneumonia effusions from 1998 to 2012 in a population of New Zealand children. *Journal of paediatrics and child health, 52*(6), 662–668 https://doi.org/10.1111/jpc.13172

McCallum J, Craig L, Whittaker I, & Baxter J. (2015). Ethnic differences in acute hospitalisations for otitis media and elective hospitalisations for ventilation tubes in New Zealand children aged 0–14 years. *New Zealand Medical Journal, 128*(1416), 10–20.

Meaney MJ. (2018). Perinatal Maternal depressive symptoms as an issue for Population health. *The American Journal of Psychiatry, 175* (11), 1084–1093. https://doi.org/10.1176/appi.ajp.2018.17091031

Ministry of Health. (2008). *Pacific Youth Health: A paper for the Pacific health and Disability Action Plan Review.* https://www.health.govt.nz/system/files/documents/publications/pacific-youth-health-may08.pdf

Ministry of Health. (2012). *Communicable disease control manual.* https://www.health.govt.nz/publications/communicable-disease-control-manual-2012

Ministry of Health. (2020). *Well Child Tamariki Ora Report.* https://www.health.govt.nz/system/files/documents/publications/well-child-tamariki-ora-review-report-2020-jul21.pdf

Ministry of Health. (2021). *Reducing Rheumatic Fever.* https://www.health.govt.nz/our-work/diseases-and-conditions/rheumatic-fever/reducing-rheumatic-fever

Moore, D. R., Zobay, O., & Ferguson, M. A. (2020). Minimal and Mild Hearing Loss in Children: Association with Auditory Perception, Cognition, and Communication Problems. *Ear and Hearing, 41*(4), 720–732. https://doi.org/10.1097/AUD.0000000000000802

Moors, J. (2016). *A Metabolic Health Study of Pacific Adolescents Investigating the metabolic health of Pacific adolescents in New Zealand: Environmental and genetic risk factors.* [Master's thesis, University of Otago]. OUR Archive. http://hdl.handle.net/10523/6208

National Research Council (US), & Institute of Medicine (US). (2004). *Children's Health, The Nation's Wealth: Assessing and Improving Child Health.* National Academies Press (US). https://doi.org/10.17226/10886

Oben, G., & Duncanson, M. (2019, November 22). *High and increasing rates of skin infection hospitalisation for Pacific children in Aotearoa* [Conference presentation]. The Paediatric Society of New Zealand 71st Annual Scientific Meeting. https://ourarchive.otago.ac.nz/handle/10523/12014

Oranga Tamariki. (2021). *Oranga Tamariki Quarterly Report June 2021*. https://www.orangatamariki.govt.nz/assets/Uploads/About-us/Performance-and-monitoring/Quarterly-report/June-2021/Oranga-Tamariki-Quarterly-Performance-Report-as-at-June-2021.pdf

Ornoy A. (2005). Growth and neurodevelopmental outcome of children born to mothers with pregestational and gestational diabetes. *Pediatric endocrinology reviews*, *3*(2), 104–113.

Pamuk, E. R., Fuchs, R., & Lutz, W. (2011). Comparing relative effects of education and economic resources on infant mortality in developing countries. *Population and Development Review*, *37*(4), 637–664. https://doi.org/10.1111/j.1728-4457.2011.00451.x

Paterson, J. E., Carter, S., Wallace, J., Ahmad, Z., Garrett, N., & Silva, P. A. (2006). Pacific Islands families study: the prevalence of chronic middle ear disease in 2-year-old Pacific children living in New Zealand. *International Journal of Pediatric Otorhinolaryngology*, *70*(10), 1771–1778. https://doi.org/10.1016/j.ijporl.2006.06.001

Paterson, J., Carter, S., Gao, W., & Perese, L. (2007). Pacific Islands Families Study: behavioral problems among two-year-old Pacific children living in New Zealand. *Journal of Child Psychology and Psychiatry, and Allied Disciplines*, *48*(5), 514–522. https://doi.org/10.1111/j.1469-7610.2006.01716.x

Paterson, J., Feehan, M., Butler, S., Williams, M., & Cowley-Malcolm, E. T. (2007). Intimate partner violence within a cohort of Pacific mothers living in New Zealand. *Journal of Interpersonal Violence*, *22*(6), 698–721. https://doi.org/10.1177/0886260507300596

Paterson, J., Iusitini, L., & Gao, W. (2011). Child developmental assessment at two-years of age: data from the Pacific Islands Families Study. *Pacific Health Dialog*, *17*(2), 51–63.

Patton, G. C., Sawyer, S. M., Santelli, J. S., Ross, D. A., Afifi, R., Allen, N. B., Arora, M., Azzopardi, P., Baldwin, W., Bonell, C., Kakuma, R., Kennedy, E., Mahon, J., McGovern, T., Mokdad, A. H., Patel, V., Petroni, S., Reavley, N., Taiwo, K., Waldfogel, J., … Viner, R. M.

(2016). Our future: a Lancet commission on adolescent health and wellbeing. *The Lancet, 387*(10036), 2423–2478. https://doi.org/10.1016/S0140-6736(16)00579-1

Perinatal Mortality Review Committee. (2021). *Fourteenth Annual Report of the Perinatal and Maternal Mortality Review Committee | Te Pūrongo ā-Tau Tekau mā Whā o te Komiti Arotake Mate Pēpi, Mate Whaea Hoki: Reporting mortality and morbidity 2018 | Te tuku pūrongo mō te mate me te whakamate 2018.* Health Quality & Safety Commission.https://www.hqsc.govt.nz/assets/PMMRC/Publications/14thPMMRCreport/report-pmmrc-14th.pdf

Perna, R., Loughan, A. R., Le, J., & Tyson, K. (2015). Gestational Diabetes: Long-Term Central Nervous System Developmental and Cognitive Sequelae. *Applied Neuropsychology. Child, 4*(3), 217–220. https://doi.org/10.1080/21622965.2013.874951

Pio, F. H., & Nosa, V. (2020). Health literacy of Samoan mothers and their experiences with health professionals. *Journal of Primary Health Care, 12*(1), 57–63. https://doi.org/10.1071/HC19026

Purdy, S. C., Taylor, S., Schluter, P. J., Tautolo, E. S., Iusitini, L., Ahmad, Z., Sundborn, G., & Paterson, J. (2019). Hearing and ear status of Pacific children aged 11 years living in New Zealand: the Pacific Islands families hearing study. *International Journal of Audiology, 58*(2), 77–86. https://doi.org/10.1080/14992027.2018.1506170

Richards, N., Reith, D., Stitely, M., & Smith, A. (2019). The Before School Check (B4SC): reporting outcomes and referral rates for all New Zealand children. *The New Zealand Medical Journal, 132*(1496), 9–19.

Roy, R., Greaves, L. M., Peiris-John, R., Clark, T., Fenaughty, J., Sutcliffe, K., Barnett, D., Hawthorne, V., Tiatia-Seath, J., & Fleming, T. (2020). *Negotiating multiple identities: Intersecting identities among Māori, Pacific, Rainbow and Disabled young people.* The Youth19 Research Group, University of Auckland and Victoria University. https://www.myd.govt.nz/documents/resources-and-reports/publications/negotiating-multiple-identities/youth19-intersectionality-report-final.pdf

Rush, E., Obolonkin, V., & Savila, F. (2013). Growth centiles of Pacific children living in Auckland, New Zealand. *Annals of Human Biology*, *40*(5), 406–412. https://doi.org/10.3109/03014460.2013.793391

Ryan, D., Grey, C., & Mischewski, B. (2019). *Tofa Saili: A review of evidence about health equity for Pacific Peoples in New Zealand.* Pacific Perspectives Ltd. https://www.pacificperspectives.co.nz/publications/

Sawyer, S. M., Afifi, R. A., Bearinger, L. H., Blakemore, S. J., Dick, B., Ezeh, A. C., & Patton, G. C. (2012). Adolescence: a foundation for future health. *The Lancet, 379*(9826), 1630–1640. https://doi.org/10.1016/S0140-6736(12)60072-5

Schluter, P. J., & Paterson, J. (2009). Relating intimate partner violence to heath-care utilisation and injuries among Pacific children in Auckland: the Pacific Islands Families Study. *Journal of Paediatrics and Child Health*, *45*(9), 518–524. https://doi.org/10.1111/j.1440-1754.2009.01554.x

Schluter, P. J., Tautolo, E., & Paterson, J. (2011). Experience of physical abuse in childhood and perpetration of physical punishment and violence in adulthood amongst fathers: findings from the Pacific Islands Families Study. *Pacific Health Dialog*, *17*(2), 148–162.

Sexton, K., Lennon, D., Oster, P., Crengle, S., Martin, D., Mulholland, K., Percival, T., Reid, S., Stewart, J., & O'Hallahan, J. (2004). The New Zealand Meningococcal Vaccine Strategy: a tailor-made vaccine to combat a devastating epidemic. *The New Zealand Medical Journal*, *117*(1200), U1015.

Sheridan, K., Haight, W. L., & Cleeland, L. (2011). The role of grandparents in preventing aggressive and other externalizing behavior problems in children from rural, methamphetamine-involved families. *Children and Youth Services Review*, *33*(9), 1583–1591. https://doi.org/10.1016/j.childyouth.2011.03.023

Simpson J., Duncanson M., Oben G., Adams J., Wicken A., Butchard M., Pierson M., Lilley R., & Gallagher S. (2017). *The Health Status of*

Children and Young People in the Northern District Health Boards 2015. New Zealand Child and Youth Epidemiology Service, University of Otago. http://hdl.handle.net/10523/6725

Sjardin, N., Reed, P., Albert, B., Mouat, F., Carter, P. J., Hofman, P., & Jefferies, C. (2018). Increasing incidence of type 2 diabetes in New Zealand children < 15 years of age in a regional-based diabetes service, Auckland, New Zealand. *Journal of paediatrics and child health*, *54*(9), 1005–1010.

Soszyn N., Cloete E., Sadler L., Stein-de Laat M., Crengle S., Bloomfield F., & Gentles T. (2019). Does Disease Severity Contribute to Disparity in Outcome Amongst Ethnic Groups in Patients with Hypoplastic Left Heart syndrome in New Zealand? *Heart, Lung and Circulation*, *28*, S348–S349. https://doi.org/10.1016/j.hlc.2019.06.499

Southwick M., Ryan D., & Kenealy T. (2012). *Primary Care for Pacific People: A Pacific and Health Systems approach*. Pacific Perspectives. https://www.health.govt.nz/system/files/documents/publications/primary-care-pacific-people-pacific-health-systems-approach.pdf

Stats NZ. (2014). *2013 Census QuickStats about culture and identity*. https://www.stats.govt.nz/reports/2013-census-quickstats-about-culture-and-identity

Stein, A., Malmberg, L. E., Sylva, K., Barnes, J., Leach, P., & FCCC team** (2008). The influence of maternal depression, caregiving, and socioeconomic status in the post-natal year on children's language development. *Child: Care, Health and Development*, *34*(5), 603–612. https://doi.org/10.1111/j.1365-2214.2008.00837.x

Stephens D. S. (2007). Conquering the meningococcus. *FEMS Microbiology Reviews*, *31*(1), 3–14. https://doi.org/10.1111/j.1574-6976.2006.00051.x

Teevale, T., Denny, S., Percival, T., Fleming, T. (2013). Pacific secondary school students' access to primary health care in New

Zealand. *The New Zealand Medical Journal, 126*(1375), 58–68. http://journal.nzma.org.nz/journal//126-1375/5680/

The Families Commission. (2011). *Teenage pregnancy and parenting: An overview*. Social Policy Evaluation and Research Unit (Superu). https://thehub.swa.govt.nz/assets/documents/teenage-pregnancy.pdf

Tin Tin, S., Woodward, A., Saraf, R., Berry, S., Atatoa Carr, P., Morton, S. M., & Grant, C. C. (2016). Internal living environment and respiratory disease in children: findings from the Growing Up in New Zealand longitudinal child cohort study. *Environmental Health, 15*(1), 1–10. https://doi.org/10.1186/s12940-016-0207-z

Trenholme, A., Vogel, A., Lennon, D., McBride, C., Stewart, J., Best, E., Mason, H., & Percival, T. (2012). Household characteristics of children under 2 years admitted with lower respiratory tract infection in Counties Manukau, South Auckland. *The New Zealand Medical Journal, 125*(1367), 15–23.

Turner N. (2019). A measles epidemic in New Zealand: Why did this occur and how can we prevent it occurring again?. *The New Zealand Medical Journal, 132*(1504), 8–12.

Twiss, J., Metcalfe, R., Edwards, E., & Byrnes, C. (2005). New Zealand national incidence of bronchiectasis "too high" for a developed country. *Archives of Disease in Childhood, 90*(7), 737–740. https://doi.org/10.1136/adc.2004.066472

UNICEF. (2003). *A League Table of Child Maltreatment Deaths in Rich Nations, Innocenti Report Card No.5, September 2003*. UNICEF, Innocenti Research Centre, Florence. https://www.unicef-irc.org/publications/pdf/repcard5e.pdf

Webb, R. H., Grant, C., & Harnden, A. (2015). Acute rheumatic fever. *BMJ: British Medical Journal, 351*(h3443), 1–8. https://doi.org/10.1136/bmj.h3443

Wilson-Costello D. (2007). Is there evidence that long-term outcomes have improved with intensive care?. *Seminars in Fetal*

& Neonatal Medicine, 12(5), 344–354. https://doi.org/10.1016/j.siny.2007.06.010

World Health Organization. (1946, July 22). *Constitution of the World Health Organization.* https://apps.who.int/gb/bd/PDF/bd47/EN/constitution-en.pdf?ua=1

World Health Organization. (2018). WHO housing and health guidelines. https://www.who.int/publications/i/item/9789241550376

Wong, W., Morris, M. C., & Zwi, J. (2009). Outcome of severe acute post-streptococcal glomerulonephritis in New Zealand children. *Pediatric Nephrology, 24*(5), 1021–1026. https://doi.org/10.1007/s00467-008-1086-5

Wong, W., Lennon, D. R., Crone, S., Neutze, J. M., & Reed, P. W. (2013). Prospective population-based study on the burden of disease from post-streptococcal glomerulonephritis of hospitalised children in New Zealand: epidemiology, clinical features and complications. *Journal of Paediatrics and Child Health*, *49*(10), 850–855. https://doi.org/10.1111/jpc.12295

Wright, N., Hammond, P., Morreau, P., & Hamill, J. (2011). Increased incidence of empyema in Polynesian children. *The New Zealand Medical Journal, 124*(1333), 32–39.

The health of women and reproductive health

Kara Okesene-Gafa

Chapter summary

The state of the health of Pacific women in Aotearoa New Zealand (AoNZ) is concerning. There is scarcity of in-depth data looking at the health issues of Pacific women in AoNZ, and like many countries globally the health of women is often low priority (World Health Organization, 2021). This chapter endeavours to collate what is currently known of the health of Pacific women in AoNZ. Counties Manukau Health in South Auckland is home to the highest proportion of Pacific women in AoNZ; hence a good proportion of this chapter is written from information available from this region.

Introduction

The health of Pacific women in Aotearoa-New Zealand (AoNZ) is concerning. Despite difficulties and health issues many Pacific women face, they are resilient and are family, church, and community oriented (Ryan et al., 2019). Women continue to rise above the challenges, making the best of their situations and forging better futures for themselves, their families, and their communities.

A high proportion of Pacific women reside in areas of socio-economic deprivation and within these contexts, obesity is highly prevalent.. One of the most concerning health issues for Pacific women in AoNZ, is living with the consequences of obesity. The obesity epidemic has continued to increase globally, in AoNZ and in the Pacific, worsening the health outcomes of Pacific women throughout their life course. The NZ health survey, 2020/2021, reported that 34% of adults and 13% of children were classified as having obesity (Ministry of Health, 2021a). Rates are highest among Pacific populations 63.4%, Māori 47.9% compared with European 29.3%, and Asian 15.9%. Te Whatu Ora, Counties Manukau in South Auckland where the highest proportion of Pacific people reside, Pacific women with overweight and obesity who birthed in their facility were 17.2% and 72.1%, respectively. The parallel rise in diabetes in pregnancy as a consequence is also concerning (Counties Manukau Health, 2020).

Obesity not only affects the lives of women, but also of their families and communities. The high rates of obesity with associated diabetes and CVD increases risks of early mortality, with reduced life expectancy. Although Pacific specific data is not well reported, it is known that obesity increases risks of many adverse gynaecological and pregnancy outcomes (Gluckman et al., 2010).

Obesity in pregnancy increases risks of the intergenerational cycle of childhood and adult obesity with increased risks of diabetes and CVD later in life (Gluckman et al., 2010). Women who develop gestational diabetes during pregnancy have a 1:2 risk of developing Type 2 diabetes within 2–10 years of the index pregnancy. Pacific women with obesity have high rates of abnormal uterine bleeding (AUB) and endometrial cancer (EC), the fastest growing cancer in Pacific women in New Zealand (Meredith et al., 2012). Although there has been improvement in reduction in breast cancer and cervical cancer in Pacific women, their rates are still higher compared to non-Pacific and non-Māori women.

The perinatal related mortality reports (PMMRC) highlighted the high rates of perinatal mortality in Pacific associated with maternal conditions, and barriers to accessing and utilising antenatal care. It also highlights the causes of perinatal related mortality in Pacific women (Perinatal and Maternal Mortality Review Committee, 2021).

Pacific women in gynaecology

Impact of obesity

Obesity is defined as a body mass index (BMI) = weight/height^2 of ≥ 30kg/m^2. This BMI has been debated by many, as Pacific people have a high nonfat mass, hence BMI for Pacific people should be higher for obesity of (≥ 32kg/m^2). A significant proportion of health issues faced by Pacific women in gynaecology are also related to the high rates of obesity. The mechanism behind high circulating exogenous estrogen, affecting the menstrual cycle is still not well known (Lash and Armstrong, 2009). It is also not known the proportion of Pacific women who suffer from Polycystic ovarian syndrome, a condition highly associated with obesity, with women demonstrating high levels of insulin resistance and insulinemia, with increased risk of metabolic dysfunction and long-term diabetes (Zore et al., 2017). These women also suffer issues with infertility.

A significant proportion of Pacific women suffer from irregular or heavy and AUB. Pacific women often do not pay attention to these symptoms and do not realise that heavy menstrual bleeding (HMB) is not normal. Excess estrogen affects feedback to the hypothalamus, resulting in irregular menstruation. Excess uncontrolled estrogen causes thickening of the lining of the uterus (endometrium) increasing risks of infertility and EC (Lash and Armstrong, 2009).

In Te Whatu Ora Counties Manukau (CM) region in South Auckland, where a significant proportion of Pacific women reside, obesity in gynaecology patients have become a major issue for provision of gynaecological services. These patients are more difficult to manage. A significant proportion of women have other co-morbidities, resulting in more complex and longer surgeries, anaesthetic difficulties, longer recovery time, and post op complications with increased risks of infections and venous thromboembolism. Counties Manukau region has the highest rates of EC driven by high rates of obesity and diabetes (Counties Manukau Health, 2020).

There are also considerable access issues to gynaecological services in South Auckland CM. There is unmet need of women in the region not accessing secondary care in a timely manner, with significant lack of resources and delays for surgical treatment due to high volumes of patients and limited access to a specialist and to theatre if needing surgery. The COVID outbreaks in 2020 and

2021 have compounded these issues with gynaecology services struggling to keep up with demand and to also fulfil requirements for the Faster Cancer Treatment (FCT) pathway for women diagnosed with cancer. Pacific women may be facing similar issues in other regions in AoNZ (Counties Manukau Health, 2020).

CM region did acknowledge equity issues with Māori and Pacific women being over-represented in gynaecological services and surgical data, due to barriers to access and lack of awareness of abnormal gynaecological signs and symptoms to seek care early. Many Pacific women with HMB are not aware that this is in fact abnormal and have learnt to live with this debilitation. There is a concern that lack of awareness of abnormal menstrual bleeding in at risk women may delay diagnosis and treatment of endometrial abnormalities including cancer (Counties Manukau Health, 2020).

Fertility

Pacific women are at risk of infertility once the menstrual cycle is affected. If there are already abnormalities in the endometrium (lining of the womb is thickened) when the woman becomes pregnant, there is increased risk of miscarriage either due to the abnormal lining of the uterus (not possible to hold a pregnancy) or abnormal conceptus or congenital abnormality (structural or chromosomal not compatible with life). Due to stringent criteria for entering fertility services in NZ, Pacific women are known to not access these services easily (Fertility Associates, 2021). There is an assumption that it is more culturally acceptable for Pacific populations to adopt children from other family members (i.e., whangai) than to undergo fertility treatment, as some of the requirements (example producing a sperm sample) may not be culturally acceptable (personal communication with fertility specialist). The BMI cutoff of 32kg/m^2 has been identified as a barrier to accessing these services by Pacific women (Fertility Associates, 2021).

There is also lack of data in Pacific women of the condition of endometriosis (lining of the endometrium transplanted outside the uterus) causing infertility which affect a proportion of young women in New Zealand.

Cancers

Endometrial cancer

The increasing rates of EC in Pacific women in NZ is concerning. A study looking at the incidence of EC in Middlemore hospital, South Auckland NZ, reported that of n = 588 women diagnosed with EC between 2000 and 2014, there was a high proportion of Pacific women (n = 242) with the highest incidence of EC; relative risk (RR) 5.11 compared with Māori RR 2.47. Pacific women had the highest overall increase incidence over 15 years with an 'annual percentage change' (APC) of 9.3 (95% confidence interval (CI) 4–14.9) compared to Māori and Other with APC of 7.2 (95% CI 0.2–14.6) and 3.4 (95% CI 0.5–6.4), respectively. Highest proportion of Pacific women with EC were in obesity class III (BMI ≥ 40kg/m^2) with most having risk factors for EC of diabetes, impaired glucose tolerance (IGT), hypertension, hyperlipidemia, and nulliparity. Fortunately, most women were diagnosed at stage FIGO Grade 1 Stage 1, amendable to surgery and treatment. Most of the treatment for Pacific women by surgery (83.9%) with 16.1% no surgery (regressed or too advanced). Concerning for Pacific women is the high APC in premenopausal women, with Pacific women acquiring EC at a much younger age (Bigby et al., 2020).

Linked cancer mortality data between 1981 and 2001 reported the increasing rates of EC in Pacific women. It was reported that in 1981–1986, EC rate for Pacific female was 22.9/100,000 with a rate difference of 11.1 (−1.7 to 239) and rate ratio 1.94 (1.10 to 3.41) compared with rates of 11.8 in European females during this time. This rate increased dramatically between 2006 and 2011 to 49.8/100,000, rate difference of 37.2 (29.1 to 45.3) *p* value (probability that the observed difference is due to chance), < 0.01 and a rate ratio of 3.95 (3.31 to 4.71) compared to European rate of 12.6 in 2006–2011 (Teng et al., 2016). Another study examined the cancer incidence rates among Pacific people living in New Zealand from 1981 to 2004 which again confirmed the markedly increased rates of EC from 37.5/100,000 in 1981–1986 to 69.7/100,00 in 2001–2004. Pooled age standardised incidence rate for EC in Pacific women was 46.7/1000 (95% CI 39.4–53.9) compared to European/Other 17.9/100,000 (17.3–18.5), with a standardised rate ratio (SRR) of 2.61 (2.22–3.05) and standardised rate difference (SRD) of 29 (21–36) (Meredith et al., 2012).

A systematic review (five studies) examining the association of increase in BMI and endometrial hyperplasia (thickened lining of the uterus) and EC in premenopausal women identified the existence of a dose response relationship between BMI and increased risk of EC. The pooled odds ratio (OR) for a BMI of ≥ 25, ≥ 30, and ≥ 40 for developing EC were 3.85 (95% CI 2.53–5.84); 5.25 (4.00–6.90); and 19.79 (11.18–35.03), respectively (Wise et al., 2016). Studies have reported increase in EC rate with increase in BMI (Scott et al., 2019) and a 2014 systematic review of 26 prospective studies found a summary RR per 5 kg/m^2 increase in BMI of developing EC of 1.56 (95% CI, 1.48–1.64) (Aune et al., 2015).

A survey of women with EC reported that they were not aware of the association between obesity with EC or reproductive health issues (Beavis et al., 2015). Women were aware of the increased risks of diabetes and CVD in association with obesity. A low proportion of women correctly identified the association of obesity with development of EC (37.4%), breast cancer (34.4%), and infertility (35.0%). Only women already diagnosed with EH and EC were more aware of the increased risk of EC, breast cancer, and infertility (53.5%, 48.8%, and 51.2%) in association with obesity compared to controls (31.7, 29.2, 29.2% [$p < 0.05$]), respectively). Only 55% of the women surveyed affirmed that their doctor discussed their weight and advising weight loss to improve their health (Beavis et al., 2015).

Other cancers

Cervical cancers in Pacific women have reduced by 64% over time, although it is still higher in Pacific than European/Other of 32.9 per 100,000 versus 16.0 per 100,000 with a pooled SRR of 2.05 (1.67–2.52), and SRD of 17 (10–24.0). Tobacco smoking may be contributing partly to cervical cancer in Pacific women (Blakely et al., 2011; Meredith et al., 2012). Lung cancer was initially lower than European but for some reason increased again by 2004 to 24 % higher than European (Blakely et al., 2011). Lung cancer rates among Pacific women have increased rapidly over time, from 16.8 per 100,000 (95 % CI, 4.9–28.6) in 1981–1986 to 57.9 per 100,000 (95 % CI, 43.5–72.3) in 2001–2004 (APC 1.9, $p = 0.02$). There were no significant trends for Pacific men (APC 0.11, $p = 0.96$) (Meredith et al., 2012).

Ovarian cancer did not appear to have any ethnic specific trends, however, pooled rates over time showed Pacific with 1.35 greater rate of ovarian cancer compared to European (Blakely et al., 2011). Thyroid cancer was elevated for Pacific females only with incidence rates for women aged 15+ of 18.5/100,000 (95 % CI, 14.6–22.4) versus 5.2/100,000 (95 % CI, 4.8–5.5) for European/Other women (SRR = 3.58; 95 % CI, 2.87–4.47) (Blakely et al., 2011). Breast cancer in Pacific overall was reported as 10% less than European/Other women in New Zealand. However, when categorised by age, the rate for those aged 25–44 years is higher for Pacific than European/Other women with a standardised rate ratio of 1.16 (95 % CI, 1.01–1.35) and a statistically significant increase (87%) in breast cancer in those > 65+ years ($p < 0.01$) (Blakely et al., 2011).

Contraception

Contraception is a fundamental human right (World Health Organization, 2020). It allows women worldwide to have choice of whether they wish to be pregnant, ability to space their pregnancies, reduce unsafe abortion practices, and have reduced maternal mortality and morbidity. Women have suffered issues with lack of understanding, access, fear of side effects, religious or cultural beliefs, and whanau or partner influence.

Different types of contraception available vary from hormonal methods to barrier methods. Hormonal methods include the oral contraceptive in pill (OCP) in tablet form to be taken daily with sugar pills at time of the menses or as an emergency contraception (EC) after unprotected sex. Others include long-acting reversible contraception (LARC) either as an intrauterine device

(Mirena or Jadess); implant under the skin in the arm (Jadelle); or an intramuscular injection (depo Provera). Copper intrauterine device is a barrier method that does not contain a hormone. Barrier methods include male and female condoms and Nuva ring. The more permanent forms of contraception are vasectomy for males and tubal ligation for females. Others include withdrawal methods and natural. Each method has effectiveness scores and failure rates.

Due to the unmet need of lack of access to contraception, there has been a conscious effort to improve women's knowledge and access to contraception for all women in AoNZ. Family planning services have been underfunded for a long time. Family Planning NZ launched an online survey to obtain information on contraceptive use in AoNZ (n = 6,764 women surveyed) (Family Planning, 2020). Limitations of the survey was its inability to represent the different women populations in AoNZ with responses from NZ European, Māori, and Pacific of 85%, 12%, and 2%, respectively. The most common age of contraceptive use was in 20–29-year old's followed by 30–39-year old's of 55% and 25%, respectively. The survey identifies the most common methods of contraception were condoms and the OCP.

The 2014/2015 New Zealand Health survey key finding reported that Pacific and those living in low socioeconomic situations were less likely to use any form of contraception (Ministry of Health, 2019). Only 52% of Pacific were using some form of modern contraception compared to 78% European/Other. Women in socioeconomic deprivation were also six times more likely to use injectable forms of contraception. Pacific women who did not want to get pregnant were less likely to have their contraception needs met. Pacific women were 0.7 times as likely to have their needs met for contraception compared to non-Pacific women. Pacific women are less likely to rely on her husband's vasectomy as a form of contraception (Ministry of Health, 2019). Jadelle implants has become the more favourable form of contraception for Pacific women. Pacific women are 1.2 times more likely to use Jadelle compared to non-Pacific women.

The Health Quality & Safety Commission NZ Atlas of health care report on contraception use by women described an almost two-fold increase in uptake of Jadelle in Pacific women (Health Quality and Safety Commisson, 2021). The acceptability of this method is possibly due to its ease of insertion under the arm, lasts 5 years, fit and forget, minimal or minor side effects, and easily reversible. The Health Quality Safety Atlas reported that Pacific women; more likely to receive a LARC after an abortion (62%) and less likely to use an intrauterine contraceptive device (IUCD) or the OCP compared to European (Health Quality and Safety Commission, 2021). This uptake of LARCs (Mirena and Jadelle) in Pacific women increased when the NZ Ministry of Health agreed to fully fund them from November 2019. Publicly funded Mirena is not only advantageous for Pacific women with AUB, but an effective form of contraception and lasts 5 years. However, there are still concerns regarding barrier to access for Pacific women needing to pay GP fees for insertion (Te Karu et al., 2021).

To overcome some of the barriers in general practice, women presenting to hospitals for gynaecological procedures or for childbirth are offered an opportunity for a LARC if suitable. In Te Whatu Ora CM region in South Auckland, more clinicians and nurse practitioners have been trained to insert postpartum

LARCs. This improved uptake due to availability, convenience, and advantages of immediate postpartum insertion (Royal College of Obstetricians and Gynaecologists, 2021). Women are counselled about the importance of spacing pregnancies at least 18 months to improve maternal and perinatal outcomes. Shorter pregnancy intervals increase risks of preterm births, low birth weight, and small for gestational age babies (Conde-Agudelo et al., 2006). There has been increased uptake of Mirena or copper IUCD insertion post caesarean sections and after abortion (Royal College of Obstetricians and Gynaecologists, 2021; Whitley et al., 2020). Women who do not consent to these are offered an opportunity for a Jadelle insertion, or other form of contraception. Robust data on the outcome of these recent methods of contraceptive use need to be collated.

The Māori Midwifery health program in Counties is developing a clinically and culturally safe process to assist Māori wahine access to contraception especially LARCs (Counties Manukau Health, 2020). A similar program could be developed for Pacific women.

Pacific women in obstetrics

Antenatal

Women booking with lead maternity carer

All pregnant women are expected to book and be registered in a maternity health care service by a health care provider, often referred to as a lead maternity carer (LMC) and usually a midwife, occasionally a private obstetrician and very rarely GPs (Ministry of Health, 2021b). Women pay for private care. The LMC will be responsible for providing maternity care antenatally, during labour, and postnatally. Some LMCs may only provide primary care, either in primary birthing units (PBU) or in hospital, meaning that if the woman needs more complex care, the LMC may hand over the care to hospital midwives and doctors. The primary care LMC will continue with care of the woman and her baby postnatally after discharge from secondary care.

Pacific women can access maternity care by booking directly with an LMC midwife. A significant proportion of Pacific women are seen by their GPs to diagnose the pregnancy and subsequently referred either directly to an existing LMC midwife who may be co-located within a GP practice or women are given written information of how to find an LMC. A proportion of women will be referred to the hospital to source care for the pregnancy through community midwifery services or if they have a high-risk pregnancy needing specialist care.

Pacific women have issues finding an LMC and as a result not accessing maternity care early. This is compounded by the severe shortages of midwives across New Zealand and very few Pacific midwives. Research in South Auckland reported Pacific women's significant struggles with finding a midwife (Moana Research, 2018). The proportion of Pacific women booking early for antenatal care with an LMC are low. Key findings from a 2020 report of maternity clinical indicator outcomes for 2018 reported that Pacific women have first trimester booking rates of 46.7% compared with European, Asian, and Indian of 83%, 76.2%, and 74.4%, respectively (Maternity report, 2020). This low rate for early booking is worse in some Auckland regions for Pacific women with Te Whatu Ora: Counties Manukau, Te Toka Tumai Auckland, and Waitemata rates of first trimester booking of 37.1%, 39.8%, and 49.8%, respectively. Effort and time have been invested into encouraging Pacific women to book early for antenatal care, however, late booking after the first trimester will continue to be a problem unless LMC workforce issues have been resolved. Difficulties finding an LMC may be a reason why Pacific women are not booking early for care among other reported socioeconomic and personal barriers to attending care in the first trimester of pregnancy (Moana Research, 2018; Corbett et al., 2014).

Early booking and screening allow identification of comorbidities that may impact on pregnancy outcomes so women could be managed and referred to secondary care early if appropriate. Antenatal booking in the first trimester is strongly recommended (Moller et al., 2017) and resulted in improved pregnancy outcomes (EBCOG Scientific Committee, 2015). Early booking allows the LMC the time to obtain the relevant history, carry out required maternal examinations, discuss important health messages, and plan the care for the rest of the pregnancy. These include organising subsequent antenatal blood tests, maternal serum screening, ultrasounds, prescription of relevant supplements, as well as informing the woman of visiting schedules and timing of other relevant screening example polycose or oral glucose tolerance test for diabetes.

To address Pacific midwifery shortages, Te Whatu-Ora CM region and other health regions in NZ have offered scholarships to encourage and support midwifery trainees through different training institutions (Ministry of Health, 2021c).

Place of birth

Pacific women have a choice as to where they would like to birth depending on whether a straightforward pregnancy with no complications and how comfortable their LMC is of providing care either in a primary birthing unit or within the hospital. Most Pacific women birth in hospitals with much lower numbers birthing in PBU. This is thought to be due to women in the Pacific region traditionally encouraged to birth in a birthing facility (mostly in hospital) by a trained health care provider. It is understandable why Pacific women tend to birth in hospitals as a high proportion have obesity and other existing co-morbidities which increases their risks of complications at the time of birth.

Due to low number of Pacific women birthing in PBU, as research carried out by Moana Research (2018) in South Auckland of Pacific women's perspectives of birthing in a PBU, reported that they do not fully understand how PBU work. Women reported of the need to be better informed of the maternity care system, any payments required (care is free but ultrasounds have a surcharge), and that their partners also needed support. The advantages of birthing in PBU were not well socialised. Some women although preferring PBU were not suitable due to pregnancy risks. Family members also interfere with women's choices to birth in a PBU. Women who managed to birth successfully in a PBU reported their positive experiences.

Research in Te Whatu-Ora CM, South Auckland NZ reported that low risk pregnant women birthing in PBUs had better birth outcomes, were less likely to experience a postpartum haemorrhage; need to go to theatre; admission to a high dependency unit/intensive care unit (HDU/ICU); and four times less likely to need birth by caesarean section compared to women presenting to secondary care (Farry, 2015). Their babies were less likely to have low Apgar scores at birth; or needed admission to neonatal intensive care unit (NICU). Low risk Pacific women are encouraged to birth in PBU if possible. Very few Pacific women may consider a homebirth.

Risk factors

Obesity

Obesity is defined as BMI ≥ 30 kg/m^2. The New Zealand health survey 2020/2021 reported that 34% of adults and 13% of children were classified as having obesity. Different ethnic groups have different rates of obesity, the highest among Pacific populations of 63.4%, Māori 47.9%, compared with European 29.3% and Asian 15.9% (Ministry of Health, 2021a). The highest number of Pacific women who birth in NZ are in Te Whatu-Ora CM region in South Auckland. Total number of births in Te Whatu-Ora CM facilities in 2020 was $n = 7{,}392$, with 25.5% overweight and 44.8% with obesity in all women and for Pacific 17.9% were overweight and 72.1% with obesity (Counties Manukau Health, 2020).

Maternal complications of obesity

Maternal obesity increases risks to the mother of miscarriage, preterm birth (Nohr et al., 2009; Torloni et al., 2009), urinary tract infection, and obstructive sleep apnoea (Nohr et al., 2009; Nuthalapaty and Rouse, 2013; Weiss et al., 2004). Labour is more likely to be induced (Nohr et al., 2009); there is increased risk of instrumental delivery (Torloni et al., 2009), perineal trauma, and markedly elevated risks of intrapartum caesarean sections due to failure to progress (Fyfe et al., 2011; Nohr et al., 2009; Poobalan et al., 2009; Sheiner et al., 2004; Weiss et al., 2004). A contributing factor may be due to obesity increasing risks of developing pregnancy complications that could result in difficulties at birth. There are also higher rates of postpartum haemorrhage and wound infections (Nuthalapaty and Rouse, 2013). Women are less likely to successfully breastfeed (Nohr et al., 2009), due to delayed lactogenesis. Hormonal changes in women with obesity are also likely to be important with increased leptin levels (reducing oxytocin levels important for milk secretion) and reduced prolactin levels in the first 48 hours postpartum (Bever Babendure et al., 2015) . In addition, elevated androgen levels in women with obesity (possibly secondary to polycystic ovarian syndrome) also delayed lactation (Bever Babendure et al., 2015). There is a likelihood of poor development of breast tissue with mammary gland hypoplasia. Other factors that may contribute include psycho-social issues with low self-image, reduced confidence in breastfeeding often due to poor baby latching; having few contacts who have breastfed before; and possibly having eating disorders. These women are therefore more likely to offer formula early and stop breastfeeding altogether (Bever Babendure et al., 2015).

Obesity and increased risk of gestational diabetes

An important complication associated with obesity during pregnancy is the development of gestational-diabetes-mellitus (GDM) which is defined as glucose intolerance first recognised during pregnancy (Alberti and Zimmet, 1998). The recorded rate of GDM is continuing to rise in NZ from 1.3% in 2001 to 4.9% in 2012 (an annual increase of 13.9%, $P < 0.01$) (Ministry of Health, 2014). Of 61,000 births/annum in NZ, approximately 3,000 of women (5%) are diagnosed with diabetes in pregnancy. The highest are among Asian (13.3%) followed by Pacific, Middle-Eastern/Latin-American/African, European, and Māori of 8.3%, 5.9%, 4.3%, and 3.9%, respectively (Ministry of Health, 2014). The increases in rates of diabetes in pregnancy is also reflected in pregnancy data from different health districts in New Zealand (National Women's Health, 2014; Winnard et al., 2011). CMH in South Auckland, increased their diabetes in pregnancy rates from 3.1% in 2006 to 8.6% in 2015 (7000 births/annum) (Counties Manukau Health, 2016). Similarly, Central Auckland's National Women's Hospital increased their rates of diabetes in pregnancy from 2% in 1994 to 10% (of 6,597 total births/annum) in 2018. Their rates of gestational diabetes for Pacific women in 2020 was 10%. It has been noted that ethnic populations (Māori and Pacific) with high rates of obesity also have high rates of diabetes in pregnancy (National Women's Health, 2018). The majority of women identified as having GDM have similar population characteristics across the Auckland region with high BMI and lower socioeconomic status (National Women's Health, 2014; Winnard et al., 2011).

GDM exposes the fetus to excess nutrients creating an abnormal metabolic intrauterine environment resulting in fetal overgrowth due to extra energy being stored as adipose tissue (Crowther et al., 2005). Large babies increase the risks to the mother of having a caesarean section or a traumatic birth with associated injuries to the baby including nerve palsy as a result of shoulder dystocia (Crowther et al., 2005), bone fractures (Landon et al., 2009), and stillbirth (Heslehurst et al., 2008). Other neonatal complications include polycythaemia resulting in jaundice and hypoglycaemia that if persistent can cause brain injury (Crowther et al., 2005; Heslehurst et al., 2008).

Both obesity and GDM unfortunately create a perpetual intergenerational cycle of 'developmental over-nutrition' (Dabelea et al., 2008). LGA babies birthed to mothers with obesity, with or without GDM, are at increased risk of having childhood obesity and metabolic syndrome (Boney et al., 2005), which continues into adulthood increasing risks of adult diabetes (Catalano and Ehrenberg, 2006). These women when they reach adult reproductive age are more likely to enter pregnancy with obesity, therefore continuing the cycle of obesity and diabetes from generation to generation (Catalano, 2003). Women who develop GDM during pregnancy have a 50% risk of developing Type 2 diabetes within 2–10 years after the affected pregnancy (Kim et al., 2002).

Obesity and increased risks of hypertensive disorders in pregnancy

There is a strong association between obesity and increased risk of hypertensive disorders in pregnancy (HDP). Unfortunately, there is scarcity of data in New Zealand regarding Pacific women's rates of HDP. Data from National Women's Annual Clinical report 2020 conveyed an increase in pregnancy induced hypertension (pre-eclampsia, superimposed pre-eclampsia, and gestational hypertension) in Pacific women from 9% in 2006 to almost 13% in 2020 (total birthing population $n = 6{,}122$ with [11.7%] Pacific) (National Women's Health, 2020). HDP in Pacific women was also slightly higher compared to European with rates of Chronic Hypertension, gestational Hypertension, and pre-eclampsia of 2%, 6%, and 8% versus 2%, 5%, and 5%, respectively.

Complications of obesity in pregnancy for the baby

Risks to the baby include increased congenital abnormalities, macrosomia (Nuthalapaty and Rouse, 2013), shoulder dystocia, meconium aspiration, fetal distress (Cedergren, 2004), stillbirth (Stacey et al., 2011), and increased risk of neuro-developmental or cognitive disorders including attention deficit hyperactivity disorder (ADHD) in childhood, eating disorders in adolescence, and psychotic disorders in adulthood (Van Lieshout et al., 2011). Children are also at increased risk of childhood obesity (Adane et al., 2018; Godfrey et al., 2017; Ruager-Martin et al., 2010), not only due to maternal obesity but also from reduced initiation and continuation of breastfeeding (Bever Babendure et al., 2015).

Other birth outcomes of note

Maternity clinical indicators trends

There are 20 New Zealand maternity clinical indicators that are evidence of data collected from different district health boards (DHBs) in New Zealand comparing outcomes between DHBs and matched against main ethnic groups of Māori, Pacific, Indian, Asian, and European (Health New Zealand, 2025). It covers a range of procedures and outcomes, mostly maternal with four baby outcomes.

Other key findings from the 2025 report of maternity clinical indicator outcomes for 2023 presented Pacific women as having lower rates of intact lower genital tract of 12% compared with Māori of 20% and European of 14.7%. It is concerning that a significant proportion of women experience trauma to the perineum at the time of birth.

Pacific women have reported higher rates of complications

Pregnancy issue and rates	Pacific	Māori	European/ Other	Asian
3rd and 4th degree tears with no episiotomy	5.6%	1.7%	3.3%	3.1%
needing a blood transfusion post birth*	5.1% (vaginal) 7.1% (caesarean)	2.8% (vaginal) 5.7% (caesarean)	2.3% (vaginal) 3.4% (caesarean)	3.1% (vaginal) 4.0% (caesarean)
General anaesthetic during a caesarean	8.8%	11.8%	7.1%	5.4%
Spontaneous vaginal birth	67%	66%	55.7%	51.6%
Assisted instrumental birth	16.7%	13.3%	18.2%	25.4%
Small for gestational age babies (SGA)**	2.3%	3.3%	2.5%	3.0%

Data are from different regions – this table focuses on Counties Manukau Health data.

*There was an overall reduction in need of a blood transfusion associated with a caesarean section from just over 6% in 2017 to 4% in 2019. This may be due to vigilance with monitoring Fe levels during pregnancy and more confidence in prescribing iron transfusion (carboxymaltose) hence reducing the need for a blood transfusion. Unfortunately this trend increased again to 7.1% in 2023.

**High BMI increases risks of HDP in pregnancy, which may result in small for gestational age (SGA) babies

Perinatal and maternal mortality review committee report 2018

The Perinatal and Maternal Mortality Review Committee Report 2018 highlighted persistent inequities in perinatal outcomes across Aotearoa New Zealand, with particular concern for Pacific women.

Counties Manukau reported the highest perinatal related mortality rate (PNMR) at 13.24 per 1,000 births, compared with lower rates in Auckland (9.07) and Waitematā (8.96). While the national perinatal mortality rate has declined since 2007, largely due to improvements among European women, no significant reduction was observed for Pacific women.

Although hypoxic peripartum deaths decreased significantly between 2007 and 2018, this improvement was driven by reductions among European mothers. Pacific women continued to experience high PNMR, particularly at the extremes of maternal age (< 20 and > 40 years). The burden of perinatal deaths was greater in Pacific and Māori communities, reflecting higher fertility rates.

Key contributors to perinatal mortality among Pacific women included maternal conditions such as diabetes, spontaneous preterm rupture of membranes, antepartum haemorrhage, perinatal infections, and unexplained stillbirth. Living in areas of highest socioeconomic deprivation (quintile 5) further increased risk, especially due to spontaneous preterm delivery. Elevated maternal BMI was also associated with higher rates of stillbirth, neonatal death, and perinatal mortality.

Importantly, barriers to access and engagement with care were identified as the most common contributory factor in avoidable perinatal deaths for Pacific babies (15.7%), compared with much lower rates among European (4.3%), Asian (1.9%), and Indian (3.3%) populations. Deprivation amplified these risks, underscoring the intersection of socioeconomic and health inequities.

The Committee's recommendations included strengthening smoking cessation support, improving antenatal care services, targeted support for mothers under 20, and developing a preterm birth prevention programme. Continued investment in SUDI prevention, culturally appropriate maternal mental health services, and fetal surveillance education was advised, alongside cultural competency and emergency obstetric training for staff. The report also called for greater uptake of full perinatal investigations, multidisciplinary management of complex medical conditions, and further research into the high PNMR in Counties Manukau, with particular attention to socioeconomic drivers.

Conclusions

Health of Pacific women in Aotearoa NZ needs to be highlighted as a priority. The health of Pacific families and communities are dependent on the health of Pacific women. This chapter touched on some of the factors affecting the health of Pacific women in New Zealand but there many others not covered including mental health and domestic violence as examples. One critically important factor impacting on the health of Pacific women in NZ is high rates of obesity. Pacific women living with the consequences of obesity are increasing, impacting on their health (chronic health diseases), the health of their babies (with in utero fetal programming), their families (intergenerational cycle of chronic diseases), and communities. Extensive research is needed to understand better the driving factors impacting the health of Pacific women in Aotearoa NZ and in the Pacific region.

Appendix

Initiatives to improve women's access to care and facilitate early booking and finding of an LMC

CMH region initiatives

Early pregnancy clinics have been set up in Otara, Mangere, and Papatoetoe region in South Auckland. These clinics are mostly stand alone, with one attached to a GP practice. The aim was to allow women direct access to a pregnancy booking service where they will be assessed and offered forms for booking bloods, and scans if required. It also facilitates women to find a carer for the rest of the pregnancy. These midwifes at times have facilitated seeing women in their homes. Women are given information of the places of birth available including the option of birthing in a primary birthing unit either Botany, Papakura, Pukekohe, or Ngahau in

Mangere if they have a low-risk pregnancy and unlikely to run into problems during the pregnancy and at birth. Other than booking for birthing, women are also offered information about healthy eating and optimal weigh gain in pregnancy, smoking cessation, and prescribed any supplements required. Should a secondary care consult be needed, these women are referred to secondary care. Women who need support from other services including social work, smoking cessation, dietary support, and to secondary care services if needed early.

Women are given first contact pregnancy information packs.

Social media channels have been generated to facilitate women with information about pregnancy.

Women are given information about healthy eating in pregnancy and healthy weight gain in pregnancy. Women are also offered a weight gain in pregnancy card which offers simple messages about drinking water and not fizzy drinks, watch portion sizes and not eating for two, eating lots of fruits and vegetables, and aim for 30 minute walk (or some sort of physical activity) per day.

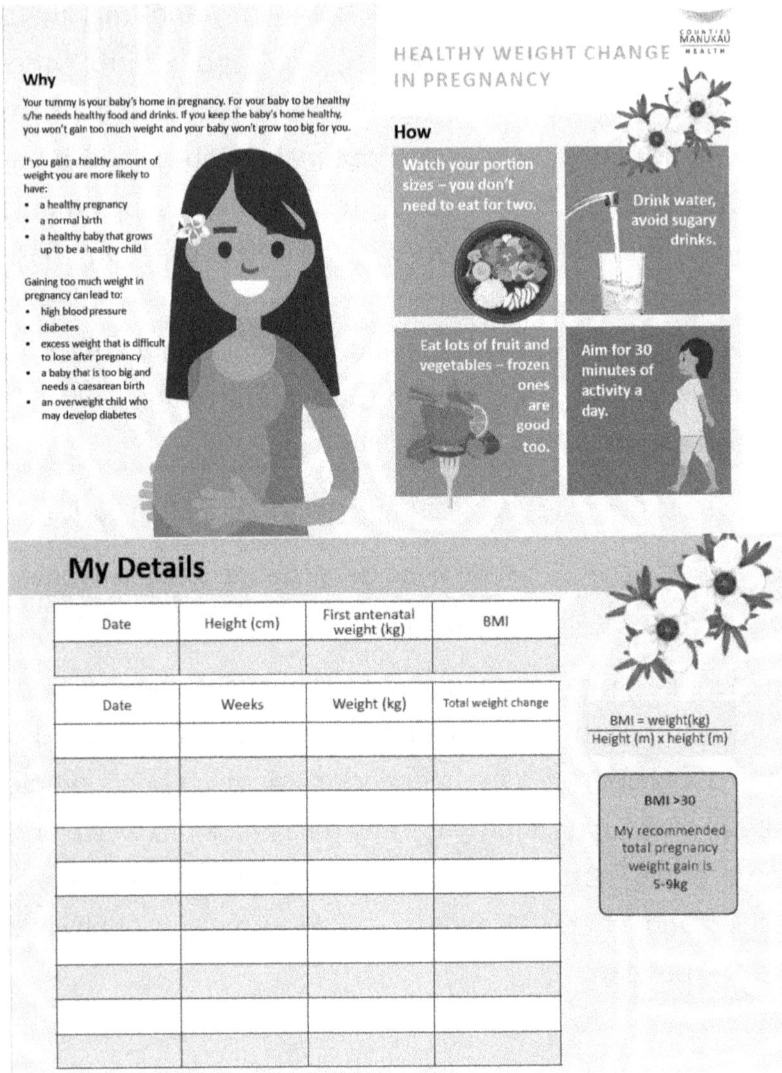

COUNTIES MANUKAU HEALTH

HEALTHY WEIGHT CHANGE IN PREGNANCY

Why

Your tummy is your baby's home in pregnancy. For your baby to be healthy s/he needs healthy food and drinks. If you keep the baby's home healthy, you won't gain too much weight and your baby won't grow too big for you.

If you gain a healthy amount of weight you are more likely to have:

- a healthy pregnancy
- a normal birth
- a healthy baby that grows up to be a healthy child

Gaining too much weight in pregnancy can lead to:

- high blood pressure
- diabetes
- excess weight that is difficult to lose after pregnancy
- a baby that is too big and needs a caesarean birth
- an overweight child who may develop diabetes

How

Watch your portion sizes – you don't need to eat for two.

Drink water, avoid sugary drinks.

Eat lots of fruit and vegetables – frozen ones are good too.

Aim for 30 minutes of activity a day.

My Details

Date	Height (cm)	First antenatal weight (kg)	BMI

Date	Weeks	Weight (kg)	Total weight change

BMI = weight(kg) / Height (m) x height (m)

BMI >30

My recommended total pregnancy weight gain is 5-9kg

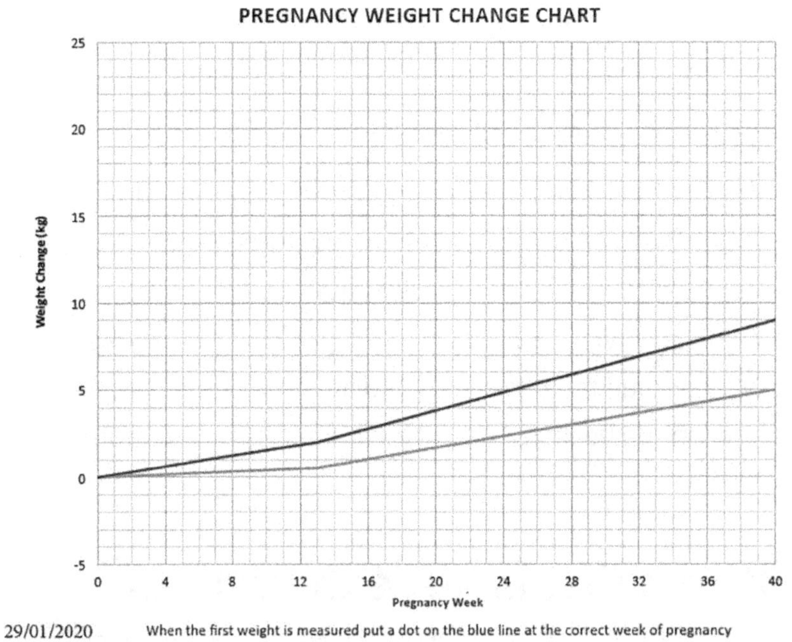

Smokefree pregnancy initiatives program continues with high success rates in assisting current smokers to quit smoking during pregnancy, with some percentage drop (3% for Pacific women from 2019).

Funding for training GPs in endometrial pipelle sampling and ability to order USS in primary care.

With the high rates of abnormal uterine bleeding and increasing rates of endometrial cancer in Pacific women, this initiative will allow access to earlier diagnosis and management.

Funding has been approved from the Ministry of Health to train more GPs to perform Pipelles and organise USS for women in the community in the CMH region and has now been approved for across Auckland region as well. This will facilitate early diagnosis and treatment, as well as early referral to secondary care for management if required. Other areas in New Zealand may wish to do the same.

Baby friendly initiatives

Despite efforts to exclusively breastfeed, exclusive breastfeeding rates have dropped to 70% in the CMH region in women discharged from Middlemore hospital. The Baby Friendly hospital initiative was developed to support women to exclusively breastfeed due to its many immediate and long-term beneficial effects on the health of the infant. It also assists the mother lose her pregnancy weight gain.

Others (list is not exhaustive)

Early prescription of folic acid to prevent neural tube defects

The small for gestational age guidelines to encourage LMCs to prescribe aspirin form 12 weeks gestation.

Hypertensive in pregnancy guidelines to prescribe Aspirin and calcium early reduce risks of superimposed pre-eclampsia in women with chronic hypertension.

Monitoring ferritin levels and optimising iron prescriptions and monitoring ferritin levels in pregnancy.

Early diagnosis of gestational diabetes in women with obesity and other risk factors so they could be diagnosed and managed early.

References

Adane, A. A., Dobson, A., Tooth, L., & Mishra, G. D. (2018). Maternal preconception weight trajectories are associated with offsprings' childhood obesity. *International Journal of Obesity, 42*(7), 1265–1274. https://doi.org/10.1038/s41366-018-0078-1

Alberti, K. G., & Zimmet, P. Z. (1998). Definition, diagnosis and classification of diabetes mellitus and its complications. Part 1: diagnosis and classification of diabetes mellitus provisional report of a WHO consultation. *Diabetic Medicine: a Journal of the British Diabetic Association, 15*(7), 539–553. https://doi.org/10.1002/(SICI)1096-9136(199807)15:7<539::AID-DIA668>3.0.CO;2-S

Aune, D., Navarro Rosenblatt, D. A., Chan, D. S., Vingeliene, S., Abar, L., Vieira, A. R., Greenwood, D. C., Bandera, E. V., & Norat, T. (2015). Anthropometric factors and endometrial cancer risk: a systematic review and dose-response meta-analysis of prospective studies. *Annals of Oncology, 26*(8), 1635–1648. https://doi.org/10.1093/annonc/mdv142

Beavis, A. L., Cheema, S., Holschneider, C. H., Duffy, E. L., & Amneus, M. W. (2015). Almost half of women with endometrial cancer or hyperplasia do not know that obesity affects their cancer risk. *Gynecologic Oncology Reports, 13*, 71–75. https://doi.org/10.1016/j.gore.2015.07.002

Bever Babendure, J., Reifsnider, E., Mendias, E., Moramarco, M. W., & Davila, Y. R. (2015). Reduced breastfeeding rates among obese mothers: a review of contributing factors, clinical considerations and future directions. *International Breastfeeding Journal, 10*, 21. https://doi.org/10.1186/s13006-015-0046-5

Bigby, S. M., Tin Tin, S., Eva, L. J., Shirley, P., Dempster-Rivett, K., & Elwood, M. (2020). Increasing incidence of endometrial carcinoma in a high-risk New Zealand community. *The Australian & New Zealand Journal of Obstetrics & Gynaecology, 60*(2), 250–257. https://doi.org/10.1111/ajo.13108

Blakely, T., Shaw, C., Atkinson, J., Cunningham, R., & Sarfati, D. (2011). Social inequalities or inequities in cancer incidence? Repeated census-cancer cohort studies, New Zealand 1981–1986 to 2001–2004. *Cancer Causes & Control, 22*(9), 1307–1318. https://doi.org/10.1007/s10552-011-9804-x

Boney, C. M., Verma, A., Tucker, R., & Vohr, B. R. (2005). Metabolic syndrome in childhood: association with birth weight, maternal obesity, and gestational diabetes mellitus. *Pediatrics, 115*(3), e290–e296. https://doi.org/10.1542/peds.2004-1808

Catalano, P. M., & Ehrenberg, H. M. (2006). The short- and long-term implications of maternal obesity on the mother and her offspring. *BJOG: an International Journal of Obstetrics and Gynaecology, 113*(10), 1126–1133. https://doi.org/10.1111/j.1471-0528.2006.00989.x

Catalano P. M. (2003). Obesity and pregnancy--the propagation of a viscous cycle?. *The Journal of Clinical Endocrinology and Metabolism, 88*(8), 3505–3506. https://doi.org/10.1210/jc.2003-031046

Cedergren M. I. (2004). Maternal morbid obesity and the risk of adverse pregnancy outcome. *Obstetrics and Gynecology, 103*(2), 219–224. https://doi.org/10.1097/01.AOG.0000107291.46159.00

Counties Manukau Health. (2016). *Maternity Quality and Safety Programme, Annual Report: 2015 - 2016.* https://www.countiesmanukau.health.nz/assets/About-CMH/Reports-and-planning/Womens-health/0b4be0966d/2015-2016-CM-Health-MQSP-Annual-Report.pdf

Counties Manukau Health. (2020). *Women's Health and Newborn, Annual Report: 2019 - 2020.* https://www.countiesmanukau.health.nz/assets/About-CMH/Reports-and-planning/Maternity/2020_CMH_maternity_Annual_Report.pdf

Conde-Agudelo, A., Rosas-Bermúdez, A., & Kafury-Goeta, A. C. (2006). Birth spacing and risk of adverse perinatal outcomes: a meta-analysis. *JAMA, 295*(15), 1809–1823. https://doi.org/10.1001/jama.295.15.1809

Corbett, S., Chelimo, C., & Okesene-Gafa, K. (2014). Barriers to early initiation of antenatal care in a multi-ethnic sample in South Auckland, New Zealand. *The New Zealand Medical Journal, 127*(1404), 53–61.

Crowther, C. A., Hiller, J. E., Moss, J. R., McPhee, A. J., Jeffries, W. S., Robinson, J. S., & Australian Carbohydrate Intolerance Study in Pregnant Women (ACHOIS) Trial Group. (2005). Effect of treatment of gestational diabetes mellitus on pregnancy outcomes. *The New England Journal of Medicine, 352*(24), 2477–2486. https://doi.org/10.1056/NEJMoa042973

Dabelea, D., Mayer-Davis, E. J., Lamichhane, A. P., D'Agostino, R. B., Jr, Liese, A. D., Vehik, K. S., Narayan, K. M., Zeitler, P., & Hamman, R. F. (2008). Association of intrauterine exposure to maternal diabetes and obesity with type 2 diabetes in youth: the SEARCH Case-Control Study. *Diabetes Care, 31*(7), 1422–1426. https://doi.org/10.2337/dc07-2417

EBCOG Scientific Committee (2015). The public health importance of antenatal care. *Facts, Views & Vision in ObGyn, 7*(1), 5–6.

Family Planning (2020). *Contraceptive Use Survey 2020.* https://www.familyplanning.org.nz/media/304436/contraception-use-survey-2020_final.pdf

Farry, A. R. (2015). *A retrospective cohort study to evaluate the effect of 'Place Presenting in Labour' and 'Model of Midwifery Care' on maternal and neonatal outcomes for the low risk women birthing in Counties Manukau District Health Board facilities 2011–2012.* [Master's thesis, Auckland University of Technology]. Tuwhera. https://openrepository.aut.ac.nz/items/7198b4aa-a827-4391-9893-c09b6b7f49f1

Fertility Associates (2021). Retrieved 17 December 2021.

Fyfe, E. M., Anderson, N. H., North, R. A., Chan, E. H. Y., Taylor, R. S., Dekker, G. A., McCowan, L. M. E., & Screening for Pregnancy Endpoints (SCOPE) Consortium (2011). Risk of first-stage and second-stage cesarean delivery by maternal body mass index among nulliparous women in labor at term. *Obstetrics and Gynecology, 117*(6), 1315–1322. https://doi.org/10.1097/AOG.0b013e318217922a

Gluckman, P. D., Hanson, M. A., & Mitchell, M. D. (2010). Developmental origins of health and disease: reducing the burden of chronic disease in the next generation. *Genome Medicine, 2*(2), 14. https://doi.org/10.1186/gm135

Godfrey, K. M., Reynolds, R. M., Prescott, S. L., Nyirenda, M., Jaddoe, V. W., Eriksson, J. G., & Broekman, B. F. (2017). Influence of maternal obesity on the long-term health of offspring. The lancet. *Diabetes & Endocrinology, 5*(1), 53–64. https://doi.org/10.1016/S2213-8587(16)30107-3

Health New Zealand. (n.d.). Maternity Clinical Indicators: The New Zealand Maternity Clinical Indicators web tool presents comparative data across a set of 19 indicators for pregnant people and their babies. https://www.tewhatuora.govt.nz/for-health-professionals/data-and-statistics/maternity/maternity-clinical-indicators

Heslehurst, N., Simpson, H., Ells, L. J., Rankin, J., Wilkinson, J., Lang, R., Brown, T. J., & Summerbell, C. D. (2008). The impact of maternal BMI status on pregnancy outcomes with immediate short-term obstetric resource implications: a meta-analysis. *Obesity Reviews, 9*(6), 635–683. https://doi.org/10.1111/j.1467-789X.2008.00511.x

Health Quality & Safety Commission. (2021). *Contraceptive use by women, 2018.* https://www.hqsc.govt.nz/our-programmes/health-quality-evaluation/projects/atlas-of-healthcare-variation/contraceptive-use/

Kim, C., Newton, K. M., & Knopp, R. H. (2002). Gestational diabetes and the incidence of type 2 diabetes: a systematic review. *Diabetes Care, 25*(10), 1862–1868. https://doi.org/10.2337/diacare.25.10.1862

Landon, M. B., Spong, C. Y., Thom, E., Carpenter, M. W., Ramin, S. M., Casey, B., Wapner, R. J., Varner, M. W., Rouse, D. J., Thorp, J. M., Jr, Sciscione, A., Catalano, P., Harper, M., Saade, G., Lain, K. Y., Sorokin, Y., Peaceman, A. M., Tolosa, J. E., Anderson, G. B., & Eunice Kennedy Shriver National Institute of Child Health and Human Development Maternal-Fetal Medicine Units Network. (2009). A multicenter, randomized trial of treatment for mild gestational diabetes. *The New England Journal of Medicine, 361*(14), 1339–1348. https://doi.org/10.1056/NEJMoa0902430

Lash, M. M., & Armstrong, A. (2009). Impact of obesity on women's health. *Fertility and Sterility, 91*(5), 1712–1716. https://doi.org/10.1016/j.fertnstert.2008.02.141

Meredith, I., Sarfati, D., Ikeda, T., & Blakely, T. (2012). Cancer in Pacific people in New Zealand. *Cancer Causes & Control, 23*(7), 1173–1184. https://doi.org/10.1007/s10552-012-9986-x

Moana Research. (2018). *Consumer Perspectives on Primary birthing: Counties Manukau.* https://www.moanaresearch.co.nz/wp-content/uploads/2019/07/Moana-Research_Primary-Birthing-Report_FINAL_online-version.pdf

Ministry of Health. (2025). *New Zealand Maternity Clinical Indicators. Key findings about births in 2023.* https://www.tewhatuora.govt.nz/for-health-professionals/data-and-statistics/maternity/report-on-maternity-web-tool https://tewhatuora.shinyapps.io/maternity-clinical-indicator-trends/

Ministry of Health. (2019). *Contraception: Findings from the 2014/2015 New Zealand Health Survey.* https://www.health.govt.nz/publication/contraception-findings-2014-15-new-zealand-health-survey

Ministry of Health. (2021). *Maternity Care.* https://www.health.govt.nz/your-health/pregnancy-and-kids/services-and-support-during-pregnancy/maternity-care

Ministry of Health. (2021). *Annual Update of Key Results, New Zealand Health Survey.* https://www.health.govt.nz/publication/annual-update-key-results-2020-21-new-zealand-health-survey

Ministry of Health. (2021). *Pacific Health Scholarships.* https://www.health.govt.nz/our-work/populations/pacific-health/pacific-health-scholarships-2022

Ministry of Health. (2014). *Screening, Diagnosis and Management of Gestational Diabetes in New Zealand: A clinical practice guideline.* http://www.health.govt.nz/publication/screening-diagnosis-and-management-gestational-diabetes-new-zealand-clinical-practice-guideline

Moller, A. B., Petzold, M., Chou, D., & Say, L. (2017). Early antenatal care visit: a systematic analysis of regional and global levels and trends of coverage from 1990 to 2013. *The Lancet: Global Health, 5*(10), e977–e983. https://doi.org/10.1016/S2214-109X(17)30325-X

National Women's Health. (2014). *National Women's Annual Clinical Report 2014.* https://nationalwomenshealth.adhb.govt.nz/healthprofessionals/annual-clinical-report/national-womens-annual-clinical-report/

National Women's Health. (2018). *National Women's Health, Annual Clinical Report 2018.* https://nationalwomenshealth.adhb.govt.nz/healthprofessionals/annual-clinical-report/national-womens-annual-clinical-report/

National Women's Health (2020). *National Women's Health 2020 Pūrongo Haumanu ā tau, Annual Clinical Report*. Auckland District Health Board. https://nationalwomenshealth.adhb.govt.nz/assets/Womens-health/Documents/ACR/Reports/2020-Annual-Clinical-Report.pdf

Nohr, E. A., Timpson, N. J., Andersen, C. S., Davey Smith, G., Olsen, J., & Sørensen, T. I. (2009). Severe obesity in young women and reproductive health: the Danish National Birth Cohort. *PloS One, 4*(12), e8444. https://doi.org/10.1371/journal.pone.0008444

Nuthalapaty, F., & Rouse, W. (2013). *The impact of obesity on female fertility and pregnancy.* http://www.uptodate.com/contents/the-impact-of-obesity-on-female-fertility-and-pregnancy

Perinatal and Maternal Mortality Review Committee. (2021). *Fourteenth Annual Report of the Perinatal and Maternal Mortality Review Committee | Te Pūrongo ā-Tau Tekau mā Whā o te Komiti*

Arotake Mate Pēpi, Mate Whaea Hoki. https://www.hqsc.govt.nz/resources/resource-library/fourteenth-annual-report-of-the-perinatal-and-maternal-mortality-review-committee-te-puro ngo-a-tau-tekau-ma-wha-o-te-komiti-arotake-mate-pepi-mate-whaea-hoki/

Poobalan, A. S., Aucott, L. S., Gurung, T., Smith, W. C., & Bhattacharya, S. (2009). Obesity as an independent risk factor for elective and emergency caesarean delivery in nulliparous women--systematic review and meta-analysis of cohort studies. *Obesity Reviews, 10*(1), 28–35. https://doi.org/10.1111/j.1467-789X.2008.00537.x

Royal College of Obstetricians and Gynaecologists. (2021). *Guidance on the provision of services after childbirth during the COVID-19 pandemic.* https://www.rcog.org.uk/globalassets/documents/guidelines/2021-02-guidance-on-the-provision-of-contraception-by-maternity-services-after-childbirth-during-the-covid-19-pandemic.pdf

Ruager-Martin, R., Hyde, M. J., & Modi, N. (2010). Maternal obesity and infant outcomes. *Early Human Development, 86*(11), 715–722. https://doi.org/10.1016/j.earlhumdev.2010.08.007

Ryan, D., Grey, C., & Mischewski, B. (2019). *Tofa Saili: A review of evidence about health equity for Pacific Peoples in New Zealand.* Pacific Perspectives Ltd. https://www.pacificperspectives.co.nz/publications/

Scott, O. W., Tin Tin, S., Bigby, S. M., & Elwood, J. M. (2019). Rapid increase in endometrial cancer incidence and ethnic differences in New Zealand. *Cancer causes & control, 30*(2), 121–127. https://doi.org/10.1007/s10552-019-1129-1

Sheiner, E., Levy, A., Menes, T. S., Silverberg, D., Katz, M., & Mazor, M. (2004). Maternal obesity as an independent risk factor for caesarean delivery. *Paediatric and Perinatal Epidemiology, 18*(3), 196–201. https://doi.org/10.1111/j.1365-3016.2004.00557.x

Stacey, T., Thompson, J. M., Mitchell, E. A., Ekeroma, A. J., Zuccollo, J. M., & McCowan, L. M. (2011). Relationship between obesity, ethnicity and risk of late stillbirth: a case control study. *BMC Pregnancy and Childbirth*, *11*, 3. https://doi.org/10.1186/1471-2393-11-3

Te Karu, L., Habib, T., & Crengle, S. (2021). The inequity of access to contraception for women in Aotearoa: an unfair, unsafe and ineffective system. *The New Zealand Medical Journal, 134*(1531), 86–88.

Teng, A. M., Atkinson, J., Disney, G., Wilson, N., Sarfati, D., McLeod, M., & Blakely, T. (2016). Ethnic inequalities in cancer incidence and mortality: census-linked cohort studies with 87 million years of person-time follow-up. *BMC Cancer*, *16*(1), 755. https://doi.org/10.1186/s12885-016-2781-4

Torloni, M. R., Betrán, A. P., Daher, S., Widmer, M., Dolan, S. M., Menon, R., Bergel, E., Allen, T., & Merialdi, M. (2009). Maternal BMI and preterm birth: a systematic review of the literature with meta-analysis. *The Journal of Maternal-Fetal & Neonatal Medicine*, *22*(11), 957–970. https://doi.org/10.3109/14767050903042561

Van Lieshout, R. J., Taylor, V. H., & Boyle, M. H. (2011). Pre-pregnancy and pregnancy obesity and neurodevelopmental outcomes in offspring: a systematic review. *Obesity Reviews*, *12*(5), e548–e559. https://doi.org/10.1111/j.1467-789X.2010.00850.x

Weiss, J. L., Malone, F. D., Emig, D., Ball, R. H., Nyberg, D. A., Comstock, C. H., Saade, G., Eddleman, K., Carter, S. M., Craigo, S. D., Carr, S. R., D'Alton, M. E., & FASTER Research Consortium. (2004). Obesity, obstetric complications and cesarean delivery rate--a population-based screening study. *American Journal of Obstetrics & Gynecology*, *190*(4), 1091–1097. https://doi.org/10.1016/j.ajog.2003.09.058

Whitley, C. E., Rose, S. B., Sim, D., & Cook, H. (2020). Association Between Women's Use of Long-Acting Reversible Contraception and Declining Abortion Rates in New Zealand. *Journal of Women's Health, 29*(1), 21–28. https://dx.doi.org/10.1089/jwh.2018.7632

Whitley, C. E., Rose, S. B., Sim, D., & Cook, H. (2020). Association Between Women's Use of Long-Acting Reversible Contraception and Declining Abortion Rates in New Zealand. *Journal of Women's Health*, *29*(1), 21–28. https://doi.org/10.1089/jwh.2018.7632

World Health Organization. (2020). *Fact Sheet: Family planning/contraception methods.* https://www.who.int/news-room/fact-sheets/detail/family-planning-contraception

World Health Organization. (2021). *Women's health.* https://www.who.int/health-topics/women-s-health/

Winnard, D., Anderson, P., Maclennan, L., & Okesene-Gafa, K. (2011). *Diabetes in pregnancy in CMDHB; Trends Over Time, a 2011 Snapshot and Service Implications.* Counties Manukau District Health Board. https://countiesmanukau.health.nz/assets/About-CMH/Reports-and-planning/Diabetes/86012bec3e/2011-Diabetes-in-Pregnancy-Trends-2011-snapshot.pdf

Wise, M. R., Jordan, V., Lagas, A., Showell, M., Wong, N., Lensen, S., & Farquhar, C. M. (2016). Obesity and endometrial hyperplasia and cancer in premenopausal women: A systematic review. *American Journal of Obstetrics & Gynecology*, *214*(6), 689.e1–689.e17. https://doi.org/10.1016/j.ajog.2016.01.175

Zore, T., Joshi, N. V., Lizneva, D., & Azziz, R. (2017). Polycystic Ovarian Syndrome: Long-Term Health Consequences. *Seminars in Reproductive Medicine*, *35*(3), 271–281. https://doi.org/10.1055/s-0037-1603096

Complex criticalities: An introduction to Pacific Rainbow+ communities health and wellbeing in Aotearoa-New Zealand and the Pacific

Malaeulu Seuta'afili Patrick Thomsen

Chapter summary

This chapter provides an introduction to the health and wellbeing challenges of Pacific Rainbow+ communities, revealing a land-scape marked by social discrimination and stigma that engender exclusion and pervasive health and wellbeing challenges. The intersectionality of heterosexist attitudes and racial/ethnic discrimination compounds the struggles faced by our communities, resulting in a complex web of poor health and wellbeing outcomes. The chapter underscores the imperative need to eradicate queer/trans phobia, advocating for a shift towards affirming positive and connected communities. Legal discrimination and violence further cast a shadow over the wellbeing of Pacific Rainbow+ peoples across the region, demanding urgent attention and redress.

Introduction

Attempts to understand the unique health and wellbeing needs of Pacific Rainbow+ communities are still relatively scant. In both Aotearoa-New Zealand (AoNZ) and in our wider Pacific region, few researchers have undertaken projects that have looked to focus specifically on this intersectional positioning within Pacific health and wellbeing research. The paucity of research on Rainbow+ communities in this country is currently being addressed by a range of recent ground-breaking studies;[1] but as Pacific communities are also underserved by our health system, the point at where these two communities meet, and those who inhabit this space have often been considered peripheral to the interests of both.

Pacific and Rainbow+ groups *are* priority equity groups, yet in research both theoretically and empirically, little space has been given to those whose experiences are impacted by what is called overlapping double-marginalisation, to voice their specific health and wellbeing needs. This chapter will provide some background into the current state of research on the health of Pacific Rainbow+ communities, detail a selected number of key issues and terminologies important to understanding our communities in Aotearoa-New Zealand, deploy two brief snapshots from Fiji and Papua New Guinea, before offering further readings and potential questions for researchers interested in carrying out work in this uniquely intersectional space. The first rule of carrying out Pacific Rainbow+ research in any field, follows the basic rules of Pacific research: ensure that Pacific Rainbow+ people are leading the research and project, not just being studied.

As a New Zealand-based researcher, I have chosen to use the term Rainbow+ for this chapter to acknowledge the purchase the term has here in our context, adding a plus sign to also denote that there is not a single Rainbow community in our country. As will be explained later in this chapter, in addition to lesbian, gay, bisexual, transgender, takatāpui, queer, intersex, asexual/agender (LGBTTQIA+) there are Pacific-specific terms that are tied to our communities, cultures, and genealogies that differentiate gender-sex divergent peoples in our own contexts that run the gambit of Pacific cultures and countries expressed as (M)āhū (V)akasalewalewa (P)alopa (F)akafafine (A)kavaine (F)akaleiti (F)a'afafine+ (Thomsen and Brown-Acton, 2021). In New Zealand, Rainbow+ communities are further differentiated by race or ethnicity, by indigeneity, by gender-sex, by sex characteristics, and by location across both urban and rural contexts. Therefore, it is more appropriate to speak of Rainbow communities as opposed to a singular Rainbow community.

The ABCs of labels and Rainbow+ health and wellbeing

Health and wellbeing researchers and social researchers generally rely on labels to cleanly draw gender and sex identity categories in their work. For Rainbow+ communities, however, labels are problematic. Theoreticians in the queer/Rainbow+ research space argue assertively against the idea of any type of static identity framework as being 'natural' (Butler, 1990; Halperin, 2003; Sedgwick, 2008; Thomsen and Iosefo-Williams, 2021). Queer theorists are reactive against notions of any truly innate queer identity or subjectivity (Eng et al., 2005). Their critique is that to be 'queer' is to diverge from the normative way of understanding your sex (biology), gender (social identity), and sexuality (desire). Therefore, not only is there no unifying label that can account for all Rainbow+ experiences, the line between gender identity, sex characteristics, and sexual orientation can somewhat be muddled. Many scholars now believe that the terms gender and sex, should be expressed as gender-sex or gender/sex, as this better captures the way that all these concepts are interrelated in the lived experiences of individuals (Fausto-Sterling, 2019).

For health researchers in particular, the opaqueness related to 'queerness' or Rainbow+ communities are important to consider. Health research and its predominant way of conducting knowledge-generating activities derives from empiricist and positivist approaches to research, which prioritise survey methods, observation, generalisability, and statistical analyses. These techniques are still useful in the Rainbow+ research space but necessitate a clear contextualisation and understanding of how each label selected is operationalised in the research process, ensuring its appropriateness to the social and cultural context the terms are derived from. Thus, qualitative research that includes talanoa, interviews, and participatory action research that tries to document the experiences of Pacific Rainbow+ communities in New Zealand is considered a necessary component to better understanding the health of our communities.

Stats NZ (2021) released a statistical standard for publishing, disseminating, and working with data around gender, sex, and variations of sex characteristics. Their report highlights the difficulty of collecting nuanced data on our communities in large surveys. The key takeaway is that data on gender and sex should only be collected when the information is absolutely needed, and their guidelines recognise the complexity of the space by suggesting that all surveys should allow for multiple gender classifications to be collected. However, although their recommendation on coding states that gender questions should be left open, their classification description in coding responses suggests a collapse of gender identities such as trans into the male female binary, with a third 'other' category left open for agender and those who select no gender. As you will see, this approach is not fit-for-purpose for Pacific Rainbow+ communities that are tied to multiple and unique cultural contexts, which projects like the Manalagi Project (Thomsen et al., 2023; Thomsen and Brown-Acton, 2021; Thomsen et al., 2021) are now attempting to address.

Heterosexism and heteronormativity

Gender is often referred to as a (powerful) social construct – one that is performed and repeated in societies, which also governs the normative way you are expected to express your gender-sex classification (Butler, 1990). A gender binary (male/female) compels, often violently, all individuals to express cross-sex desire, while simultaneously pathologising and rejecting same-sex desire as abnormal. Queer theorists not only make known how the process of normalising heterosexuality takes place in society, but they also often study the impact this has on individuals who do not experience gender-sex and sexual desire in a "normative" way. Rainbow+ health researchers, although few in New Zealand, build on this and focus their work toward revealing how heterosexism and societal discrimination is built into all our institutions, heightening the importance for us to understand this as a key social determinant to health and wellbeing for Rainbow+ communities.

All societies have normative expectations that are translated into socially constructed roles in behaviour including gender. For example, men are expected to dress in particular ways, and so, too, are women, and the opposite sexes are meant to desire each other. All our societies' institutions are built around the perpetuation of these normative visions of the world, committed to reinforcing the gender binary and heterosexual desire as our societies' ideas of normalcy (Castro Varela et al., 2011). The societal practices which reinforce sexuality between men and women (think marriage up until recently) as the only natural way to experience desire is termed a heteronormative way of seeing the world. Practices that continue to privilege this way of seeing and working in shaping the institutions we are all embedded in as people is referred to as heterosexism. Heterosexism exists because male-female relationships are considered the predominant norm in society and therefore treated as the default-superior-form of relationship coupling.

LGBT and the QIA+

A term that many are more likely to be familiar with is LGBT, an acronym that stands for (L)esbian, (G)ay, (B)isexual, and (T)ransgender. This acronym exists as a convenience for sorting and categorising purposes and does not represent a homogenous community who have a singular focus or experience. Much like how the term Pasifika emerged in New Zealand as a concerted collective response by many different peoples of the Moana to represent themselves politically in pushing back against our communities' perpetual marginalisation (Thomsen and Iosefo-Williams 2021), LGBT has roots in similar coalitional politics. Marsha P Johnson, a transgender woman, is famous for throwing the first brick at Stonewall, considered the birthplace of Gay activism in the United States (Brockell, 2019).

Emerging in the 1990s and coinciding with movements in literary scholarship, the term (Q)ueer was added to the acronym, to push past the binary and essentialist logics that scholars of gay and lesbian studies had tended to work through. A divide emerged at this point, where gay and lesbian scholars often tied their work to interrogating gender/sex categories to the gender binary (male and female) and transgressive behaviours of it (transsexual; transvestitism; transgender), while queer, advanced the notion of disrupting normalcy, and introducing concepts of liminality and often a complete rejection of the gender binary. Many queer identifying folks celebrate the way their own experiences highlight the mismatches between gender/gender-sex and sexuality, in living their lives.

Since then, however, trans women have often been subjected to transphobia from gay men, trans men from lesbian women, and lesbian women often lament how the interests of gay men have dominated representation in the 'queer' community, side lining queer women's experiences and concerns. Recently the rise of Trans Exclusionary Radical Feminists, also known as TERFs, have targeted, often violently, trans women by attempting to reinforce an essentialist notion of gender tied to biology (Lu, 2020). Their claim is that trans women should not be considered women (Mckinnon, 2018); a notion all specialists of gender and sexuality reject as transphobic sentiment (Lu, 2020), as gender and even sex characteristics and identities has been found to be non-binary (Garofolo and Garvin, 2020). TERFs engage in attempts to silence and exclude trans women, which can have deadly consequences and should be seen as a major health and hauora concern. As such, health research into Rainbow+ communities must be cognisant of these shades of difference especially as many of the members of Pacific Rainbow+ communities are coded as trans in this literature.

Illustrative of this complexity is the fact that a man, for example, can have sex with another man, often abbreviated in health and sexuality research as MSM. However, this does not necessarily mean that they claim a gay identity/subjectivity. Rather it suggests that they partake in homosexual sexual acts. As with all identities, to be gay or lesbian – or bisexual for that matter – is not an essentialist and immutable category. One's sexuality (desire) and sexual preferences do not always determine a sexual 'identity' and does not define one's gender. These concepts require social agreement through the process of a shared discursive meaning-making. In simple terms, how we understand gender and how we represent it shifts by culture, context, and time and functions to dictate what acceptable notions of behaviour are in a society.

MVPFAFF+

The term MVPFAFF+ has its origins in a speech delivered by Phylesha Brown-Acton MNZM at the 2nd Asia-Pacific Outgames Human Rights Conference held in Wellington in 2011 (Brown-Acton, 2011).[2] At this conference, Brown-Acton on behalf of approximately 50 advocates and delegates from across the Pacific made known to queer delegates from all across the Asia-Pacific region, that Pacific-specific terminologies exist in our region for queer, Rainbow, trans, and non-binary individuals tied to our unique cultural context. And that terms like LGBTQI did not have exclusive cultural relevance in our differentiated contexts.

MVPFAFF+ stands in place for Māhū (Hawai'i and Tahiti), Vakasalewalewa (Fiji), Palopa (Papua New Guinea), Fakafifine (Niue), 'Akavaine (Kuki 'Āirani), Fakaleitī/Leitī (Tonga), Fa'afafine (Sāmoa), with the + acknowledging that there are 22 Pacific countries, territories, cultures, and languages that express gender diversity in their unique local context in different ways. Although the mnemonic has been taken by many to be the Pacific version of the LGBTQIA+ label and variations of it, this was not its originally intended function. For Brown-Acton, the idea was to demonstrate that the universalist tendencies of global queer activism and movements, bore a quality of erasure that did not respect our unique contexts in the Pacific. As such, Pacific Rainbow+ communities have struggled with getting recognition and space for Pacific indigenous expressions in mainstream

Rainbow+ communities *and* within mainstream Pacific communities for their unique wellbeing needs.

Speaking at a regional-wide, international conference, Brown-Acton's speech was crucial in acknowledging the role culture plays in Pacific Rainbow+ communities' health and wellbeing. This has major implications on health research for our Rainbow+ communities in Aotearoa-New Zealand and in the region. Brown-Acton references in her speech, the words spoken by Fuimaono Karl Pulotu-Endemann, a renowned fa'afafine scholar, who delivered a keynote at the same conference prior to Brown-Acton's address. Recognised as the architect of the Fonofale Model of Pacific Wellbeing, Pulotu-Endemann related the LGBTQI term to the medical pathologisation of difference, designed to exclude queer/Rainbow+ folk from society, denying us rights by way of framing us as unnatural and deviant. However, it is more accurate to understand MVPFAFF+ identities as speaking specifically within and from the context of Pacific worlds.

So, although both groups and communities share political urgencies – in fact it is common for many of us to even identify as being part of both groups – MVPFAFF+ is also a framework of relational belonging, it intentionally ties us from the Pacific and of Pacific heritage to the cultures, practices, and traditions of our families, villages, clans, communities, and nations. Meaning we know ourselves as Rainbow+ but our specific Pacific contexts connect our understanding of identity and social identities/roles to the norms and customs of our cultural communities. This also means that our experiences as Rainbow+ people in New Zealand and other diaspora contexts, is tied to the racialised experience of otherness our Pacific communities have faced while migrating to diaspora locations, like New Zealand for various reasons.

Intersectionality

The term intersectionality was coined by the Black feminist scholar-activist and lawyer Kimberlé Crenshaw (1989) in her famous essay 'Demarginalising the intersection of race and sex'. Since then, intersectionality has become a vitally important framework for highlighting intersecting experiences of marginalisation and is also relevant to understanding Pacific Rainbow+ health and wellbeing. The idea Crenshaw put forward in her articulation of intersectionality is that because society sees identity frameworks often as singular (gender-sex, race, class, culture, religion, dis/ability etc.) categories, we have constructed systems that must always sort people into these single classifications. Surveys in health research, as an example, often create binary gender or sex category to choose from even if you do not feel they fully capture your essence as a person. Crenshaw used the legal system to demonstrate how this can lead to erasure, specifically for Black women in the US, which allows violence to be enacted on their specific bodies, positioned at the edges of where marginalisation exists and erased by both marginalised groups, they are members of.[3]

For Pacific Rainbow+ communities in New Zealand, our experience of this country's social, political, economic, educational, health and wellbeing institutions, intersects at the edges of gender-sex discrimination and racial/ethnic discrimination as well as experiences of dis/ability for others. This means that efforts to better understand and support health and wellbeing outcomes for Rainbow+ communities, will not fully capture the needs and critical issues for our Pacific Rainbow+ communities without an intentional intersectional and indigenous Pacific lens. Moreover, mainstream Pacific concerns and experiences around racism in our health system is not going to fully account for the experiences of Pacific Rainbow+ communities either, as exclusion, discrimination based on our non-normative gender-sex positioning, can come from within our Pacific communities as well.

But because our health system and social, political, and public institutions still treat race/ethnicity and gender-sex, sexuality, and sexual orientation as singular categories, we are likely to have our concerns lost at the margins. Intersectionality shows that these categories of marginalisation are not meant to be separate or additive, but mutually constitutive. Our communities' experiences of racism and navigating heterosexism are (ultimately) intertwined and inseparable. The role that mutually enforcing forms of discrimination play in Pacific Rainbow+ health in New Zealand and increasingly within our region is now being acknowledged as a critical factor in understanding how we can improve the health and wellbeing of our multiply marginalised groups.

The role of discrimination in the health and wellbeing of Pacific Rainbow+ communities in Aotearoa-New Zealand

According to Stats NZ (2024), data from the 2023 census where gender and sexuality identity data was collected for the first time in AoNZ, 4.9% of New Zealanders identified as non-heterosexual.

While this is lower than previous estimates of between 6%-15% in other studies for AoNZ's Rainbow+ populations, in general, research shows that marginalisation and discrimination *is* linked to the overrepresentation of Rainbow+ peoples in NZ with poorer health outcomes (Oranga Tāngata, 2018). In this context, discrimination is more than just treating someone differently, or excluding them (sometimes violently) due to how they identify and are coded in terms of race, gender, sex, dis/ability, and so on, discrimination is more capaciously understood as a socially structured and sanctioned phenomenon, justified by ideology (white supremacy, colonialism. racism, heterosexism, transphobia) and expressed in interactions among and between individuals and institutions; maintaining privileges for members of dominant groups at the cost of deprivation for others (Dovidio et al., 2010). In simple terms, and within this context, discrimination is both an interpersonal and system-level phenomenon that intentionally seeks to reinforce the privilege and power of dominant groups. The way structural and interpersonal discrimination is linked, means Pacific Rainbow+ researchers often focus their research on understanding the relationship between both.

So when we speak about discrimination in the Pacific Rainbow+ communities context in New Zealand, we are referring to actions, behaviours, words, statements, laws, and exclusionary norms experienced by our communities at both an interpersonal and systemic level, which are sanctioned by heterosexist, heteronormative, *and* racist as well as classist institutions that pathologieses gender-sex, race/ethnicity, citizenship, and place of birth; constructing us as less worthy of rights, less worthy of respect, and leads to our often violent exclusion from New Zealand society.

Discrimination is positively associated with poorer mental health and physical health, which impacts members of our communities and their decisions around seeking out support from the New Zealand health system (Cormack et al., 2018).

The Manalagi Project (Health Research Council, 2020) is the first Health and Wellbeing Project that will intentionally address the way intersecting forms of discrimination impact hauora for Pacific Rainbow+ communities in New Zealand in accessing the New Zealand health system. According to Manalagi Data, about 60% of their survey respondents from Pacific Rainbow+ communities in AoNZ reported experiencing some kind of discrimination when visiting a healthcare setting in the past (Thomsen et al., 2023). In addition to this, the project also found that experiencing just one instance of discrimination in a healthcare setting for Pacific Rainbow+ was associated with a 60% increase in likelihood of Pacific Rainbow+ avoiding healthcare services in the future (Thomsen et al., 2026).

Overall Rainbow+ people in New Zealand are 19% less likely to report being satisfied with life, while experiencing an increased likelihood of moderate to severe anxiety, depression, and/or psychological distress; this starts early, with Youth 12 survey reporting same-sex or both sex attracted students as three times more likely to experience symptoms of depression, self-harm, suicidal ideation, and attempts as non-Rainbow+ students (Lucassen et al., 2014). Furthermore, what the Youth 12 survey refers to same/both-sex attracted youth are more likely to be bullied, be physically harmed, and to be afraid that someone would hurt or bother them at school. Additionally, 59.4% of same/both-sex attracted students had deliberately self-harmed, 41.3% had significant depressive symptoms, 18.3% had attempted suicide in the last 12 months, and 35.7% had difficulty getting help for their emotional concerns (Lucassen et al., 2014). One of the major issues being the lack of mental health services in our country attuned to the specific needs of Rainbow+ individuals. Rather than being Rainbow+ affirmative, mainstream services tend to reinforce heteronormativity and heterosexism, framing our communities as abnormal (Fraser, 2020; Semp, 2011; Semp and Read, 2015)

For Pacific Rainbow+ youth in particular, the Youth 19 survey found that most Pacific Rainbow+ young people reported positive family and school environments, high levels of volunteering, and moderate or good health. However, they also reported major inequities compared to others, including significantly higher food and housing insecurity, poorer healthcare access, and higher discrimination by healthcare providers than Pākehā counterparts and higher levels of mental health concerns than non-Rainbow+ peers. In total, they reported more challenges than students who were Pacific and non-Rainbow+, those who were Pākehā and Rainbow+, and those who were Pākehā and non-Rainbow+ (Tiatia-Seath et al., 2021). For Pacific trans and non-binary individuals, the Counting Ourselves survey found that transgender and non-binary Pacific people were at a higher risk of experiencing gender-based violence (GBV) within the domestic sphere, at an increased risk of engaging in risk related behaviours, while also being more likely to be treated unfairly at a hotel, restaurant, or theatre and avoid essential services like the bank or the doctor (Veale et al., 2019). Thus, despite the lack of research that exists on our communities in New Zealand, what currently exists demonstrates that our communities face many challenges to achieving positive and resilient health and wellbeing outcomes.

Rainbow health and wellbeing research in Pacific contexts

From within the Pacific region there is also the same paucity of research that afflicts our communities in AoNZ. There are, however, more and more localised studies beginning to emerge, which are highlighting the role of discrimination in Pacific societies that impact Rainbow+ communities, especially those who are trans and also identify as part of the MVPFAFF+ umbrella. For many locations in the region, the role of discrimination and a lack of safety for Rainbow+ communities expressed as violence, as well as surveys on sexual health is where most of the data on our communities' wellbeing can be gleaned. Local NGOs in places like Fiji and Papua New Guinea as an example, demonstrate the resistance and work local Rainbow+ organisations are engaging in to improve the wellbeing and safety of Pacific Rainbow+ peoples.

Snapshot: Fiji

In 2016, Fiji's Prime Minister, Frank Bainimarama stated that all LGBTQ Fijians should move to Iceland and get married there if that was their desire (D'Angelo, 2016). In 2018, Jone Kata, the leader of the opposition Social Democratic Liberal Party of Fiji, posted a statement that suggested all members of the LGBTQ community in Fiji should be sent to four isolated islands in hopes of making them extinct (Waqairadovu, 2018). This climate of fear and threats of violence are not just limited to discriminatory statements by politicians. In 2018, on the International Day against transphobia, trans woman Akuila Salavuki was found lying in a pool of blood on the Suva foreshore. Nicknamed Lucky, her murder is suspected to have been motivated by transphobia. Also, the murder of gay student Iosefo Magnus, illustrates the danger that trans, sexual, and gender diverse people face in Fiji (Fox, 2018).

Haus of Kameleon a Fijian social justice organisation devoted to ending discrimination and violence against transgender people, in their study titled 'Every Breath a Transgender Women Takes is an Act of Revolution: Fighting for Intersectional Justice in Fiji' reported that 70% of transgender women in Fiji experience violence, 63% experiencing physical violence and 36.8% experiencing sexual violence; 73.7% reported experiencing emotional or verbal abuse since coming out (Kumar, 2020). It is also thought that transgender women who do not conform to societal expectations of sexuality and gender presentation are at heightened risk of violence based on their sexuality or gender identity. Reliable statistics on violence against transgender people are scarce, as large numbers of victims do not report the crimes to law enforcement because of well-founded fear and distrust (Bavinton et al., 2011).

A community-based study by the AIDS taskforce of Fiji (Bavinton et al., 2011) highlighted the lack of safety for trans women in Fiji. Trans women were targeted for abuse; with 40% previously forced to have sex against their will. This study also found that MSM and transgender specific services were limited. Most respondents (approximately 67%–70%) had never been approached by HIV outreach workers or been given condoms or lubricant by outreach workers. Less than half (43.0%) could name one or more organisations working with Rainbow+ communities in Fiji. This is important. The report also found that these populations are at high risk of HIV. Only 21.6% of respondents consistently used condoms during anal sex with a male or transgender partner in the previous 6 months at the time the survey was held. More than one in five reported never using them. Only 10% had taken an HIV test in the preceding 12 months and knew the results. Barriers to testing included confidentiality and privacy issues as well as respondents reporting judgmental attitudes by clinic staff. Unsurprisingly, many of the study participants had experienced some form of stigma and discrimination. About two-thirds felt unsafe and uncomfortable expressing their sexuality or gender. About 57% reported experiencing verbal abuse and a third had been physically hurt in the previous 6 months.

Considering the lack of trans specific data and clear discrimination faced by Fiji's trans and gender diverse community, several trans affirming NGOs are engaging in advocacy in Fiji. Founded in 2011, DIVA for Equality is a radical feminist collective, currently the only one of its kind in the region formally constituted by lesbians, gender non-conforming women, and trans masculine people. It is currently conducting the first Lesbian, Bisexual, Transgender, and Intersex (LBTI) human rights and social justice research, developed, carried out, and analysed by the LBTI community, for the LBTI community (Diva for Equality, n.d.). House of Colours is an LGBTQI organisation based in Labasa, northern Fiji, who work with stakeholders and communities raising awareness on sexual orientation and gender identity and expression (House of Colours, n.d.). The Rainbow Pride Foundation is a non-profit organisation that advocates for the human rights of LGBTI people so that they can live free from discrimination, persecution, and violence. They work with policy makers in providing advice on more LGBTI inclusive policies. They also provide legal advocacy services for LGBTI individuals, HIV prevention awareness, mental health service navigation, and provide training and workshops for employers, service providers, and community organisations to develop more inclusive and safer spaces for LGBTI (Rainbow Pride Foundation Fiji, n.d.).

Founded in 2010, the Drodrolagi Movement, aims to create and celebrate a culture of equality, respect, dignity, and pride for the LGBTI and queer community in Fiji (Drodrolagi Movement, n.d.). 'DroMo' is a social support and educational network that is based at the University of the South Pacific (Sauvakacolo, 2011). Survival Advocacy Network was established in 2009 through the Scarlet Alliance Programme. They aim to empower the lesbian, gay, bisexual, and trans sex workers community in Fiji, to ensure their ability to work and live in a safe environment and work toward the elimination of stigma and discrimination against sex workers (Fiji Women's Fund, n.d.).[17] Strumphet Alliance Network as detailed by the Global Network of Sex Work Projects is an organisation led by former sex workers who are trans inclusive. Strumpet opposes the criminalisation and other legal oppression of sex work and advocates for universal access to health services, including primary health care, HIV, and sexual and reproductive health services (Strumphet Alliance Network, n.d.). Other trans affirming organisations working in Fiji include (but are not limited to): Youth Champs 4 Mental Health (n.d), the Red Cross, and femLINK (femLINK Pacific – Fiji, n.d.)

Snapshot: Papua New Guinea

Papua New Guinea (PNG) is one of the most culturally diverse countries in the world with more than 800 native languages (One World Nations Online, n.d.). Main spoken languages are English (official) and Tok Pisin (an English-based Creole). Western terms – Lesbian, Gay, Bisexual, Transgender, and so on – carry heavy stigma in PNG (Rainbow Papua New Guinea, 2016). As a result, trans and gender diverse communities in PNG face major obstacles in being able to live their lives free of discrimination. In recent years, a Tok Pisin term Palopa was coined by gay and transgender Papua New Guineans of Port Moresby (Stewart, 2014). Palopa is the 'P' of the MVPFAFF+ framework articulated by Brown-Acton (2011). There is also a documented identity of the Sambian people kwolu-aatmwol (male thing-transforming-into-female thing) (Hubbard, 1998), which indicates that gender diversity has an Indigenous reference point in PNG. It is also important to note here that in PNG gay men are often approached by heterosexual men for sexual encounters, and this is not considered a homosexual encounter, being 'gay' is more tied to feminine roles in wider society (Sokhin, n.d.).

Although no relevant laws criminalise transgender or Rainbow+ peoples in PNG, they are noticeably absent in important legislative and policy frameworks, for trans and gender diverse communities in PNG there are a suite of legal provisions that clearly restrict their freedoms and represents attempts to criminalise and pathologise them. The PNG Criminal Code, Section 210 criminalises sexual penetration described as carnal knowledge 'against the order of nature'. If found guilty, this carries a maximum sentence of 14 years (Criminal Code 1974 of Papua New Guinea, n.d.). Attempts to commit this offence are subject to a penalty of up to 7 years imprisonment. Only such acts between men are criminalised by this law. In addition, Section 212 prohibits acts of 'gross indecency' between men, or the procurement or attempted procurement thereof, with a penalty of up to 3 years imprisonment (Criminal Code 1974 of Papua New Guinea, n.d.).

In terms of wider support for transgender and gender diverse communities in PNG, there is no mention of any Rainbow+ in the National Health Plan that guides health provision and strategy in PNG from 2011 to 2020 (Government of Papua New Guinea, 2010).[10] Much like AoNZ and in other locations throughout the Pacific, surveys show that MSM and transgender persons are more likely than other groups to face stigma and discrimination in accessing health services in PNG (Carroll, 2016). MSM and transgender persons are particularly stigmatised when presenting for check-ups, tests, and treatment in relation to possible sexually transmitted diseases. These impediments to accessing health care services not only disproportionately affect these vulnerable populations, but generally increase the high prevalence of the HIV epidemic among LGBTI people in PNG (Carroll, 2016).

In 2017, it was estimated that roughly 47,795 (0.89%) people lived with HIV in PNG. This is the highest rate of prevalence in the Pacific at the time (Kora, 2017). HIV prevalence among MSM and transgender individuals in Port Moresby and Lae are 8.5% and 7.1%, more than seven times the population average (Kelly-Hanku et al., 2018). In terms of other sexually transmitted infections, the prevalence of hepatitis B, syphilis, chlamydia, and gonorrhoea was high with 34.0% of MSM and transgender populations in Port Moresby and 42.0% in Lae diagnosed with one or more STI (excluding HIV). Despite this higher rate for MSM and transgender individuals, two in three did not see a health care worker (62.3%–63.0%) (Kelly-Hanku et al., 2018). Thus, the absence of a focus on the Rainbow+ community in the country's health plan demonstrates the danger of heterosexist approaches to health interventions, when marginalised groups such as transgender and gender diverse communities are more likely to be placed at risk of HIV and other STI infections.

A qualitative survey into GBV against MSM and transgender people in PNG, conducted between April and May 2011, found that almost half of participants were unemployed (FHI 360, 2013). It also reported the type of GBV against MSM and transgender persons most commonly experienced by participants has been categorised as 'other types of GBV,' including stigma, discrimination, stealing from MSM transgender people, social exclusion, police refusing to file cases for MSM and transgender people, clinic staff refusing services, and familial rejection (FHI 360, 2013). Perhaps even more distressing is that 19 out of 23 (83%) surveyed MSM and transgender persons reported having experienced physical violence and 15 out of 23 (65%) reported having experienced sexual violence (FHI 360, 2013). Alarmingly, trans people also reported a reluctance to report GBV to police because of fear of further violence, lack of action by police or even being charged by police for violating laws against same-sex relations (FHI 360, 2013).

Considering the precarious position Rainbow+ people occupy in PNG, there are now organisations that advocate for the rights and humanity of this marginalised community. Kapul Champions was established by local MSM and transgender community members to represent the interests of these communities across the country and to better contribute to the national HIV response. Kapul Champions highlight a lack of research on specific practices and cultures in PNG; that there is a lack of strong existing formal MSM and transgender networks; violence by police and family members; alcohol misuse among MSM and transgender; and coercive sex all impacting the lives and dignity of Rainbow+ people (Tyne and Australian Federation of AIDs Organizations, 2013). In addition to identifying these issues, the consultations that formed Kapul Champions (which included over 100 MSM and transgender community members), called for the formation of a national organisation, while acknowledging the existence of informal networks across the country already (Tyne and Australian Federation of AIDs Organizations, 2013). Hannuabada Village in Port Moresby is one of the few safe havens for LGBT Papua New Guineans. About 30 gay men live in the village, in a collection of traditional Papuan houses built on stilts. Other gay PNG men have moved there from around the country (Sokhin, n.d.).

Conclusion

Pacific Rainbow+ communities face immense challenges to their health and wellbeing. Predominantly, these issues are tied to social discrimination and stigma that is used to exclude us. This chapter has attempted to introduce the complex terminologies and concepts that impact the way we must understand Pacific

Rainbow+ health and wellbeing as intersectional, impacted by complex and interconnected issues. Heterosexist attitudes intersect with racial/ethnic discrimination to make life for our communities difficult as health and social agencies perpetuate heterornormative, and exclusionary practices. To understand the health and wellbeing of Pacific Rainbow+ communities is to understand the need to remove queer/trans phobia and affirm the positive and connected nature of Pacific communities, including our Rainbow+ peoples. Pacific Rainbow+ peoples within our region are also subjected to legal discrimination and visceral violences that governs their wellbeing. Both contexts require Pacific communities and leaders to engage the heterosexist nature of our community structures and societal norms more meaningfully.

Further Reading

Manalagi Website

Home. The Manalagi Project. (n.d.). https://www.manalagi.org/

Thomsen, P., McLean-Orsborn, S., Ainea, H., & Verner-Pula, A. (2021). Examining the State of Health Research on Pacific Rainbow Communities in New Zealand; Literature Review. *Pacific Health Dialog, 21*(7), 449–457. https://doi.org/10.26635/phd.2021.111

Thomsen, P., & Brown-Acton, P. (2021). Manalagi Talanoa A Community-Centred Approach to Research on the Health and Wellbeing of Pacific Rainbow LGBTIQA+ MVPFAFF Communities in Aotearoa New Zealand. *Pacific Health Dialog, 21*(7), 465–471. https://doi.org/doi.org/10.26635/phd.2021.117

Survey reports from across the Pacific

Carroll, A. (2016). State Sponsored Homophobia 2016: A World Survey of Sexual Orientation Laws: Criminalisation, Protection and Recognition.International Lesbian, Gay, Bisexual, Trans and Intersex Association. https://ilga.org/downloads/02_ILGA_State_Sponsored_Homophobia_2016_ENG_WEB_150516.pdf

Ravulo, J., Hollier, J., & Waqa, M. (2024). *Experiences of LBTQ+ women across the Pacific: A report commissioned by the Pacific Sexual and Gender Diversity Network (PSGDN)*. University of Sydney.

Ravulo, J., Hollier, J., & Waqa, M. (2024a). *The lived experiences of PIDSOGIESC+ communities: A report commissioned by the Pacific Sexual and Gender Diversity Network (PSGDN)*. The University of Sydney.

Queer theory and health research

Butler, J. (1990). *Gender Trouble: Feminism and the subversion of identity*. Routledge.

Oranga Tāngata, Oranga Whānau. (2018). *Rainbow communities, mental health and addictions a submission to the Government Inquiry into Mental Health and Addiction*. https://www.mentalhealth.org.nz/assets/Our-Work/policy-advocacy/Rainbow-communities-and-mental-health-submission-to-the-Inquiry-into-Mental-Health-and-Addiction-08062018.pdf

Fraser, G. (2020). *Rainbow Experiences of accessing mental health support in Aotearoa New Zealand: A community-based mixed methods study*. [Doctoral thesis, Victoria University of Wellington]. Victoria University of Wellington Research Archive. http://researcharchive.vuw.ac.nz/xmlui/handle/10063/9042

Youth' 12

Lucassen, M., Clark, T., Moselen, E., Robinson, E., & The Adolescent Health Research Group. (2014). *Youth' 12: The health and wellbeing of secondary school students in New Zealand*. The University of Auckland. https://www.researchgate.net/publication/271138377_Youth'12_the_health_and_wellbeing_of_secondary_school_students_in_New_Zealand_Results_for_young_people_attracted_to_the_same_sex_or_both_sexes

Youth 19

Tiatia-Seath, J., Fleming, T., Sutcliffe, K., Fenaughty, J., Roy, R., Greaves, L., & Clark, T. (2021). *A Youth19 Brief: Pacific Rainbow young people.* The Youth19 Research Group, Victoria University of Wellington and the University of Auckland. https://static1.squarespace.com/static/5bdbb75ccef37259122e59aa/t/60dd11a05fc4a74bf0de3e7a/1625100708894/Pacific+Rainbow+Youth19+Brief.pdf

Counting Ourselves

Veale, J., Byrne, J., Tan, K. K. H., Guy, S., Yee, A., Nopera, T. M.-L., & Bentham, R. (2019). *Counting Ourselves: The health and wellbeing of trans and non-binary people in Aotearoa New Zealand.* Transgender Health Research Lab. https://researchcommons.waikato.ac.nz/handle/10289/12942

Honour Project Aotearoa

Pihama, L., Green, A., Mika, Carl, Roskruge, M., Simmonds, S., Nopera, T., Skipper, H., Laurence, R., Te Kotahi Research Institute, & Te Whariki Takapou (Organisation). (2020). *Honour Project Aotearoa.* https://natlib-primo.hosted.exlibrisgroup.com/primo-explore/fulldisplay?docid=NLNZ_ALMA11356009630002836&context=L&vid=NLNZ&search_scope=NLNZ&tab=catalogue&lang=en_US

References

Bavinton, B., & UNDP Pacific Centre. (2011). *Secret Lives, Other Voices: A Community-Based Study Exploring Male-to-Male Sex, Gender Identity and HIV Transmission Risk in Fiji.* AIDS Task Force of Fiji. http://www.undp.org/content/dam/undp/library/hivaids/English/SecretLivesOtherVoices.pdf

Brockell, G. (2019, June 12). The transgender women at Stonewall were pushed out of the gay rights movement. Now they are getting a statue in New York. *The Washington Post.* https://www.washingtonpost.com/history/2019/06/12/transgender-women-heart-stonewall-riots-are-getting-statue-new-york/

Brown-Acton, P. (2011, March 18). Phylesha Brown-Acton transcript. http://www.pridenz.com/apog_phylesha_brown_acton_transcript.html

Butler, J. (1990). *Gender Trouble: Feminism and the subversion of identity*. Routledge.

Castro Varela, M. D. M., Dhawan, N., & Engel, A. (Eds.). (2011). *Hegemony and Heteronormativity: Revisiting 'The Political' in Queer Politics* (1st ed.). Routledge. https://doi.org/10.4324/9781315586496

Cormack, D., Stanley, J., & Harris, R. (2018). Multiple forms of discrimination and relationships with health and wellbeing: Findings from national cross-sectional surveys in Aotearoa/New Zealand. *International Journal for Equity in Health*, *17*(1), 26. https://doi.org/10.1186/s12939-018-0735-y

Crenshaw, K. (1989). Demarginalizing the Intersection of Race and Sex: A Black Feminist Critique of Antidiscrimination Doctrine, Feminist Theory and Antiracist Politics. *University of Chicago Legal Forum*, *1989*(1), 139–168.

Criminal Code 1974 of Papua New Guinea. https://ihl-databases.icrc.org/applic/ihl/ihl-nat.nsf/0/04c49944817d24c8c12576fd00438671/$FILE/Papua%20New%20Guinea-%20Criminal%20Code.pdf

D'Angelo, C. (2016, January 6). Fiji Prime Minister Tells Gay Couples To Move To Iceland. *HuffPost*. https://www.huffpost.com/entry/fijis-prime-minister-calls-same-sex-marriage-rubbish_n_568d6b34e4b0a2b6fb6e6155

Diva for Equality. (n.d.). *Profile*. https://www.spc.int/diva-equality

Dovidio, J., Hewstone, M., Glick, P., & Esses, V. (2010). Prejudice, stereotyping and discrimination: theoretical and empirical overview. In J. F. Dovidio, M. Hewstone, & P. Glick (Eds.), *The SAGE handbook of prejudice, stereotyping and discrimination* (1st ed., pp. 3–28). SAGE Publications Ltd, https://www.doi.org/10.4135/9781446200919.n1

Drodrolagi Movement. (n.d.). *About*. Facebook Page. https://www.facebook.com/pg/Drodrolagi.Movement/about/?ref=page_internal

Eng, D. L., Halberstam, J., & Muñoz, E. J. (2005). What's Queer about Queer Studies Now? *Social Text*, *23*(3–4), 1–18.

Fausto-Sterling, A. (2019). Gender/Sex, Sexual Orientation, and Identity Are in the Body: How Did They Get There? *The Journal of Sex Research*, *56*(4–5), 529–555. https://doi.org/10.1080/00224499.2019.1581883

femLINK Pacific - Fiji (n.d.). *Our Mission, Vision and Values*. https://www.femlinkpacific.org.fj/index.php/en/about-us/mission-vision

FHI 360. (2013). *Exploring Gender-Based Violence Among Men Who Have Sex with Men, Male Sex Worker and Transgender Communities in Bangladesh and Papua New Guinea*. p22–23 https://www.fhi360.org/sites/default/files/media/documents/GBV%20Study%20report_Final.pdf

Fiji Women's Fund. (n.d.). *Survival Advocacy Network*. https://fijiwomensfund.org/project/survival-advocacy-network-san/

Fox, L. (2018, July 23). Murdered on International day against Transphobia: Fears Fiji killing is a hate crime. *ABC News*. https://amp.abc.net.au/article/10026188?pfmredir=sm

Fraser, G. (2020). *Rainbow Experiences of accessing mental health support in Aotearoa New Zealand: A community-based mixed methods study*. [Doctoral thesis, Victoria University of Wellington]. Victoria University of Wellington Research Archive. http://researcharchive.vuw.ac.nz/xmlui/handle/10063/9042

Garofalo, E. M., & Garvin, H. M. (2020). The Confusion Between Biological Sex and Gender and Potential Implications of Misrepresentation. In A. R Klales (Ed.), *Sex Estimation of the Human*

Skeleton (1st ed., pp. 35–52). Academic Press. http://doi.org/10.1016/B978-0-12-815767-1.00004-3

Government of Papua New Guinea. (2010). *National Health Plan 2011–2020*. www.health.gov.pg/publications/PNGNHP%20Vol1_2014.pdf

Halperin, D. M. (2003). The Normalization of Queer Theory. *Journal of Homosexuality, 45*(2–4), 339–343. https://doi.org/10.1300/J082v45n02_17

Health Research Council. (2020). *Manalagi: Aotearoa Pacific Rainbow/Queer/LGBTIQA+ MVPFAFF Health and Wellbeing Project*. https://hrc.govt.nz/resources/research-repository/manalagi-aotearoa-pacific-rainbowqueerlgbtiqa-mvpfaff-health-and

House of Colours. (n.d.). *Facebook Page*. https://www.facebook.com/pg/House-of-Colours-Labasa-1054706194599269/about/?ref=page_internal

Hubbard, R. (1998). Gender and genitals: Constructs of sex and gender. In D. Denny (Ed.), *Current concepts in transgender identity*. Garland Pub.

Carroll, A. (2016). *State Sponsored Homophobia - A World Survey of Sexual Orientation Laws: Criminalisation, Protection and Recognition*. International Lesbian, Gay, Bisexual, Trans and Intersex Association. https://ilga.org/downloads/02_ILGA_State_Sponsored_Homophobia_2016_ENG_WEB_150516.pdf

Kelly-Hanku, A., Willie, B., Weikum, D. A., Boli Neo, R., Kupul, M., Coy, K., Hou, P., Aeno. H., Ase, S., Gabuzzi, J., Nembari, J., Narakobi, R., Amos-Kuma, A., Gare, J., Dala, N., Wapling, J., Toliman, P., John, L., Nosi, S., … Hakim, A. (2018). *Kauntim mi tu: Multi-Site Summary Report from the Key Population Integrated Bio-Behavioural Survey, Papua New Guinea*. Papua New Guinea Institute of Medical Research Kirby Institute. https://www.aidsdatahub.org/sites/default/files/publication/PNG_Kauntim_mi_tu_Multi-Site_Summary_Report_from_the_Key_Population_IBBS_2018.pdf

Kora, A. (2017, October 18). PNG Tops Pacific's HIV Prevalence List. *Loop Pacific*. http://www.looppng.com/lifestyle/%E2%80%8Bpng-tops-pacifics-hiv-prevalence-list-68139

Kumar, R. (2020, November 21). Research by Haus of Khameleon says 70% of transgender women in Fiji have experienced some form of violence Wali says Fiji's transgender community must always be protected. *Fiji Village*. https://www.fijivillage.com/news/Research-by-Haus-of-Khameleon-says-70-of-transgender-women-in-Fiji-have-experienced-some-form-of-violence-r5fx84/

Lu, C. T. (2020). *A computational approach to analyzing and detecting trans-exclusionary radical feminists (TERFs) on Twitter*. [Undergraduate thesis, Dartmouth College]. Dartmouth College Undergraduate Theses. https://digitalcommons.dartmouth.edu/senior_theses/165

Lucassen, M., Clark, T., Moselen, E., Robinson, E., & The Adolescent Health Research Group. (2014). *Youth' 12: The health and wellbeing of secondary school students in New Zealand*. The University of Auckland. https://www.researchgate.net/publication/271138377_Youth'12_the_health_and_wellbeing_of_secondary_school_students_in_New_Zealand_Results_for_young_people_attracted_to_the_same_sex_or_both_sexes

McKinnon, R. (2018). The Epistemology of Propaganda. *Philosophy and Phenomenological Research*, *96*(2), 483–489. https://doi.org/10.1111/phpr.12429

One World Nations Online. (n.d.). *Country Profile - Papua New Guinea*. https://www.nationsonline.org/oneworld/papua_new_guinea.htm

Oranga Tāngata, Oranga Whānau. (2018). *Rainbow communities, mental health and addictions a submission to the Government Inquiry into Mental Health and Addiction*. https://www.mentalhealth.org.nz/assets/Our-Work/policy-advocacy/Rainbow-communities-and-mental-health-submission-to-the-Inquiry-into-Mental-Health-and-Addiction-08062018.pdf

Pihama, L., Green, A., Mika, Carl, Roskruge, M., Simmonds, S., Nopera, T., Skipper, H., Laurence, R., Te Kotahi Research Institute, & Te Whariki Takapou (Organisation). (2020). *Honour Project Aotearoa.* https://natlib-primo.hosted.exlibrisgroup.com/primo-explore/fulldisplay?docid=NLNZ_ALMA11356009630002836&context=L&vid=NLNZ&search_scope=NLNZ&tab=catalogue&lang=en_US

Rainbow Papua New Guinea. (2016, October 28). *Reclaiming our Rainbow Cultural Identities.* https://rainbowpng.wordpress.com/2016/10/28/reclaiming-our-rainbow-cultural-identities/

Rainbow Pride Foundation Fiji. (n.d.). *What We Do.* https://rainbowpridefoundation.org/

Sauvakacolo, S. (2011, October 2). Drodrolagi Movement Celebrates 1st Year. *Fiji Sun.* https://fijisun.com.fj/2011/10/02/drodrolagi-movement-celebrates-1st-year/

Sedgwick, E. K. (2008). *Epistemology of the closet.* University of California Press.

Semp, D. (2011). Questioning heteronormativity: Using queer theory to inform research and practice within public mental health services. *Psychology & Sexuality, 2*(1), 69–86. https://doi.org/10.1080/19419899.2011.536317

Semp, D., & Read, J. (2015). Queer conversations: Improving access to, and quality of, mental health services for same-sex-attracted clients. *Psychology & Sexuality, 6*(3), 217–228. https://doi.org/10.1080/19419899.2014.890122

Sokhin, V. (n.d.). *Being Gay in Papua New Guinea.* Vlad Sokhin. http://www.vladsokhin.com/work/being-gay-in-papua-new-guinea/#1

Stats NZ. (2021). *Statistical Standard for Gender, Sex, and Variations of Sex Characteristics.* https://www.stats.govt.nz/methods/data-standard-for-gender-sex-and-variations-of-sex-characteristics/

Stewart, C. (2014). *Name, shame and blame: Criminalising consensual sex in Papua New Guinea*. Australian National University Press. http://doi.org/10.22459/NSB.12.2014

Thomsen, P., Brown-Acton, P., Manuela, S., Tiatia-Seath, J., Greaves, L., & Sluyther, J. (2023). *The Manalagi Survey Community Report: Examining the Health and Wellbeing of Pacific Rainbow+ Peoples in Aotearoa-New Zealand*. The Manalagi Project Team. https://www.manalagi.org/_files/ugd/b7eedf_7a214bf6e78349f084581c5f2b68bf2d.pdf

Thomsen, P., & Brown-Acton, P. (2021). Manalagi Talanoa A Community-Centred Approach to Research on the Health and Wellbeing of Pacific Rainbow LGBTIQA+ MVPFAFF Communities in Aotearoa New Zealand. *Pacific Health Dialog*, *21*(7), 465–471. https://doi.org/doi.org/10.26635/phd.2021.117

Thomsen, P., & Iosefo-Williams, J. (2021). Disruptions, Decolonial Desire and Diaspora: A Provocation Toward a Pacific Queer World-Making Scholarly Practice in Aotearoa-New Zealand. *Journal of New Zealand Studies*, *NS* (33).

Thomsen, P., McLean-Orsborn, S., Ainea, H., & Verner-Pula, A. (2021). Examining the State of Health Research on Pacific Rainbow Communities in New Zealand; Literature Review. *Pacific Health Dialog*, *21*(7), 449–457. https://doi.org/10.26635/phd.2021.111

Thomsen, P., Tan, K., Brown-Acton, P., Manuela, S., Enari, D., Sisifa, S., McLean-Orsborn, S., Ng Shiu, R., & Wong Z. (2026). Investigating the Association Between Experiencing Discrimination in Healthcare Settings and Avoidance of Healthcare Services among Pacific Rainbow+ in Aotearoa-New Zealand. *New Zealand Medical Journal*, *139*(1629).

Stats NZ. (2024). *2023-census-shows-1-in-20-adults-belong-to-aotearoa-new-zealands-lgbtiq-population*. https://www.stats.govt.nz/news/2023-census-shows-1-in-20-adults-belong-to-aotearoa-new-zealands-lgbtiq-population/

Strumphet Alliance Network. (n.d.) *Global Network of Sex Work Projects*. (n.d.). https://www.nswp.org/members/strumphet-alliance-network

Tyne, M., & Australian Federation of AIDs Organizations. (2013). Regional Feature: Kapul Champions a Proud New Voice in Papua New Guinea. *Health Equity Matters*. https://www.afao.org.au/article/regional-feature-kapul-champions-proud-new-voice-papua-new-guinea/

Veale, J., Byrne, J., Tan, K. K. H., Guy, S., Yee, A., Nopera, T. M.-L., & Bentham, R. (2019). *Counting Ourselves: The health and wellbeing of trans and non-binary people in Aotearoa New Zealand*. Transgender Health Research Lab. https://researchcommons.waikato.ac.nz/handle/10289/12942

Waqairadovu, A. (2018, November 20). Kata's statement about LGBTQ community is discriminatory and he should be held accountable for it. *Fiji Village*. https://www.fijivillage.com/news/Katas-statement-about-LGBTQ-community-is-discriminatory-and-he-should-be-held-accountable-for-it---Wali-5rsk92/

Youth Champs 4 Mental Health. (n.d.). *About Us*. https://youthchampsfiji.wixsite.com/yc4mh/about-us

Tagata Sa'ili Malo: The story of the Pacific disability community

Tunumafono Faamoetauola Avaula Colenso Faamoe, MNZM

Chapter summary

The story of the Pacific disability community (now termed tagata sa'ilimalo) is an important one to tell. This chapter provides a case study of the evolution of the tagata sa'ilimalo community and sector over the last two decades. The background describes three key relationships with the disability community, the wider Pacific community, and with other New Zealanders including Māori as tangata whenua. The impact of two key shifts in disability policy is then outlined: The New Zealand Disability Strategy and the Enabling Good Lives approach. The latter approach is being used in the development of a new Pacific disability model of support by the Tangaroa Disability Collective, a project co-led with tagata sa'ilimalo that originated as part of a push for greater pandemic resilience. The role of the Tōfā Mamao Collective is explored, along with their new vision for Pacific disability (Tagata

Sa'ilimalo), term of identity (tagata sa'ilimalo), and vision-in-action (Soalaupule).

Introduction

> *... always remember that having a disability is not a personality and it will never define who you become in life.*
> (Rachel, Tōfā Mamao Collective)

Two decades ago, the voice of a young disabled Pacific person (tagata sa'ilimalo) expressing a view of this type in the public domain was unheard of. For Rachel is part of a community that at that point was largely invisible to the mainstream disability sector. This situation changed in the early 2000s following the emergence of leadership from tagata sa'ilimalo and better access to services through a new regional Needs Assessment and Service Coordination system.

Instrumental to this change was the shift in government policy to reflect international trends in the rights of disabled people. A central policy was the New Zealand Disability Strategy ('the Strategy'), launched in 2001 by the Ministry of Health. This cross-government collaboration aims to remove societal barriers, promote inclusion, and improve participation of disabled people. In this respect, the Strategy is relatively unique because of its overarching framework to drive wide-ranging outcomes. In 2016, the Strategy, now under the Office of Disability Issues (ODI), was refreshed to reflect a stronger focus on choice, control, and self-determination, reinforce Te Tiriti o Waitangi obligations and endorse a twin track approach to inequalities.

Good progress in policy aside, the patterns of use of disability support services today tell their own story. Compared to the general population, tagata sa'ilimalo overuse some services, underuse others, rework others to make these fit their needs, or opt out of usage of others altogether. There are, however, significant opportunities in the disability system to improve the response and by extension outcomes for Pacific people.

This paper provides a case study of the evolution of the tagata sa'ilimalo community and sector over the last two decades. It largely centres on Ministry of Health funded disability support services because that is where the first initiatives arose. The background is framed as 'Whakawhanaungatanga', describing three key relationships and the interconnections between the disability community, the wider Pacific community, and that with other New Zealanders including Māori as tangata whenua.

The impact of two key shifts in disability policy in the last two decades and their impact on tagata sa'ilimalo are then outlined. The first shift stems from the launch of the New Zealand Disability Strategy in 2001 and the subsequent beginnings of Pacific disability sector capability. The second relates to adoption of the Enabling Good Lives approach that informs the New Model of Disability to be implemented from 2021 (Enabling Good Lives, n.d.).

It is this second shift in policy that offers real opportunity to the Pacific community, and this is discussed at the end of this chapter. In particular, the shift from a service-oriented system to one that operates from within the context in which a person lives is arguably a game-changer. The potential is evident when this shift is considered alongside the 2020 Ola Manuia Project currently underway in Auckland to create a Pacific disability model of support.

Background: Whakawhanaungatanga

The COVID-19 global pandemic has shifted our focus towards the state of health and wellbeing in New Zealand and the resilience of our communities. This has led to a closer look at whakawhanaungatanga (a Māori term for relating well to others) for the disability community.

Mainstream disability community

The civil rights movement of the 1960s was a seminal time for the global disability community, providing the momentum to tackle discrimination, oppression, and exclusion. Today's gains stem from subsequent adoption of international conventions that have seen governments around the world increasingly accept responsibility for all members of society, regardless of disability.

Despite these changes there remains a long way to go while 'the remnants of tradition and past belief influence present-day practices' (Munyi, 2012). A core historical influence has been the 'premise that people with disabilities are not fully human' (Kendrick, 2010). From the time of the Greeks, the sick were considered inferior (Barker et al., 1953), with Plato recommending that people with disabilities be put away in some 'mysterious unknown places' (Goldberg & Lippman, 1974), a belief still evident up until the latter half of last century.

In the sixteenth century, Christians such as Luther and John Calvin indicated that the mentally retarded and other persons with disabilities were possessed by evil spirits (Lukoff & Cohen,

1972). These beliefs also traversed into the twentieth century, courtesy of the prevalence of Christianity in the western world. Negative attitudes also prevailed in non-Christian and non-Western communities. Many examples abound of disabled people being rejected and considered disposable economic burdens. But there are also contradictions. For example, Lukoff and Cohen (1972) note that some communities banished or ill-treated the blind while others accorded them special privileges.

In response to international changes, the New Zealand government has proactively provided leadership through legislation and policies. Through transformation of the disability system, it aims to better align the public system to its goals. One of these alignments relates to the funding of disability support services, currently managed by the Ministry of Health. This is a source of tension due to concerns about the impact of the 'medical model' within the disability community. Following community advocacy, disability policy was transferred to the newly created ODI within the Ministry of Social Development in 2012.

It is undeniable that health interventions are fundamental to improving lives. But the 'medical model' reinforces historic labels and attitudes that cast disabled people as a problem to be fixed, disabled and unequal compared to able bodied people. Contrast this approach with disability's 'social model', one that initially drew on 'a human rights discourse, defining disabled people as an excluded or oppressed social group. It distinguishes between the impairments that people have and the barriers to social participation that they experience' (Office for Disability Issues, 2019).

What constrains the disability sector's performance are the limitations of a service system designed for another era. As with other human service sectors, this sector mainly comprises a mix of post-colonial non-government providers and a proliferation of for-profit providers contracted following major growth of support and residential services from the 1990s onwards. These 'mainstream' organisations evolved around a 'monocultural' one-size-fits-all paradigm (Salahshour, 2021).

The disability sector's limitations were tested most in Auckland from the 2000s, when rapid population growth fuelled by immigration accelerated demographic changes. By the 2010s, this region had achieved 'super-diversity' (Vertovec, 2007) status. At that time, over half the adult population was born overseas and the majority of children in South Auckland were non-Pākehā/European. The changes to Auckland's population challenged the traditional assumptions of 'mainstream' culture.

Pacific people and disability

On the importance of social connectedness within the Pacific community: '*Super important, most Pacific Island families do not know these services are available to them, sometimes you'll find they are either too proud or too humble to ask for help. In most cases Pacific families do not want to trouble anyone*' (AJ, Tōfā Mamao Collective).

Pacific identity is central to the lives of most tagata sa'ilimalo; disability is a subset of cultural identity. While the Pacific community is highly diverse, there are enough commonalities based on shared heritage, migration histories, active diasporas, and cultural and social norms to bring this broad group under one umbrella of 'Pacific' for the purposes of describing a cultural context.

"Pacific' is not just a word that describes Pacific Island migrants now residing in New Zealand; it is a term that describes a behaviour, a way of viewing the world (around us) and the way in which we operate within it' (Thomsen et al., 2018, p 1). The foundations for describing the Pacific world through models and worldviews are well established and solidified in government policy. The Ministry of Pacific Peoples has identified, for example, several values that need to be acknowledged, including family, collectivism and communitarianism, spirituality, reciprocity, and respect.

The following table contrasts the fundamental values of Pākehā/European and Pacific Peoples/Māori in a way that brings into sharp relief the differences in paradigms.

It is this contrast in worldviews that has propelled Pacific development to create Pacific models that incorporate a Pacific worldview, as part of a contemporary 'mainstream' system.

The notion of 'disability' is one that is relatively new to the Pacific community. At the same time there is evidence that some of the limiting attitudes found elsewhere towards disabled people also prevail in the Pacific community. As the Pacific disability community evolved, there was a receptiveness among the wider community to improve attitudes, but the opportunity to do so in a Pacific cultural setting has been limited. It is important in these next steps of development to resolve this tension so that the dual experience of being Pacific and also disabled is dignified.

The journey ahead is even more crucial given the extent of disability issues confronting the Pacific community. Approximately

Table 1: Fundamental values – Pākehā vs Pacific peoples/ Māori (Tamasese et al., 2003), cited by New Zealand Treasury Report: A Pacific Perspective on the Living Standards Framework and Wellbeing, 2018)

Pākehā	**Pacific Peoples/Māori**
• Individual	• Communal
• Secular	• Spiritual
• Consumer	• Ecological
• Conflictual	• Consensual

24% of New Zealanders indicated that they have more than one disability in the 2013 census. While it is difficult to determine exact figures on the rates of impairment across disability types and ages in the Pacific community, it is known that the rate of disability is slightly higher than the general population (Stats NZ, 2014).

Particular issues are revealed for example in the lower employment rates of Pacific younger disabled people (9% versus 5%). There is also a higher incidence of chronic disease in the Pacific community as well as the associated impairments – this creates pressure on households.

> *I think it is important for the caregivers to have the group here, the older generation do not have the knowledge of technology, but caregivers will be able to reach out. A lot of caregivers do not know what support is out there is for them, can get a bit daunting. If it is just them coping with whoever they are looking after. It is important for them to get connected because sometimes if your family are not supporting you, that can be a lot to put on one person or*

> *one family member. I know this from experience.* (Leutu, Tōfā Mamao Collective, Wellington)

Also of relevance is the impact of poverty on children – another area of concern. While specific figures are not available in New Zealand, it is known that 'there is a two-way relationship between disability and poverty in childhood. Disabled children are among the most likely to experience poverty and poor children are more likely to become disabled than those who are better off.' (Pillai et al., 2007, p 6).

In terms of the use of services, as mentioned earlier, tagata sa'ili-malo overuse some services, underuse others, rework others to make these fit their needs, or opt out of usage of others altogether. An example is the proportionately higher use of home care services than the general population; here, there is a Pacific provider of home care services, and individuals and families can receive funding to engage their own carers at home including family members.

These patterns highlight the struggle of the Pacific disability community to use a service system that was not well designed to meet their needs.

> *"We can look for solutions, to have that purpose helps me to reach out to families. It has helped me and my family knowing the connections that is available. Seeing what works and what does not. It helps me to help my family understand my situation."* (Naomi, Tōfā Mamao Collective)

As the disability support system is centred on individual and family support and the existence of natural supports, thinking how supports can be more appropriately designed is important. The following 'operating model' provides an example of a tool for this purpose.

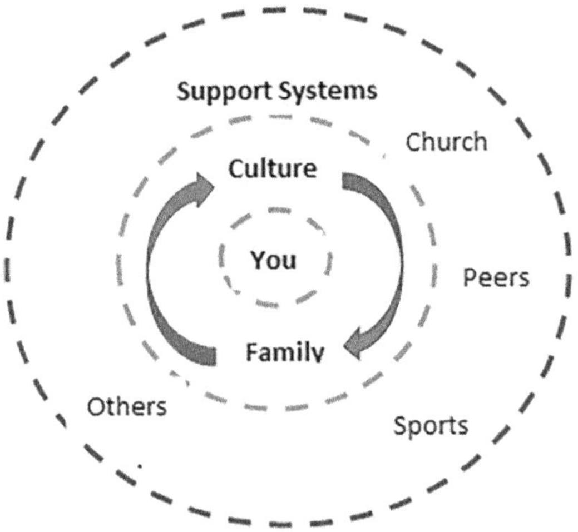

Figure 1: Adapted from Pacific Operating Model, NZ Treasury, 'A Pacific Perspective on the Living Standards Framework', 2018

Te Ao Aotearoa

The third relationship is with Te Ao Aotearoa, the world within which Pacific New Zealanders live. In this world, Te Tiriti o Waitangi and the partnership between Māori and the Crown is central. At the same time, Pacific people have a longstanding political, social, and economic history with New Zealand. Its relationship with Māori as tangata whenua predates colonisation – the kinship ties between Indigenous peoples of the Pacific region distinguishes Pacific peoples from other migrant New Zealanders.

Shift one: New Zealand disability strategy, 2001

In 2001, the New Zealand Disability Strategy ('the Strategy'), spearheaded by the then Associate Minister of Health and Minister of Disability Issues, Ruth Dyson was launched. An update in 2008 captured New Zealand's ratification of the United Nations Convention on the Rights of Persons with Disabilities. The Strategy's vision is:

> *New Zealand is a non-disabling society – a place where disabled people have an equal opportunity to achieve their goals and aspirations, and all of New Zealand works together to make this happen (Office for Disability Issues, 2001).*

The response of the Ministry of Health's Auckland ODI was to review the adequacy of its contracting coverage of disability support services.

Its first action was to set up a partnership with disabled people and the Ministry of Health, an innovation to provide a disability perspective into local policy. At that time, the Auckland Office's mainstream contracting team had a strong presence of Māori and Pacific staff and a management committed to ensuring the partnership was representative. Alongside this initiative, a new service was established – the DIASS or Disability Information and Advisory and Support Service. Rather than one mainstream service, four providers were contracted, each governed by tagata sa'ilimalo: one for the general disability population, one for the general family and carers group, one for Māori, and one for Pacific peoples. The latter service was PIASS Trust.

Soon after, a new regional Needs Assessment and Service Coordination service was contracted to improve responsiveness to the diverse Auckland population. The new provider was Taikura Trust, the first Māori and Pacific governed mainstream service in the disability sector. Following a review of home-based support, two Pacific providers were contracted, Pacific Homecare, an existing provider, and Pasifika Integrated Healthcare. PIASS Trust went on to engage Pacific disabled people and their families and carers, surfacing the previously 'invisible' community. The outcome of all the changes was the emergence of the fledgling but important Pacific disability community and sector.

Shift two: New Zealand disability strategy 2016–2022

In 2016, the Strategy, now located under the auspices of the ODI in the Ministry of Social Development was refreshed. It states:

- "The principles and approaches will help make sure the disabled community is visible, acknowledged and respected on an equal basis with others, and that disabled people can live a life with dignity and feel valued.
- The three principles are: Te Tiriti o Waitangi, the Convention on the Rights of Persons with Disabilities, and ensuring disabled people are involved in decision-making that impacts them.
- The two approaches are: Investing in our whole lives – a long-term approach, and Specific and mainstream services – a twin-track approach."

The Ministry of Health also released Faiva Ora 2016–2021 National Pasifika Disability Action Plan, aligned to the Strategy. The Strategy incorporates principles identified in the Enabling Good Lives approach. Trials of this approach began from 2012 onwards in Wellington, Christchurch, and Waikato. Its knowledge base brings together advances in disability and person-directed services, centred on key principles of 'choice, control and self-determination'. The emphasis is on using natural as well as formal supports. Funding is pooled from the Ministries of Health, Social Development, and Education.

A key influence was the Hon. Tariana Turia, Minister of Disability Issues in 2011, and also the Minister responsible for the Whānau Ora Programme. Her involvement continued the interplay of knowledge between Māori and Disability that began in the early 2000s.

Adopting the Enabling Good Lives approach is arguably transformational, because it turns on its head a support system that was firmly service-oriented to one that is person-directed, operating within the contexts of people's actual lives (Enabling Good Lives, n.d.). This approach presents a significant opportunity for Pacific peoples. By 2019, Pacific disability sector capability had grown and matured from its formative roots in the early 2000s, making it well positioned to uptake further development. An opportunity presented itself the following year.

The opportunity

In 2020, in recognition of the disproportionate impact the second outbreak had on Pacific communities, the Government released funds, as part of Ola Manuia: the Pacific Health and Wellbeing Action Plan, to ensure the Pacific health and disability sector has the capacity to respond to the ongoing resurgence during the Pandemic. Part of this funding was tagged to the disability sector as a flexible pool of funding to assist the disability support services response and ensure that those who are at higher risk of infection have the support they need. The Hon. Jenny Salesa, then Associate Minister of Health, played an important role securing funding to be managed by the Ministry of Health's Pacific Health Team.

The funding was provided for a new Auckland-based project, the Ola Manuia Disability 'Model of Support' ('the Project') centered on the Enabling Good Life approach. Service coverage of only tagata sa'ilimalo in Tāmaki Makaurau provides a unique opportunity to build a for-Pacific-by-Pacific service underpinning the project. The Project contract is with the Tangaroa Disability Collective comprised of Pacific Homecare (lead provider), Taikura Trust, Vaka Tautua, PIASS Trust, and the Tōfā Mamao Collective.

Shaping a Pacific model of disability support

To create a Pacific Disability Model of Support, the project is able to draw on the rich body of knowledge and experience that has evolved in other areas of Pacific development and supplement this knowledge in ways that incorporate the disability experience. It also has the benefit of a history of collaboration within the Pacific disability and wider Pacific sectors.

The tagata sa'ilimalo perspective is provided by PIASS Trust and the Tōfā Mamao Collective (Tōfa Mamao, n.d). *Tōfā Mamao* means 'navigating the future, guided by the past'. Tōfā Mamao was set up in 2018 in Auckland, nurtured by Taikura Trust and PIASS Trust, as an 'independently unique grassroots collective made up of Pacific disabled people, their families, and carers' to influence change in the disability sector. Two further social hubs were established in 2021 in Wellington and Christchurch, funded by the Ministry of Health through the Pacific Health Directorate under the 'Valuing Lived Experience Project', a collaboration between PIASS Trust, Tōfā Mamao Collective, and Vaka Tautua.

Tōfā Mamao has shared its vision with the Tangaroa Disability Collective to support development of the Ola Manuia Pacific Disability Model of Support, a summary of which is outlined below.

Activation life-giving vision

> *A shared vision is not an idea…it is rather, a force in people's hearts…at its simplest level, a shared vision is the answer to the question 'What do we want to create?'* (Senge, 2006)

The Strategy's vision has limitations for a Pacific disability vision because it evolved at a time when the focus was on a disabling society. Responsibility for change rests with others, casting the disabled person in the role of passive recipient and reinforcing the culture of diminished expectations and dependency. In setting its own vision, Tōfā Mamao focused on two areas.

The first was the need for a vision that spoke to them as Pacific people, with a disability, living in Aotearoa, one that stretched them to achieve their potential. Māori have similarly seen this need and have shaped the term *Tāngata Whaikaha* to reflect a Kaupapa Māori approach. *Tāngata whaikaha* describes two or more Māori people with a disability. The term tāngata whaikaha shares the optimism and future focus of Whāia Te Ao Mārama – whaikaha means 'to have ability' or 'to be enabled'. *Tāngata whaikaha* means people who are determined to do well, or is certainly a goal that they reach for (Ministry of Health, 2018).

The second was to provide a vehicle for leadership within the Pacific community where limiting expectations and attitudes can restrict growth.

Two concepts make up the vision. At the same time the vision is not static, it requires shaping with communities to gain ownership and thereby commitment to act. Over time it is anticipated that, as with Māori, a body of knowledge will evolve to support further development of a uniquely Pacific disability model. The concepts are initially expressed in Samoan terms that are likely to be modified over time as the wider Pacific community engages with the disability concept.

The first concept is the vision of ***Tagata Sa'ilimalo***, which acts as both a vision and a term for identity. It is intended to be aspirational to motivate and engage people in a journey towards successful lives in their cultural settings.

Vision: Tagata Sa'ilimalo – The pursuit of success, the celebration of achievement, of individual, and collective vitality.

> "Tagata Sa'ilimalo (*tagata* = people or person, *sa'ilimalo* = pursuit of success) is a new vision of Pacific disability in Aotearoa and also a term of identity to replace "Pacific disabled people, their families, and carers/supporters." Tagata sa'ilimalo are one and many. Tagata sa'ilimalo refers not only to an individual, but also to the family and community who surround them.
> Tagata Sa'ilimalo is an aspirational vision of the pursuit of success underpinned by sheer determination and sustained by the collective vitality of Pacific peoples. It is a vision that reflects the hopes of the Pacific disability community to imagine better for their future. The Tagata Sa'ilimalo vision is inclusive of all Pacific peoples in

> Aotearoa and all disability types. The name derives from a Samoan phrase, but we anticipate additional names will be developed in other Pacific languages to describe the same underlying vision.
>
> The origin of the name is a phrase used to acknowledge an individual or group's victory or achievement: *malo le sa'ili malo, malo le finau, malo le tauivi*. In English this means: well done for pursuing success; well done for raising and arguing the point; well done for persevering with the struggle. This expression allows those who have witnessed or taken part in the successful journey to recognize everything it took to get there." (Tōfā Mamao Collective, n.d).

Tōfā Mamao's vision embraces the potential of people, is congratulatory of the sheer determination it takes to overcome obstacles. It seeks to create expectations of disabled people that are the same as their able-bodied peers, in their families and in their communities.

The second concept is ***Soalaupule***, the vision-in-action, that aims to help steer both the individual experience and the experience of the collective.

Vision in action: Soalaupule – self-determination, shared decision making, shared accountabilities, and shared outcomes

> *"Soalaupule (shared authority) is the name of our vision in action that will guide changing practices. Soalaupule is a group decision-making process in which participants share both the decision and accountability for the outcomes.*

Soalaupule allows self-determination while intertwining the lives of everyone who takes part." (Tōfā Mamao Collective, n.d).

This concept also makes the shift towards expectations of active participation in the process of life building. It applies at both individual and collective levels of experience.

Conclusion

The story of the evolution of a defined Pacific disability community and sector is the story of a social movement, one that is uniquely Pacific. Embodied in this development is a collaboration of Pacific people and their supporters, from the community upwards to the service sector, public administrators, and politicians behind a common vision. For-Pacific-by-Pacific is not a separate system. Rather it can be viewed as a key human service sector competence of cultural intelligence, connectedness, and shared values, that when applied can generate creative solutions to complex issues that the traditional 'mainstream' struggles with. Within the COVID-19 context, the communitarianism displayed by all the actors in this story overcame the 'invisibility' of Pacific disability, bringing it into sharper relief for ongoing attention. The legacy of the Pacific disability movement is the existence today of strong Pacific disability community and sector capability, a presence that will contribute to better outcomes for all Pacific people and New Zealanders in the future.

Post-script

On Friday 29 October, 2021, the day this chapter was completed, the Hon. Carmel Sepuloni, Minister of Social Development and Minister for Disability Issues announced a suite of transformative changes to the disability system. A new independent agency will be established, for now called the Ministry of Disabled People. She also stated that 'partnership with disabled people and whanau will be a 'top table' issue for the new Ministry' and that 'most recently a compelling case was put to me from the Pacific Disability via the Tōfā Mamao Collective.'

References

Barker, R.G., Wright, B.A., Meyerson, L., & Gornick, M.R. (1953). *Adjustment to physical handicap and illness: a survey of the social psychology of physique and disability*. New York Social Science Research Council.

Enabling Good Lives. (n.d.). 1. How Enabling Good Lives Started — the August 2011 Report. https://www.enablinggoodlives.co.nz/about-egl/enabling-good-lives-context/1-how-enabling-good-lives-started-the-august-2011-report/

Goldberg, I.I & Lippman, L. (1974). "Plato had a word for it". *Exceptional Children*, *40*(5), 325–334. https://doi.org/10.1177/001440297404000501

Lukoff, I.F., & Cohen, O. (1972). *Attitudes Towards Blind Persons*. Amer Foundation for the Blind.

Kendrick, M. J. (2010). Historical contributors towards increasing respect for the voices of people with disabilities in Western societies. *International Journal of Disability, Community and Rehabilitation, 9*(1).

Ministry of Pacific Peoples. (2022). *Yavu, Foundations of Pacific Engagement*. Ministry of Pacific Peoples. https://www.mpp.govt.nz/assets/Resources/Yavu-Booklet.pdf

Ministry of Health. (2017). *Faiva Ora 2016–2021 National Pasifika Disability Action Plan*. https://www.health.govt.nz/system/files/documents/publications/faiva-ora-2016-2021-national-pasifika-disability-plan-aug17_0.pdf

Ministry of Health. (2018). *Whāia Te Ao Marama 2018 to 2022: The Māori Disability Action Plan.* https://www.health.govt.nz/system/files/documents/publications/whaia-te-ao-marama-2018-to-2022.pdf

Ministry of Health. (2020). *Ola Manuia: Pacific Health and Wellbeing Action Plan 2020–2025.* https://www.health.govt.nz/system/files/documents/publications/ola_manuia-phwap-22june.pdf

Munyi, C.W. (2012). Past and present perceptions towards disability: A historical perspective. *Disability Studies Quarterly, 32*(2).

Office for Disability Issues. (2001). *The New Zealand Disability Strategy, Making a World of Difference.* Ministry of Health. https://www.odi.govt.nz/assets/New-Zealand-Disability-Strategy-files/nz-disability-strategy.pdf

Office for Disability Issues. (2016). *New Zealand Disability Strategy 2016–2026.* https://www.odi.govt.nz/nz-disability-strategy/about-the-strategy/new-zealand-disability-strategy-2016-2026/

Office for Disability Issues. (2017). *Enabling Good Lives.* https://www.odi.govt.nz/nz-disability-strategy/other-initiatives/enabling-good-lives/

Office for Disability Issues. (2019). *Guidance for Policy Makers.* https://www.odi.govt.nz/guidance-and-resources/guidance-for-policy-makes

Pillai, R., Rankin, J., Stanley, K., Bennett, J., Hetherington, D., Stone, L., & Withers, K. (2007). *Disability 2020: Opportunities for the full and equal citizenship of disabled people in Britain in 2020.* Institute for Public Policy Research. https://www.ippr.org/files/images/media/files/publication/2011/05/Disability_2020_full_1568.pdf

Salahshour, N. (2021). A Critique of New Zealand's Exclusive Approach to Intercultural Education. *New Zealand Journal of Educational Studies, 56*(1), 111–128. https://doi.org/10.1007/s40841-020-00179-9

Senge, P. (2006). *The Fifth Discipline: The Art and Practice of The Learning Organization* (1st ed.). Doubleday/Currency.

Stats NZ. (2014). *The New Zealand Disability Survey 2013*. https://www.stats.govt.nz/assets/Uploads/Disability-survey/Disability-survey-2013/Disability-survey-2013-additional-documents/Disability-Survey-2013.pdf

Tamasese, T.K., Parsons, T.L., Sullivan, G., & Waldegrave, C. (2003). *A qualitative study into Pacific perspectives on cultural obligations and volunteering: a research project*. The Family Centre Social Policy Research Unit.

Thomsen, S., Tevita, J., & Levi-Teu, Z. (2018). *A Pacific Perspective on the Living Standards Framework*. New Zealand Treasury.

Tōfā Mamao Collective. (n.d.). *About*. https://tofamamao.com/about

Vertovec, S. (2007). *Reading 'super-diversity'*. Max Planck Institute for the Study of Religious and Ethnic Diversity. https://www.mmg.mpg.de/38383/blog-vertovec-super-diversity

Manato'a: The health of Pacific males

Edmond Fehoko

David Taufui Mikato Fa'avae

Chapter summary

A recent study affirmed the significance of socio-ecological factors in capturing the changing nature of health and wellbeing for Pacific peoples in Aotearoa New Zealand (Lilo et al., 2020). With high Pacific representations in health-related statistics both nationally and regionally, heightened by the current global pandemic, the ecological conditions and socio-cultural contexts that shape Pacific men's health captures aspects of resilience and wellbeing. Unpacking such aspects require relevant tools for analyses. We employ talanoa–vā, a socio-relational theoretical framework to articulate Tangata moana and the interconnections with masculinities that shape Pacific men's understanding of resilience and wellbeing. Integrating talanoa–vā and the case study approach, we capture and synthesise a variety of data sources collected from research studies, statistics, alongside self-reported data to highlight resilience and wellbeing in NZ and the Pacific. Tangata moana and manato'a provides an understanding of Pacific-centred masculinities that empowers agentic meaning-making across places and spaces for Pacific males in New Zealand and the Pacific.

Introduction

Pacific males and health and wellbeing in Aotearoa New Zealand and the Pacific region continues to be a concern. Pacific people are overrepresented in negative health-related statistics linked to diabetes and obesity (Pulu et al., 2021). Their sense of resilience and wellbeing is not always clearly articulated in the literature. Our paper seeks to draw from a socio-ecological understanding of men's health and masculinities, relying on health-related statistical data as well as descriptive case studies. We provide a way of articulating Pacific masculinity within Tangata Moana, unpacking the holistic nature of Pacific personhood.

In a 2015 study on Pacific identity and wellbeing by psychologists Sam Manuela (of Cook Island heritage) and Chris Sibley, they affirm 'the extent to which one feels they are able to participate and express their self within a Pacific cultural context is positively associated with personal satisfaction with health' (p. 153). Lilo et al (2020) also claim the significance of the societal, familial, and communal contexts in synthesising Pacific wellbeing. However, few studies have unfolded the social layers that encapsulate Pacific understandings of masculinities, that is, the socio-cultural behaviours and characteristics that embody the Pacific person (Fehoko, 2015, 2020; Marsters et al., 2021; Tautolo, 2011). To capture widely the diverse layers linked to Pacific men's health in society and across social contexts, we position 'tangata moana' (loosely defined as people of the Pacific) as an individual and collective construct which aligns Pacific health to aspects of gender, masculinities, and cultural as well as sexual identities across NZ and the Pacific. Tangata moana symbolises men's health through 'Pacific personhood', shaped by the diverse specificities inherent in our social, ethnic, and gendered roles and responsibilities across national boundaries which are fluid and mobile (Fa'avae et al., 2021; Te Punga Somerville, 2012; Thomsen & Iosefo-Williams, 2021).

The notion of 'Self' and 'Others' are constructed within social psychology through the self-construal theory based on how individuals construe or interpret herself/himself/themselves within social situations in relation to the collective. Within cultural psychology, one of the central claims is that an 'individual's representations of self and others are influenced by that individual's culture of origin' (Ray et al., 2010, p. 318). Triandis (1995) articulate two models of self- and other- construal – independence and interdependence. Both Triandis (1995) and Ray et al. (2010) note, individualistic cultures, the US for instance, promote independent self construals which emphasise 'internal attributes, the uniqueness of the self and independence from close others' (p. 318).

Contrastingly, collectivist cultures, for instance Tonga, Samoa, Niue, or Cook Islands, are believed to foster interdependent self-construals that emphasise 'relatedness, or the interdependence of self with close others' (Ray et al., 2010, p. 318). Cook Islands scholar Sam Manuela draws from the self-construal theory in his chapter within this book and makes connection with the

Polynesian-centred notion of vā – socio-relational connections. From a dominant western social psychology perspective, the self-construal theory is a consequence of empirical and tested research and the development of research-related discourses in the western academe over time (Hofstede, 1980; Ray et al., 2010; Triandis, 1995; Stojcic, 2020).

Peoples' diverse interpretations of the 'self' in relation to 'others' are two variables that have been tested, constructed, and measured across the social psychology discipline for their validity and reliability within set research conditions and boundaries (Hofstede, 1980; Markus & Kitayama, 1991; Nisbett et al., 2001; Ray et al., 2010; Stojcic, 2020). From an Indigenous Pacific lens, similar to Sione Tu'itahi's chapter in this book which looks at the holistic and interconnected nature of Indigenous bodies of knowledge in relation to the environment, fonua (land), moana (ocean), and langi (sky), we provide a socio-relational interpretation of tangata moana and its connection to notions of self in relative to others using vā as a socio-relational framework of understanding Pacific men's health across social, cultural, spiritual, and sacred inter-connections.

Indigenous Pacific bodies of knowledge and socio-cultural practices have sustained and continued our communities and societies for generations (Thaman, 1995). Notions of wellbeing from indigenous Māori in Aotearoa New Zealand are linked to balancing their daily work life and cultural and collective responsibilities. The study by Warbrick et al. (2016) claim that, although Māori men have a desire to be active and understand the importance of physical activity, 'balancing their cultural obligations to community and whānau (immediate and wider family)' (p. 1) is a struggle. Pacific males also share similar challenges. To capture Pacific men's wellbeing and resilience from a socio-ecological approach, it is necessary to unfold what this looks like through the gender and masculinities lenses.

Gender and indigenous masculinities in relation to men's health

Researchers of Pacific ancestry have positioned colonialism as a key factor in the way Pacific masculinities are portrayed and understood (Hokowhitu, 2004; Tengan, 2002). According to Hokowhitu (2008), there is not one authentic form of Māori (or Pacific) masculinity, rather there are many representations of them. For instance, Pacific masculinities can be embodied in the form of a grandfather, father, brother, manual labourer, sportsman, to name a few. Within Pacific (or Māori) men, they embody various forms of Pacific masculinities based on their responsibilities and roles within kin, clan, extended families, or iwi (tribe), or hapu (sub-tribe).

Health is a context that shapes the Pacific person. Like the way in which clothing and illness became tropes for new attitudes toward the 'self', an example of missionaries' arrival in the Pacific – diabetes and obesity have provided ways to perceive, express, and symbolise Pacific men's health. Body politics and the muscular physique of an elite sportsman, for instance, has also influenced the way society and communities think about the ideal Pacific male bodies (Tengan & Markham, 2009), ignoring other body forms as being authentic representations of Pacific personhood (Hokowhitu, 2008; Thomsen & Brown-Acton, 2021). Therefore, when thinking about Pacific men's health, there is a tendency to focus on a deficit view linked to disease and illness. To widen our perspectives, conceptualising the health of Pacific males, it requires a socio-ecological view of Pacific masculine subjectivities (Hokowhitu, 2008) that privileges indigenous framings of men's health across disciplines, time, places, and spaces. This involves unpacking traditional and local socio-cultural as well as contextual health-related statistics and forms of representing Pacific men's health in NZ and the Pacific.

Health statistics

Pacific male health-related statistics feature more significantly among many of the major causes of mortality and morbidity than they should (Blakely et al., 2005; Dearie et al., 2021). The lives of Pacific males are shaped by unique historical, socio-cultural, economic, environment, political, and health factors that impact on their social, psychological, physical, and collective wellbeing (Fehoko, 2015). Data suggests that Pacific peoples are at the low end of the health spectrum (Health Promotion Agency, 2018), especially Pacific males who are at higher risk of dying by suicide, engaging with the criminal justice system, drug, and alcohol related illnesses, excessive smoking, developing problem gambling behaviours, premature and severe cardiovascular disease, Type 2 diabetes with associated complications.

What is clear is the extent to which inadequate utilisation of health services contributes to the problems experienced by Pacific males (Kitione et al., 2005). Further, Pacific males are one of the lowest users of primary health care services and tend to

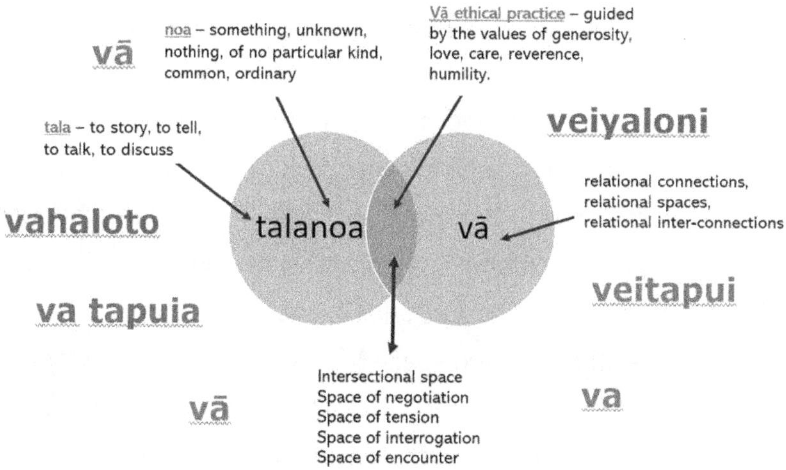

Figure 1: Talanoa-vā framework

delay care, often presenting when their situation has significantly progressed, and their illness is serious (Kapeli et al., 2020). The barriers that exist for Pacific males in the Pacific region and abroad in many places are complex and not easy to identify or even to rectify. Our focus in this chapter is to hone in on the socio-ecological and socio-relational descriptions that conceptualise men's health beyond the negative health statistics and to capture the complex layers of meanings that relate to resilience and wellbeing.

Talanoa-vā an integrated approach

Building on the cultural traditions of indigenous knowledges and practice and the traditions of research inquiry, talanoa–vā is a theoretical framework used to interrogate and unpack the critical relational spaces in which ideas, constructs, and practices intersect and encounter (Fa'avae et al., 2021). As a practice, 'talanoa' is associated with conversations and dialogue. It is a practice familiar to communities from Niue, Samoa, Fiji, Tokelau, and Tonga. However, the meanings and practice of talanoa across each can vary based on the context and purpose of the engagement and the people involved. Vā is a concept linked to socio-relational connections and relational spaces and grounded in Te Gagana Tokelau. Vā is also found in Lea faka-Tonga and its derivative veitapui which relates to sacred space. Va and its derivative va tapuia (sacred space) are common to Samoa (Refiti, 2014; Suaalii-Sauni, 2017). In Niue however, vahaloto is a concept used to refer to the space in between (see Togiatama-Otto, 2015), whereas veiyaloni is used to describe relationships and relational connections in Fijian contexts (Aporosa & Fa'avae, 2021).

The approach is a method used to synthesise multiple data sources. The sources of data synthesised in this chapter are collected from research studies, reports, statistics, as well as self-reported narratives. The key themes (re)presented in the case studies were triangulated using the (1) existing literature on Pacific health, the (2) analysis of documents and reports, and the (3) ongoing talanoa conversations, storying, and reporting of our experiences with Pacific males and their wellbeing within NZ and the Pacific.

Weaving together indigenous Pacific and western-centric research approaches can seem problematic in research especially when it comes to decolonisation aspirations. It is a good way for Pacific researchers to inquire into the limitations and boundaries of indigenous methods and methodologies in dominant spaces like higher education which does not always value Pacific knowledges and practices (Smith & Wolfgramm-Foliaki, 2020) and identify generative possibilities. Nonetheless, one needs to tread this space carefully and with guidance. Integrating and implementing both talanoa–vā and the case study approach, from indigenous Pacific and Western knowledge traditions, provides an appropriate way to capture and synthesise how the notions of Pacific men's health can be understood through the multiple layers of socio-cultural, socio-political, socio-economic, and socio-spiritual framings. It is also important to note that such framings can also be carried across places/contexts, such as NZ and the Pacific region.

Case study 1: Masculine behaviours and social activities in the Pacific and abroad

Gambling is a social activity that can often lead to harmful affects' over one's psychological, physical, mental, and emotional health, which impacts families and communities. Gambling is an activity that is a foreign concept yet has existed in the Pacific region for years. For example, Papoutsaki (2008) described the Micronesian region as the largest 'gambling haven' in the Pacific. That gambling was promoted as attracting high-spending foreigners, boosting tourism and foreign exchange. However, in recent years, there have been a number of referendums that have attempted to address and reduce the proliferation of gambling venues in the region. A 1998 Guam referendum rejected by three to one a proposal to allow casino gambling. A similar experience occurred in the Marshall Islands in 1998. According to Pickles (2014, p. 208), there is no archaeological evidence of indigenous gambling in Melanesia prior to nineteenth and twentieth century colonialism.

In 1907, the British Colonial government made it illegal for 'natives' of PNG to gamble (Murray, 1925). However, the introduction by visiting traders of card gambling in PNG swept through the country in the 1950s. The introduction of Chinese traders in PNG also saw a multitude of gaming houses opening up (Hogbin, 1951). According to Pickles (2014), card gambling swept through the country from its earliest iterations in heavy contact areas in the late 19th and early 20th centuries, along the developing inland trade routes and across the land surrounding coastal plantations, and then up through the Highlands from east to west in the 1950s and 1960s (p. 209). Zimmer (1987, p. 34) explored young men's involvement in three card games in Papua New Guinea, which include attracting a network of supporters among older men and women, the establishment of relations of mutual assistance with other youths, distinguishing oneself as the possessor of attributes or powers, laying the foundation for future prestige and success and attracting a mate. Gambling activities such as bingo, casinos, card and dice games, Lotto, and betting are now evident in a number of Polynesian island nations such as Tonga, Samoa, Tuvalu, Tokelau, Cook Islands, French Polynesia, and Niue (Papoutsaki, 2008). In 2010, the Samoan Government introduced the Casino and Gambling Bill 2010 which made casino gambling legal in Samoa. The casino was introduced on the grounds that it would serve as a tourist attraction. In line with this, legislation in Samoa will allow only holders of foreign passports to enter casinos.

Fehoko (2020) conducted an exploratory study on the Tongan male experiences and perceptions of gambling and problem gambling in New Zealand. Given their central place in Tonga's hierarchical and monarchical systems and as head of the family, and their role in holding and passing on family knowledge, it was important to have a Tongan male elder and youth perspective. A total of 28 Tongan male elders and 18 Tongan male youth participated through focus group talanoa and individual talanoa. Fehoko found that the gambling behaviours of Tongan elders originated in Tonga through social and familial activities. It is important to note that all Tongan male elders were born and raised in Tonga before migrating to New Zealand in search of prosperous opportunities. While it was not perceived as gambling, the introduction of rewards impacted on the health and wellbeing of their families and villages. For example, some Tongan male elders shared how they would spend the majority of their money and time on gambling with other villagers in activities such as card games, darts, and billiards. All Tongan male elders migrated to New Zealand in the 1980s. At this time, horse-race betting (affectionately known as the TAB) became the space for Tongan males to win money, but more importantly to socialise with other Pacific males. The introduction of casinos and other gambling activities saw the rise of Tongan males engaging in these activities. Gambling participation in New Zealand also contributed to increased blood pressure, loss of sleep and migraines, increased alcohol, tobacco or drug consumption, acts of self-harm, and attempted suicide. A community approach needs to be employed to address the gambling behaviours of Pacific males in New Zealand, in particular from a family, community, church, service provider, and policy perspective.

Case study 2: Resilience and wellbeing in the Pacific region

Tagata o le moana is a Samoan phrase that affirms and appreciates the subjectivities of indigenous peoples in the moana (ocean, Oceania). Matapo (2021) describes such subjectivities as likened to a Moana-collective-assemblage, reflecting the sacred kinship and shared histories and genealogies within the moana. From a Tongan perspective, Tangata moana is symbolic of the vā ethical–relational inter-connections inherent in the collective subjectivities of Tongan people and their ancestral and genealogical ties to the ocean including the aba/fonua/āina/vanua/fanua/whenua (land in the vernacular of Kiribati, Tongan, Hawaiian, Fijian, Samoan, Māori). Mila's (2014) use of 'mana moana' reflects the potent spiritual power manifested in the embodied inspirations, resilient practices, and sense of wellbeing across their places and spaces. The coupling of mana-to'a is a representation of mana moana, another way to infuse a sense of mālie (uplifting spirit and energy) and māfana (heart-warming, inwardly warmth) for Pacific males.

The global and local demands implicate how local people in the Pacific practice their sense of resilience and wellbeing (Dousset & Nayral, 2019). Dousset & Nayral (2019) claim the 'global modes of thinking and doing are embedded in renewed perceptions of local and regional specificities' (p. 11). With the introduction of western schooling and Eurocentric ways of thinking and doing in the classroom is interpreted as resulting in a 'loss of cultural or ethnic specificity' (ibid). A study by Nayral (2018) purports the gender relations in Kanak society within New Caledonia have undergone deep transformations (p. 126). Kanak women now have easier access to a better and longer education. The number of Kanak women earning salaries and occupying highly qualified positions has increased (Nayral, 2018). Although Western schooling and education has given females across the Pacific access to educational opportunities and leadership responsibilities, customary and tribal status continue to privilege men. Highlighting such tensions and shifts will help capture the changes in the practices of gender relations within schooling and the community contexts.

International organisation, The United Nations Educational, Scientific and Cultural Organisation (UNESCO) funded regional projects to achieve gender equity and access. In 2017, UNESCO funded a study based in Tonga, which explored school related gender-based violence (SRGBV) and its implications on students and teachers in schooling and the community (Fa'avae et al., 2017). The SRGBV studies generally focus on physical, sexual, and emotional violence towards minority groups within schooling. The SRGBV study in Tonga undertook a multiple methods approach using a questionnaire tool and focus group talanoa and found that females, fakaleiti, and disability are often marginalised in Tongan schooling. In the Niue context, a study by Thomas (2020) explored the manifestation of gender relations that inflict harm disproportionately on women and girls. 27 informant interviews were conducted alongside 14 family-tree mapping interviews using blended narrative-Talanoa methods. The study found that interpersonal relationships are significant to understanding gender-based violence (GBV) incidents and that family spaces provide opportunities to transform and change practice.

Conclusion

In recognition of the projected growth of the Pacific population in New Zealand, Pacific males are overrepresented in terms of adverse outcomes, from exposure to many social and health indicators concerning deprivation and morbidity in New Zealand. Pacific men need to realise that they need to start taking hold of their responsibilities and obligations and control of their direction to improve their self-image and take up their rightful place within their family structure, social structure, and communities. Pacific male elders and youth health is an issue, which has become increasingly important for health researchers and policy makers. There is a need to address the range of health access issues and conditions for Pacific males not only in a strategic fashion but also in a sensitive and effective manner (Masters et al., 2021). There are many Pacific male health issues that need to be addressed, among these are: the health status of Pacific males in prison, injecting drug use among young Pacific males, the alarming rate at which family violence is occurring as well as the continued high rates of suicide in the Pacific region and abroad. Removing barriers to good quality health care is also a fundamental need that requires close consideration for Pacific males. It is important to note that if Pacific males are not healthy, their role in families, villages, communities, and cultures would be diminished with many other issues, which in turn, could not be addressed (Fehoko, 2020). While in the recent past there have been some improvements in male health, there is however, still substantial work that needs to be done to improve the health status of males in the Pacific region and abroad (Lilo et al., 2020). Future research needs to be conducted in collaboration with Pacific males so that sensitive health issues can be handled with care and understanding.

Suggested further readings

Biersack, A. (2016). Introduction: Emergent masculinities in the Pacific. *The Asia Pacific Journal of Anthropology, 3–4*, 197–212. https://doi.org/10.1080/14442213.2016.1186215

Manuela, S., & Sibley, C. (2015). The Pacific identity and wellbeing scale-revised (PIWPS-R). *Cultural Diversity and Ethnic Minority Psychology, 21*(1), 146–155.

Marsters, C., & Tiatia-Seath, J. (2019). Young Pacific male Rugby players perceptions and experiences of mental wellbeing. *Sports, 7*(4), 83. https://doi.org/10.3390%2Fsports7040083

Ofanoa, M., Buetow, S., Ofanoa, S., Huggard, P., Paynter, J., & Nosa, V. (2020). Reasons for and impacts of kava use by Tongan men in kava clubs in Auckland and Tonga. *Social Sciences, 9*(2)56–60. https://doi.org.10.11648/j.ss.20200902.13

Patton, G., Darmstadt, G., Petroni, S., & Sawyer, S. (2018). A gender lens on the health and wellbeing of young males. *Journal of Adolescent Health, 62*, 56–58, http://doi.org/10.1016/j.jadohea lth.2017.06.020

Tautolo, E. (2015). Pacific father involvement and early child behaviour outcomes: Findings from the Pacific Islands families study. *Journal of Child and Family study, 24*(12), 3497–3505. https://doi.org/10.1007/s10826-015-0151-5

Tukuitonga, C.F., & Bindman, A.B. (2002). Ethnic and gender differences in the use of coronary artery revascularisation procedures in New Zealand. *The New Zealand Medical Journal, 115*(1152):179–182.

Vaka, S., Neville, S., & Holroyd, E. (2020). An ethnic interpretation of mental distress from the perspective of Tongan men and community leaders. *International Journal of Mental Health Nursing, 29*, 953–961. https://doi.org/10.1111/inm.12732

References

Aporosa, S. A., & Fa'avae, D. T. M. (2021). Grounding Pacific practice: Fono at the fale and veiqaraqaravi vakavanua. *Waikato Journal of Education, 26*, 35–43. https://doi.org/10.15663/wje.v26i1.852

Blakely, T., Tobiasb, M., Robsonc, B., Ajwanid, S., Bonne, M., & Woodwarde, A. (2005). Widening ethnic mortality disparities in New Zealand 1981–99. Social Science and Medicine, 61. 2233–2251. doi:10.1016/j.socscimed.2005.02.011

Dearie, C., Linhart, C., Rafai, E., Nand, D., Morrell, S., & Taylor, R. (2021). Trends in mortality and life expectancy in Fiji over 20 years. BMC Public Health, 21, 1185. https://doi.org/10.1186/s12889-021-11186-w

Dousset, L., & Nayral, M. (2019). Pacific realities: Changing perspectives on resilience and resistance. Berghahn Books.

Fa'avae, D., Otunuku, M., Robyns, R., & Siale, L. (2017). *School related gender based violence: a case study in Tonga*. United Nations Educational, Scientific and Cultural Organisation (UNESCO).

Fa'avae, D. T. M., Tecun, A., & Siu'ulua, S. (2021). Talanoa vā: indigenous masculinities and the intersections of indigeneity, race, and gender within higher education. *Higher Education Research & Development*. https://doi.org/10.1080/07294360.2021.1882402

Fehoko, E. S. (2015). Social space and cultural identity: The faikava as a supplementary site for maintaining Tongan identity in New Zealand. *New Zealand Sociology, 30*(1), 131–139.

Fehoko, E. S. (2020). *From Games to Gambling: An Exploratory Study of Tongan-born and New Zealand-born Male Perceptions and Experiences of Gambling and Problem Gambling in New Zealand.* [Doctoral Thesis, Auckland University of Technology]. Tuwhera. http://hdl.handle.net/10292/13818

Hofstede, G. (1980). Culture and Organizations. *International Studies of Management and Organization*, *10*(4), 15–41. http://doi.org/10.1080/00208825.1980.11656300

Hogbin, I. (1951). Transformation scene: The changing culture of a New Guinea village. London, UK: Routledge.

Hokowhitu, B. (2004). Tackling Māori Masculinity: A Colonial Genealogy of Savagery and Sport. *The Contemporary Pacific*, *16*(2), 259–284.

Hokowhitu, B. (2008). The Death of Koro Paka: "Traditional" Māori Patriarchy. *The Contemporary Pacific*, *20*(1), 115–141.

Kapeli, S., Manuela, S., & Sibley, C. (2020). Understanding Pasifika mental health in New Zealand: A review of literature. *MAI Journal*, *9*(3), 249–271. https://doi.org/10.20507/MAIJournal.2020.9.3.7

Kitione, L., Ryan, D., Tanuvasa, A., & Gray, B. (2025). Pacific people in Aotearoa New Zealand and the treatment of long-term conditions: A narrative literature review about Pacific people's understandings of health and wellbeing. Journal of Primary Health Care, 17(4), 372–378. doi:10.1071/HC24151

Lilo, L. S., Tautolo, E., S., & Smith, M. (2020). Health literacy, culture and Pacific peoples in Aotearoa-New Zealand: A review. *Pacific Health, 3*, 1–11. https://doi.org/10.24135/pacifichealth.v3i0.4

Markus, H.R., & Kitayama, S. (1991). Culture and the self: Implications for cognition, emotion, and motivation. *Psychological Review*, *98*(2), 224–53. https://doi.org/10.1037/0033-295X.98.2.224

Marsters, C. P. E., Tiatia-Seath, J., & Uperesa, L. (2021). Young Pacific Male Athletes' Attitudes Toward Mental Health Help-Seeking in Aotearoa New Zealand. *Asia Pacific Journal of Public Health*, *33*(6–7), 789–791. https://doi.org/10.1177/10105395211022944

Matapo, J. (2021). *Tagata o le Moana - The people of Moana: Traversing Pacific Indigenous philosophy in Pasifika education research*. [Doctoral Thesis, Auckland University of Technology]. Tuwhera. https://openrepository.aut.ac.nz/server/api/core/bitstreams/488301d0-86a3-41c5-ab3e-e054b1fde87e/content

Mila, K. (2014). Theorising advantage in a context of disparity: Pacific peoples who grow up in New Zealand. In P. Fairbairn-Dunlop & E. Coxon (Eds.), *Talanoa: Building a Pasifika research culture* (1st ed., pp. 32–52). Dunmore Publishing Ltd.

Murray, H. (1925). Papua of to-day or an Australian colony in the making. P. S. King & Son.

Nayral, M. (2018). Resisting UN Ideals to Make Men and Women Equal in Politics: When a Humanist Concern Turns into Arithmetic in Ouvea (New Caledonia). In L. Dousset & M. Nayral (Eds.), *Pacific Realities: Changing Perspectives on Resilience and Resistance* (pp 89–106). Berghahn Books.

Nisbett, R., Peng, K., Choi, I., & Norenzayan, A. (2001). Culture and systems of thought: Holistic versus analytic cognition. *Psychological Review, 108*(2), 291–310. https://doi.org/10.1037/0033-295X.108.2.291

Papoutsaki, E. (2008). South Pacific Islands communication: Regional perspectives, local issues. Asian Media Information Communication Centre. ISBN: 9789814136082, 9814136085

Pickles, A. (2014). Introduction: Gambling as analytic in Melanesia. Oceania, 84(3). 207–211. DOI:10.1002/ocea.5057

Pulu, V., Tiatia-Seath, J., Borman, B., & Firestone, R. (2021). Investigating principles that underlie frameworks for Pacific health research using a co-design approach: learnings from a Tongan community based project. *Pacific Health Dialog, 21*(7), 399–406. http://www.doi/10.26635/phd.2021.115

Ray, R. D., Shelton, A. L., Hollon, N. G., Matsumoto, D., Frankel, C. B., Gross, J. J., & Gabrieli, J. D. E. (2010). Interdependent self-construal and neural representations of self and mother. *Social Cognitive and Affective Neuroscience, 5*(2–3), 318–323. https://doi.org/10.1093/scan/nsp039

Refiti, A. L. (2014). *Mavae and Tofiga: spatial exposition of the Samoan cosmogony and architecture.* [Doctoral Thesis, Auckland

University of Technology]. Tuwhera. https://openrepository.aut.ac.nz/bitstreams/33cf1a81-c3e0-4e5b-af87-7e02b4c854bc/download

Stojcic, I., Wei, Q., & Ren, X. (2020). Historical Sustenance Style and Social Orientations in China: Chinese Mongolians Are More Independent Than Han Chinese. *Frontiers in Psychology*, *11*, 864. https://doi.org/10.3389/fpsyg.2020.00864

Suaalii-Sauni, T. (2017). The va and kaupapa Māori. In T. Hoskins & A. Jones (Eds.), *Critical conversations in kaupapa Māori* (1st ed., pp. 168–171). Huia Publishers.

Tautolo, E. (2011). *Pacific fathers cultivating the future: The health of Pacific fathers and their influence upon and involvement with their children*. [Doctoral Thesis, Auckland University of Technology]. Tuwhera. https://openrepository.aut.ac.nz/items/f7329e73-0ca7-4f2c-9d43-a55657f8da37

Tengan, T. P. K. (2002). (En)gendering Colonialism: Masculinities in Hawai'i and Aotearoa. *Journal for Cultural Research*, *6*(3), 229–238.

Tengan, T. P. K., & Markham, J. M. (2009). Performing Polynesian Masculinities in American Football: From 'Rainbows to Warriors'. *The International Journal of the History of Sport*, *26*(16), 2412–2431. http:// doi.org/10.1080/09523360903466768

Te Punga Somerville, A. (2012). *Once Were Pacific: Māori connections to Oceania*. University of Minnesota Press.

Thaman, K. H. (1995). Concepts of learning, knowledge and wisdom in Tonga, and their relevance to modern education. *Prospects: quarterly review of comparative education, 25*(4), 723–733. http://doi.org/b9h7wq

Thomas, E. (2020). *Gender-based Violence in Niue: Challenges and Opportunities in Small Pacific Islands* [Master's thesis, The University of Auckland]. http://hdl.handle.net/2292/53469

Thomsen, S. P., & Iosefo-Williams, J. (2021). Disruptions, Decolonial Desire and Diaspora: A Provocation toward a Pacific Queer

Worldmaking Scholarly Practice in Aotearoa-New Zealand. *Journal of New Zealand Studies, 33*, 94–109. https://doi.org/10.26686/jnzs.iNS33.7385

Thomsen, P., & Brown-Acton, P. (2021). Manalagi Talanoa A Community-Centred Approach to Research on the Health and Wellbeing of Pacific Rainbow LGBTIQA+ MVPFAFF Communities in Aotearoa New Zealand. *Pacific Health Dialog, 21*(7), 465–471. http://doi.org/10.26635/phd.2021.117

Togiatama-Otto P. V. (2015). Through My Brown Eyes. *Midwifery Today with International Midwife*, (115), 44–48.

Triandis, H. C. (1995). *Individualism & collectivism*. Westview Press.

Warbrick, I., Wilson, D., Boulton, A. (2016). Provider, father, and bro - Sedentary Māori men and their thoughts on physical activity. *International Journal for Equity in Health, 15*(22), 1–11. http://doi/10.1186/s12939-016-0313-0

Zimmer, L. (1987). Gambling with cards in Melanesia and Australia: An introduction. Oceania, 58(1), 1–5.

Mental health

Siale Foliaki

Brittany Stanley-Wishart

Chapter summary

This chapter presents and discusses the mental health status of Pacific peoples within New Zealand. It also highlights the interplay between psychological and physical health. This chapter aligns with Pacific values and understandings acknowledging that each individual Pacific community has their own unique perspectives on mental illness and mental wellbeing. Some of these mental health aspects have been touched on within preceding chapters in the book, including certain priority areas, such as suicide, so they will not be covered here.

Introduction

Historically the prevalence of mental disorders in Pacific peoples was poorly quantified but over the last 20 years major research initiatives have improved our understanding of the prevalence and severity of mental disorders in Pacific peoples. In 2006, Te Rau Hinengaro, the first national study on the prevalence of mental disorders in New Zealanders undertaken addressed this issue (Wells et al., 2006). It was the first and remains the largest mental health study in New Zealand, with responses from 12,992 New Zealanders, including 2,374 Pacific respondents. Of these, 49.2% were Samoan; 20.7% were Cook Island Māori; 16.5% were Tongan; and 17.5% were other Pacific peoples (Foliaki et al., 2006; Wells et al., 2006). This was largely representative of the ethnic distribution of Pacific peoples within New Zealand at the time (Stats NZ, 2008).

The Te Rau Hinengaro study found that almost half of the New Zealand population met the criteria for a mental illness at some point in their lives. Demographic patterns showed that the likelihood of experiencing a mental illness was highest for young people, those who were women, had lower educational qualifications, lower income, lived in areas of higher deprivation, or were of Māori or Pacific ethnicity (Wells et al., 2006). Ongoing research has found that these findings have remained relatively

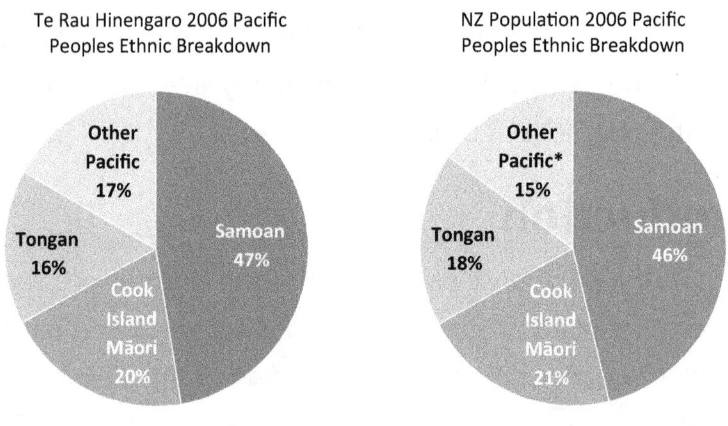

Graph 1: Ethnic breakdown of Pacific respondents in Te Rau Hinengaro vs ethnic breakdown of Pacific peoples within New Zealand as at 2006

*Other Pacific inclusive of 8% Niuean, 4% Fijian, 3% Tokelauan, and 1% Tuvaluan. Available at https://statsnz.contentdm.oclc.org/digital/collection/p20045coll20/id/420

stable over time; reiterated within the New Zealand Mental Health Survey Monitor (previously known as the New Zealand Mental Health Survey – Hudson et al., 2017) conducted in 2015. Further, Te Rau Hinengaro showed that higher levels of anxiety and depression, specifically, were also seen in women, those aged between 25 and 44 years and those of Māori and Pasifika descent experience higher levels of anxiety and depression (Stats NZ 2015; Kapeli et al., 2020).

In terms of the perception of and management of mental well-being, New Zealand-based and international research findings show that cultural beliefs can influence many aspects of mental health. This includes how service users express their symptoms, their style of coping, their family and community support, their understanding of mental health, and their willingness to seek treatment. Likewise, the cultures of the service provider and the service system can influence diagnosis, treatment, and service delivery (Jimenez et al., 2012; U.S. Department of Health and Human Services, 2001). Various studies have also demonstrated that Pacific beliefs regarding mental health can and do differ from Western beliefs due to their contrasting perspectives regarding mental distress, cultural identity, and social and familial connection and obligation (Canfield & Cunningham, 2004; Culbertson, 1999; Hezel, 1994; Tiatia-Seath, 2014; Vaioleti, 2006; Vaka, 2014).

Te Kaveinga, a Health Promotion Agency highlighted key findings regarding mental health and wellbeing of Pacific peoples in 2015 and 2016 from two population surveys (Ataera-Minster & Trowland, 2018): The New Zealand Mental Health Monitor and the Health and Lifestyles Survey which indicated that:

- "Pacific peoples are well connected socially and culturally
- Cultural connectedness is weaker in multi-ethnic Pacific peoples and Pacific peoples whose heritage is from Pacific nations where there is a constitutional agreement with New Zealand (i.e., Cook Islands Māori, Niueans and Tokelauans).
- Pacific peoples, on average, report higher psychological distress and depressive symptoms over the past 2 to 4 weeks than the Others (i.e., non-Māori, non-Pacific people).
- The stigma surrounding mental health issues is high among Pacific peoples.
- Some Pacific peoples don't know where to get help for mental distress and awareness of national mental health websites is low."

The resulting suggestions for mental health promotion as a result of the above included diversifying 'culturally appropriate' health promotion, increasing awareness of mental health pathways, reducing stigma and removing barriers to care, strengthening the Pacific mental health and addictions workforce and increasing research around the relationship between Pacific mental health and cultural identity.

As a youthful, diverse, and growing population, understanding Pacific peoples' experiences of mental illness within New Zealand (including risk and protective factors), is one of the first steps to developing solutions that can lead to more equitable mental health outcomes for future generations of Pacific people.

Intergenerational trauma

There are a number of risk factors associated with poorer mental health outcomes which precede birth and/or are external to an individual. The Pacific and New Zealand have both been affected by colonisation (Kjellgren, 2004; Fraenkel, 2012) and the impact of this can be felt by future generations, through a process called intergenerational trauma. This is a type of trauma which is passed between individuals and communities through both psychosocial and biological (epigenetics) factors as well as societal and systemic structures (Lev–Wiesel, 2007; Lehrner & Yehuda, 2018, Alhassen et al., 2021).

Symptoms experienced by future generations experiencing intergenerational trauma can include impaired self-esteem, increased aggression, increased likelihood of sleep disturbances, guilt, hypervigilance, rumination, tendency towards catastrophising. All of these factors can contribute to poorer mental health outcomes, and can contribute to higher rates of emotional distress, increased rates of anxiety and depressive disorders, higher rates of suicide, increased rates of substance disorder, and higher prevalence of Post Traumantic Stress Disorder (PTSD) (Menzies, 2010; Kirmayer et al., 2014).

Intergenerational trauma that effects populations may not only result from colonisation, but other large scale traumas including war, massacres, removal of children, gentrification, spread of deadly diseases, eradication of social, cultural, and spiritual practices, as well as other significant events (Wesley-Esquimaux & Smolewski, 2004; Menzies, 2010). Of note, all of these can occur within the process of colonisation or as discrete occurrences. Regarding Pacific peoples in New Zealand, and acknowledging the on-going effects of colonisation, other significant events that could result in the transmission of trauma throughout generations include both contemporary events such as, the Measles outbreak in 2019, and the COVID-19 pandemic and historical events such as the Dawn Raids of the 1970s and the 1918 influenza pandemic in Samoa (Ministry for Culture and Heritage, 2020). These events should be taken into consideration when reviewing and discussing mental health outcomes for Pacific peoples.

Environmental determinants

Explanation for the cause of differing mental health outcomes has often oscillated between nature and nurture. While several disorders have a hereditary component (Cross-Disorder Group of the Psychiatric Genomics Consortium, 2013), environmental factors and social determinants are also an important contributor in the development of mental disorders (Compton, 2015). These include increased rates of deprivation, reduced access to education, lower household incomes, and increased housing difficulties (Compton, 2015). As has already been highlighted in preceding chapters, this is an important consideration in the assessment and management of Pacific peoples given the increased rates of deprivation, reduced access to housing, lower rates of tertiary education certificates (Bachelor's degree or higher), and lower household incomes experienced by Pacific peoples in New Zealand compared to the total population (Wells et al., 2006).

Antenatal period

Pregnancy can be a complex and often challenging time in relation to the psychological wellbeing of the individual and their intimate relations. Antenatal psychopathology is associated with poorer health and social outcomes for mother and the unborn child and Pacific women in New Zealand have higher rates of antenatal depressive symptoms (ADS) than women from other ethnic groups. The Growing Up in New Zealand Study (McDaid et al., 2019) attempted to identify factors that were significantly associated with depression in pregnant Pacific women living in New Zealand.

Data was collected from 5,657 pregnant women, 727 of whom identified their ethnicity as Pacific Island. Antenatal depression symptoms were measured using the Edinburgh Depression Scale with scores above 12 indicating elevated antenatal depression symptoms. The results indicated that 23% of pregnant Pacific women experiencing ADS, which was a significantly higher rate compared to non-Pacific women, whilst ADS affected one in three Pacific women aged < 25 years. Factors associated with ADS in Pacific women included age <25 years, moderate to severe nausea during pregnancy, perceived stress, family stress, and relationship conflict as well as not seeing the importance of maintaining one's Pacific culture and traditions and negative feelings towards New Zealand culture. Pregnant Pacific women without a family general practitioner (GP) before their pregnancy were also 4.5-fold more likely to experience ADS than non-Pacific women with a regular GP (McDaid et al., 2019)

Postnatal

Maternal psychopathology has a significant impact on the emotional wellbeing of a new-born child and increases the incident of mental disorders throughout their lifetime.

The Pacific Island Families Study (Paterson et al., 2008) was the largest study of postnatal depression among Pacific mothers undertaken in New Zealand. They interviewed 1,376 mothers of Pacific Island infants aged 6 weeks old residing in Auckland, New Zealand, using the Edinburgh Postnatal Depression Scale (EPDS).

The study found that 16.4% of mothers were assessed as probably experiencing depression with prevalence rates varying from 7.6% for Samoans to 30.9% for Tongans. In addition to ethnicity, other risk factors identified by stepwise multiple logistic regression included low Pacific Island acculturation, first birth, stress due to insufficient food, household income less than $40,000, difficulty with transport, dissatisfaction with pregnancy, birth experience, baby's sleep patterns, partner relationship, and home. A large prevalence difference between Tongans and other groups remained when the effects of other risk factors were controlled statistically. The study concluded that the prevalence of depressive symptoms among Pacific mothers is at the upper end of the range typically reported. However, the overall rate and risk factors identified were generally similar to those found in previous research (Abbot & Williams, 2006).

Children and adolescents

Pacific peoples within New Zealand have a young population with children (14 and under) making up more than two-thirds of the Pacific population. This means that the mental health and wellbeing of children and adolescents is essential for Pacific peoples as a whole. Data from Pacific peoples and Mental Health Report (Ministry of Health, 2008) as well as the Youth 2000 survey (Helu et al., 2009) showed that young Pacific peoples were more likely to experience a serious mental disorder compared to older Pacific peoples; this was consistent with the New Zealand population. This same report highlighted that 20% of Pacific secondary school students experienced symptoms of depression that would be classified as serious or needing professional assistance compared to 16.2% of Māori and 11.7% of the total NZ population. Despite this, young Pacific people from 0 to 19 years old made up only 2.9% of mental health clients of the same age.

Of interest, young people of Cook Island Māori descent had the highest 12-month prevalence of mental disorders at 29.3% compared to Samoan young people at 24.5% and Tongan young people at 19.6%. However, these results from the Pacific Peoples and Mental Health Report were not statistically significant (Ministry of Health, 2008).

Adulthood

Pacific peoples in New Zealand experience higher levels of mental disorders compared to the general population as mentioned above. The 12-month prevalence of mental disorders is 25% and the lifetime prevalence is 46.6% compared to 20.7% and 39.5% of the total New Zealand population, respectively (Oakley Browne et al., 2006; Foliaki et al., 2006). Most interestingly, results from Te Rau Hinengaro showed that of New Zealand born Pacific peoples, the 12-month prevalence for any mental disorder was significantly higher for those who migrated to NZ before the age of 18 compared to those who migrated after the age of 18 (31.4% vs 15.0%, respectively) (Oakley Browne et al., 2006; Foliaki et al., 2006).

Pacific peoples were more likely to be affected by a serious mental disorder over their lifetime compared to the total New Zealand population (5.9% vs 4.7%, respectively). Furthermore,

Pacific peoples were also more likely to experience anxiety disorders and mood disorders over a 12-month period compared to the total NZ population. The rates of eating disorders were similar (Foliaki et al., 2006).

Both the 12-month and lifetime prevalence of comorbid disorders were also higher for Pacific peoples compared to the total New Zealand population:

Of Pacific peoples who experienced a mood disorder, 34.9% had a comorbid anxiety disorder and 16.8% had a comorbid substance use disorder.

Gender discrepancies have also been identified with Pacific women more likely to experience certain anxiety disorders, major depression, and eating disorders and less likely to experience substance dependence compared to Pacific men (Foliaki et al., 2006; Ataera-Minster & Trowland, 2018). However, this data does not appear to take into account gender diverse Pacific peoples.

Substance abuse and addictions

Substance abuse and addictions are a significant issue impacting Pacific peoples in New Zealand with higher levels of substance disorder (4.9% compared to 2.7% in the total New Zealand population), alcohol abuse and/or dependence (4.2% compared to 2.2%), and marijuana use and/or dependence (1.3% compared to 1.0%) (Foliaki et al., 2006). Despite this, findings from Te Rau Hinengaro highlighted that Pacific peoples were less likely to use alcohol or other drug services compared to the total population and Pacific peoples aged 15–19 years old accessed these services at a similar rate to

Table 1: Rate of specific mental disorders within the pacific population.

	12-Month Prevalence		**Lifetime Prevalence**	
	Pacific	**Total NZ Pop**	**Pacific**	**Total NZ Pop**
Any disorder*	25%	20.7%	46.5%	39.5%
Anxiety disorders	16.2%	14.8%	27.7%	24.9%
Mood disorders	8.6%	7.9%	19.0%	20.2%
Substance use disorders	5.3%	3.5%	17.7%	12.3%
Eating disorders	1.5%	1.5%	4.4%	1.7%

*as classified by *DSM-IV CIDI 3.0 mental disorder*

other New Zealanders of the same age (Oakley Browne et al., 2006; Ministry of Health 2008).

However, Pacific people are also more likely to be non-drinkers (46% compared to 19%), yet of those who do drink, they are more likely to have consumed more than ten glasses on the last drinking occasion (27% compared to 8% of the total New Zealand population) (Foliaki et al., 2006; Oakley Browne et al., 2006). In any 12-month period, 34.3% of Pacific peoples with alcohol dependence also reported drug abuse problems, while 28.6% met criteria for drug dependence compared to 28.1% of the total New Zealand population (Foliaki et al., 2006).

Table 2: Comorbid mental disorders among Pacific peoples compared to the total New Zealand population.

	12-Month Prevalence		**Lifetime Prevalence**	
	Pacific	**Total NZ Pop**	**Pacific**	**Total NZ Pop**
1 Disorder	16.6%	13.0%	23.4%	20.0%
2 Disorders	5.1%	4.4%	12.4%	9.9%
3+ Disorders	3.3%	3.3%	10.7%	9.7%

Excess substance use is not only associated with increased rates of socioeconomic deprivation which can be a contributor to poorer mental health outcomes (Kim & Kim, 2017), but there is also an increased rate of concurrent substance dependence as well as a direct association with increased rates of mental illness. Te Rau Hinengaro identified that 53.7% of Pacific peoples with a drug dependence also reported alcohol abuse symptoms in the past 12 months. It was also noted that 27.6% of Pacific people who had a substance use disorder also had a mood disorder while 41.8% met criteria for an anxiety disorder. However, Pacific peoples with a mood or anxiety disorder, were less likely to experience a comorbid substance disorder compared to the general population (Foliaki et al., 2006; Oakley Browne et al., 2006).

Old age

A recently published study looking at the care received by Māori and Pacific peoples living with dementia compared to those of

New Zealand Europeans showed that Pacific peoples are more likely to develop dementia at a younger age compared to NZ Europeans (75.5 years vs 80.1 years) are more likely to have moderate-severe dementia at time of diagnosis (48% vs 31% in New Zealand Europeans), have higher rates of impairment (as per the CIS-G Index > 1.5) at 77% compared to 69% for New Zealand European people, and are less likely to be receiving home-based service supports (33% vs 45%). However Pacific peoples are much less likely to be living alone at time of diagnosis (8% vs 31%) (Ma'u et al., 2022). The overall prevalence rates for dementia in New Zealand among Pacific peoples in the 60+ population are 6.3% compared to 3.7% for European and in the 80+ population are 22.2% compared to 13.6% for New Zealand Europeans (Cheung et al., 2022).

Limited data exists regarding the prevalence of mental disorders in Pacific adults over the age of 65. Te Kaveinga briefly mentions that the rates of psychological distress in Pacific people is higher in young people aged 15–24 years (38%) and older adults aged 45–64 years (35%) (Ataera-Minster & Trowland, 2018), but does not reference those over 65 years and a previous study from the UK sampling over 3,000 people has highlighted relatively high prevalence rates of mental disorders in those over the age of 65 years (Andreas et al., 2017). Combined with data that indicates New Zealand's Pacific population is ageing at a faster rate than the national average (Stats NZ, 2020), further data in this area is a priority.

Use of mental health services

Pacific peoples are more likely to be admitted to an inpatient psychiatric unit (198 per 100,000 compared to 170 per 1000,000) with Pacific men utilising this at a 40% higher rate compared to Pacific women (Ministry of Health, 2005). If Pacific peoples are admitted to an acute inpatient unit, then their length of stay is higher than the total NZ population by approximately 4 days, they incur higher treatment costs per head in mental health care compared to New Zealand Europeans, and their rates of seclusion (involuntary containment and isolation within an acute mental health facility) are also higher in comparison to the general population (Ministry of Health, 2005). Community Treatment Orders are an aspect of the Mental Health Act which means that patients are required to comply with treatment recommendations as ordered by the court, and research indicates Pacific peoples are more likely to be placed under a CTO than New Zealand European people (Stats NZ, 2020; Beaglehole et al., 2021).

Higher rates of mental distress among Pacific populations in New Zealand may reflect greater barriers to accessing mental health services, greater burden of economic inequality and cultural differences in mental health beliefs. Previous findings indicate that 85% of New Zealand Europeans were more likely to say that they were able to identify anxiety and depression, compared with 51% of Pasifika (Hudson et al., 2017).

Despite the higher overall prevalence of mental disorders, the rate of Pacific peoples receiving mental health treatment has previously been identified as 35% lower than the rate for the total New Zealand population (Ministry of Health, 2005). This was further corroborated in Te Rau Hinengaro and updated data from the Ministry of Health, which showed that, in those with a serious mental disorder, Pacific peoples accessing health services for any mental health reason was less than half that of the total

New Zealand population in those with a serious mental disorder (Foliaki et al., 2006; Ministry of Health, 2008):

These results were adjusted for age, sex, educational qualifications, and household income indicating reasons outside of these which account for reduced access and contact with mental health services (Folikai et al., 2006). The evidence base concerning Pacific mental health in New Zealand suggests lower recognition and service use, which further suggests that mental health literacy is lower for Pacific peoples than for non-Pacific (Kapeli et al., 2020).

Conclusion

The research evidence indicates that the mental health status of Pacific peoples within New Zealand is poorer overall compared to non-Māori, non-Pacific populations. Pacific peoples have higher rates of mental disorders, with higher rates of severity, and higher rates of comorbidity. Despite this, Pacific peoples also experience reduced access to mental health services, and when they do access services, they are more likely to be impacted by involuntary treatment.

Table 3: Rate of access to any health service for a mental health reason in the past 12 months.

	Pacific Peoples	**Total NZ Population**
Any	25%	41%
Serious	25%	58%
Moderate disorder	26.5%	35.5%

It is clear that there are contributors that have not been fully identified and the data from Te Rau Hinengaro regarding migration and mental disorders highlights this. Prioritising the identification of these factors will be one of the most important steps that can highlight our direction, hone our focus, and drive problem-solving that can ultimately lead towards improving the mental wellbeing of all Pacific peoples in New Zealand for generations to come.

Worthwhile questions in the context of COVID-19

For postgraduate students reading this chapter – to think about pacific mental health within the context of COVID-19

1. Why is there such a significant difference in prevalence of mental disorders between NZ born and Pacific born Pacific people.
2. How has the impact of COVID affected the mental health and wellbeing of Pacific people within New Zealand?
3. What would be some outcomes related to COVID and mental health that may be beneficial to measure in the Pacific population in New Zealand and how would this help our communities in the future?

Key readings

- Te Rau Hinengaro, 2006
- Foliaki, S., Kokaua, J., Schaaf, D., & Tukuitonga, C. (2006). Twelve-month and lifetime prevalences of mental disorders and treatment contact among Pacific people in Te Rau Hinengaro: The New Zealand Mental Health Survey. *Australia*

& *New Zealand Journal of Psychiatry*, 40(10), 924–934. https://doi.org/10.1080/j.1440-1614.2006.01912.x

- Understanding Pasifika Mental Health in New Zealand (Literature Review), 2020
- Kapeli, S., Manuela, S., & Sibley, C. (2020). Understanding Pasifika mental health in New Zealand: A review of literature. *MAI Journal*, 9(3), 249–271. https://doi.org/10.20507/MAIJournal.2020.9.3.7

References

Abbott, M. W., & Williams, M. M. (2006). Postnatal depressive symptoms among Pacific mothers in Auckland: prevalence and risk factors. *Aust N Z J Psychiatry*, 40(3):230–238. doi: 10.1080/j.1440-1614.2006.01779.x. PMID: 16476150.

Alhassen, S., Chen, S., Alhassen, L., Phan, A., Khoudari, M., De Silva, A., Barhoosh, H., Wang, Z., Parrocha, C., Shapiro, E., Henrich, C., Wang, Z., Mutesa, L., Baldi, P., Abbott, G. W., & Alachkar, A. (2021). Intergenerational trauma transmission is associated with brain metabotranscriptome remodeling and mitochondrial dysfunction. *Communications Biology*, *4*(783). https://doi.org/10.1038/s42003-021-02255-2

Andreas, S., Schulz, H., Volkert, J., Dehoust, M., Sehner, S., Suling, A., Ausín, B., Canuto, A., Crawford, M., Da Ronch, C., Grassi, L., Hershkovitz, Y., Muñoz, M., Quirk, A., Rotenstein, O., Santos-Olmo, A. B., Shalev, A., Strehle, J., Weber, K., Wegscheider, K., … Härter, M. (2017). Prevalence of mental disorders in elderly people: the European MentDis_ICF65+ study. *The British Journal of Psychiatry, 210*(2), 125–131. https://doi.org/10.1192/bjp.bp.115.180463

Ataera-Minster, J., & Trowland, H. (2018). *Te Kaveinga: Mental health and wellbeing of Pacific peoples. Results from the New Zealand Mental Health Monitor & Health and Lifestyles Survey.* Health Promotion Agency. https://www.hpa.org.nz/sites/default/files/FinalReport-TeKaveinga-Mental%20health%20and%20wellbeing%20of%20Pacific%20peoples-Jun2018.pdf

Beaglehole, B., Newtown-Howes, G., & Frampton, C. (2021). Compulsory Community Treatment Orders in New Zealand and the provision of care: An examination of national databases and predictors of outcome. *The Lancet Regional Health – Western Pacific, 17* (100375). https://doi.org/10.1016/j.lanwpc.2021.100275

Canfield, S., & Cunningham, J. (2004). Cross-Cultural Considerations in Counseling Clients of Samoan Heritage. *Issues in Religion and Psychotherapy, 29*(1), 4.

Cheung, G., To, E., Rivera-Rodriguez, C., Ma'u, E., Hai Yan Chan, A., Ryan, B., & Cullum, S. (2022). Dementia prevalence estimation among the main ethnic groups in New Zealand: a population-based descriptive study of routinely collected health data. *BMJ Open, 12*(9), e062304. https://doi.org/10.1136/bmjopen-2022-062304

Compton, M. (2015). The Social Determinants of Mental Health. *Psychiatry and Society: Global Mental Health, 13*(4), 419–425. https://doi.org/10.1176/appi.focus.20150017

Cross-Disorder Group of the Psychiatric Genomics Consortium. (2013). Identification of risk loci with shared effects on five major psychiatric disorders: a genome-wide analysis. *The Lancet, 381*(9875), 1371–1379. https://doi.org/10.1016/S0140-6736(12)62129-1

Culbertson, P. (1999). Listening Differently with Māori and Polynesian Clients. *Ata: Journal of Psychotherapy Aotearoa New Zealand, 5*(1), 64–82. https://doi.org/10.9791/ajpanz.1999.09

Foliaki, S., Kokaua, J., Schaaf, D., & Tukuitonga, C. (2006). Twelve-month and lifetime prevalences of mental disorders and treatment contact among Pacific people in Te Rau Hinengaro: The New Zealand Mental Health Survey. *Australia & New Zealand Journal of Psychiatry, 40*(10), 924–934. https://doi.org/10.1080/j.1440-1614.2006.01912.x

Fraenkel, J. (2012). *'Pacific Islands and New Zealand - Colonisation and trade in the Pacific'.* Te Ara - the Encyclopedia of New Zealand.

http://www.TeAra.govt.nz/en/pacific-islands-and-new-zealand/page-3

Helu, S.L., Robinson E., Grant, S., Herd, R., & Danny S. (2009). *Youth '07 The Health and Wellbeing of Secondary School Students in New Zealand; Results for the Pacific Young People*. The University of Auckland. https://www.fmhs.auckland.ac.nz/assets/fmhs/faculty/ahrg/docs/2007-initial-findings.pdf

Hezel, F. (1994), What can we do to prevent suicide in the Pacific? *Pacific Health Dialog*, *1*(1), 59–62.

Hudson, S., Russell, L., & Holland, K. (2017). *Indicators of mental health and wellbeing of adults: Findings from the 2015 New Zealand Mental Health Monitor*. Health Promotion Agency. https://www.hpa.org.nz/sites/default/files/726033_2%20NDI%20Report%2001%20August.pdf

Jimenez, D., Bartels, S., Cardenas, V., Dhaliwal, S., & Alegria, M. (2012). Cultural Beliefs and Mental Health Treatment Preferences of Ethnically Diverse Older Adult Consumers in Primary Care. *The American Journal of Geriatric Psychiatry*, *20*(6), 533–542. https://doi.org/10.1097/JGP.0b013e318227f876

Kapeli, S., Manuela, S., & Sibley, C. (2020). Understanding Pasifika mental health in New Zealand: A review of literature. *MAI Journal*, *9*(3), 249–271. https://doi.org/10.20507/MAIJournal.2020.9.3.7

Kim, J., & Kim, H. (2017). Demographic and environmental factors associated with mental health: A cross-sectional study. *International Journal of Environmental Research and Public Health*, *14*(4), 431. https://doi.org/10.3390/ijerph14040431

Kirmayer, L., Gone, J., & Moses, J. (2014). Rethinking Historical Trauma. *Transcultural Psychiatry*, *51*(3), 299–319. https://doi.org/10.1177/1363461514536358

Kjellgren, E. (2004). European Exploration of the Pacific, 1600–1800. *Heilbrunn Timeline of Art History, The Metropolitan Museum of Art*. http://www.metmuseum.org/toah/hd/expa/hd_expa.html

Lehrner, A., & Yehuda., R. (2018). Cultural trauma and epigenetic inheritance. *Development and Psychopathology*, *30*(5) 1763–1777. https://doi.org/10.1017/S0954579418001153

Lev–Wiesel, R. (2007). Intergenerational Transmission of Trauma across Three Generations: A Preliminary Study. *Qualitative Social Work*, *6*(1), 75–94. https://doi.org/10.1177/1473325007074167

Ma'u, E., Saeed, F., Yates, S., Oulaghan, B., Whittington, R., Coomarasamy, C., Cheung, G., & Cullum, S. (2022). Do Māori and Pacific Peoples Living with Dementia in New Zealand Receive Equitable Long-Term Care Compared with New Zealand Europeans? *Journal of Long-Term Care, 33*(8), 1098–1104. http://doi.org/10.31389/jltc.148

Menzies, P. (2010). Intergenerational Trauma from a Mental Health Perspective. *The Native Social Work Journal*, *7*, 63–85.

McDaid, F., Underwood, L., Fa'alili-Fidow, J., Waldie, K., Peterson, E., Bird, A., D'Souza, S., & Morton, S. (2019). Antenatal depression symptoms in Pacific women: evidence from Growing Up in New Zealand. *Journal of Primary Health Care*, *11*(2), 96–108. https://doi.org/10.1071/HC18102

Ministry for Culture and Heritage. (2020). *'Influenza in Samoa'.* https://nzhistory.govt.nz/culture/1918-influenza-pandemic/samoa#:~:text=The%20disease%20spread%20rapidly%20through,ceremonies%20for%20their%20loved%20ones

Ministry of Health. (2005). *Te Orau Ora: Pacific Mental Health Profile. Wellington: Ministry of Health.* https://www.moh.govt.nz/notebook/nbbooks.nsf/0/9f56f480f030606acc2570180070fc77/$FILE/pacificmentalhealthprofile.pdf

Ministry of Health. (2008). *Pacific Peoples and Mental Health: A paper for the Pacific Health and Disability Action Plan Review.* https://www.moh.govt.nz/notebook/nbbooks.nsf/0/CA1AD1F6E5015A82CC2574490074B4C9/$file/pacific-peoples-mental-health-feb08.pdf

Oakley Browne, M., Wells, J., Scott, K., & Mcgee, M. (2006). Lifetime Prevalence and Projected Lifetime Risk of DSM-IV Disorders in Te Rau Hinengaro: The New Zealand Mental Health Survey. *Australian & New Zealand Journal of Psychiatry, 40*(10), 865–874. https://doi.org/10.1080/j.1440-1614.2006.01905.x

Paterson, J., Percival, T., Schluter, P., Sundborn, G., Abbott, M., Carter, S., Cowley-Malcolm, E., Borrows, J., Gao, W., & the PIF Study Group. (2008). Cohort Profile: The Pacific Islands Families (PIF) Study. *International Journal of Epidemiology, 37*(2), 273–279. https://doi.org/10.1093/ije/dym171

Stats NZ. (2008). *Pacific Profiles: 2006.* https://statsnz.contentdm.oclc.org/digital/collection/p20045coll20/id/420

Stats NZ. (2020). *Ethnic group summaries reveal New Zealand's multicultural make-up.* https://www.stats.govt.nz/news/ethnic-group-summaries-reveal-new-zealands-multicultural-make-up/

Stats NZ. (2015). *New Zealand General Social Survey: 2014.* http://infoshare.stats.govt.nz/browse_for_stats/people_and_communities/Households/nzgss_HOTP2014.aspx#gsc.tab=0

Tiatia-Seath, J. (2014). Pacific peoples, mental health service engagement and suicide prevention in Aotearoa New Zealand. *Ethnicity and Inequalities in Health and Social Care, 7*(3), 111–121. https://doi.org/ghgvr2

U.S. Department of Health and Human Services. (2001). *Mental Health: Culture, Race, and Ethnicity—A Supplement to Mental Health: A Report of the Surgeon General.* U.S. Department of Health and Human Services, Substance Abuse and Mental Health Services Administration, Center for Mental Health Services. https://portal.ct.gov/-/media/DMHAS/OMHE/mhethnicitypdf.pdf

Vaioleti, T. (2006). Talanoa research methodology: A developing position on Pacific research. *Waikato Journal of Education, 12*(1), 21–34. https://doi.org/c6mj

Vaka, S. (2014). *A Tongan talanoa about conceptualisations, constructions and understandings of mental illness* [Doctoral thesis, Massey University]. Massey Research Online. https://mro.massey.ac.nz/handle/10179/5777

Wells, J., Oakley Browne, M., Scott, K., McGee, M., Baxter, J., & Kokaua, J., New Zealand Mental Health Survey Research Team. (2006). Te Rau Hinengaro: the New Zealand Mental Health Survey: overview of methods and findings. *The Australian and New Zealand Journal of Psychiatry, 40*(10), 835–844. https://doi.org/10.1080/j.1440-1614.2006.01902.x

Wesley-Esquimaux, C., & Smolewski M. (2004). *Historic Trauma and Aboriginal Healing*. Aboriginal Healing Foundation. https://www.ahf.ca/downloads/historic-trauma.pdf

Addiction: Alcohol, tobacco, and other drug use in Pacific communities across Aotearoa-New Zealand and the Pacific region

Vili Nosa

Chapter summary

This chapter describes alcohol, tobacco, and other drugs among Pacific Islands peoples in the Pacific region and in New Zealand, where many Pacific people live. This chapter demonstrates that Pacific people are at risk of substance use and addiction, and that this can have significant consequences for individuals, families, and communities. It describes services set up to address alcohol and substance use among Pacific people in New Zealand and considers how to improve services and support for Pacific communities.

Introduction

Addiction involves compulsive engagement in an activity, despite negative consequences. Addiction has been linked to genetics, age, environmental factors such as low socioeconomic status, and feelings of powerlessness.

Addictions to tobacco, alcohol, drugs, food, and gambling can harm the health and wellbeing of individuals and significantly affects their family and communities. It has been estimated that the economic cost of addiction in some countries is higher than the cost of diabetes and cancer combined (International Narcotics Control Board, 2014).

Addictions can impact on people's physical and mental health, affect their relationships, increase the use of medical services, lead to long-term complications, reduce productivity, increase welfare costs, and be associated with crime and incarceration (Merikangas & McClair, 2012). Therefore, there is an increasing focus on understanding the causes and consequences of addiction and potential solutions.

Health and justice services have identified problematic substance use and addiction as an issue in the Pacific region and in countries where high numbers of Pacific people have migrated. Understanding an issue is key to tackling it, so this chapter summarises what we know about the use of alcohol, tobacco, and other drugs among Pacific peoples in the Pacific region and in New Zealand.

Alcohol, tobacco, and other drugs use in the Pacific region

It is difficult to get robust figures about the proportion of people in the Pacific Islands who use substances such as alcohol, tobacco, and other drugs versus those who are addicted. There are also likely to be differences across the various Pacific Islands. In this section, we summarise the sparse research evidence to showcase that more work in this area is needed.

Early European contact from sailors, missionaries, and others brought about significant changes in Pacific social structure, lifestyle, diet, and behaviours (Power et al., 2015). This included the use of alcohol, tobacco, and some drugs which were not traditionally part of Pacific Islands cultures (Nosa et al., 2018). Over the past 400 years, Pacific peoples have begun to use these substances more heavily.

Alcohol

The proportion of men and women with problematic or addictive drinking is unknown because records are not kept consistently, and definitions differ for each Pacific country. However, the data varies for each country as most information is not regular, reliable, and routine monitoring of patterns and trends is a concern. What is known is that there appear to be evidence of high levels of alcohol and risky alcohol consumption in some Pacific Islands Countries and Territories. Binge drinking is reported to be common among men and boys in the Pacific Islands and there has also been an increase in prevalence among Pacific women (Power et al., 2015, Nosa et al., 2018, Warren et al., 2006).

Homebrew

Homebrew involved brewing alcohol for non-commercial purposes. It can be cheaper than buying commercially available alcohol. In the Pacific this is sometimes created from methylated spirits and harmful substances. Homebrew use is common in the Marshall Islands, Papua New Guinea, Tonga, and Tuvalu, among other places. Men are the main drinkers, often those with low socioeconomic status. Research has found that negative impacts from homebrew include aggression, losing control, unconsciousness, stomach aches, heartburn, and feeling sick (Nosa et al., 2018).

Kava

Kava is a drink formed by straining the roots and stump of the Piper mythisticum plant through water. Kava acts as a relaxant and does not have the euphoric effects and loss of inhibition commonly associated with alcoholic drinks (Aporosa, 2015). It has been consumed for centuries across the Pacific region.

Different countries use it in different ways, including in ceremonies. For instance, in Fiji kava or 'yaqona' is used in rituals at ceremonial gatherings. In Vanuatu there are kava clubhouses for men only, including over 200 kava bars in one city, which shows its popularity. Tonga has various kava ceremonies. Here only women can serve kava while the men drink it. In Samoa, the 'ava' (kava) is first given to the highest chief and then to the senior-most hosts and so forth according to rank. In Hawai'i, there are approximately 13 types of kava domestically grown and both women and men can drink it (Aporosa, 2015). In Tonga kava is used as a fundraising activity to raise funds for projects such as building a new church (Ofanoa et al., 2020).

Whilst it has traditional uses, there is emerging evidence that kava can be addictive and harmful. For instance, a study in Tonga found that heavy kava sessions resulted in a lack motivation and energy among participants, who often ended up not going to their paid jobs. This resulted in a lack of income to support their families. Kava consumption was also linked to family violence, perhaps due to the associated stress and financial hardship (Ofanoa et al., 2021).

Tobacco

Tobacco was first introduced to the Pacific Islands during visits by Europeans in the sixteenth and seventeenth centuries (Marshall, 2013). It quickly became one of the most sought-after goods merchants offered to Pacific Islanders to entice them into trade relations (Linhart et al., 2017). Some studies have found particularly high rates of smoking among Pacific women in Tokelau and Nauru (Kessaram et al., 2015).

Over 3 million deaths linked to tobacco smoking in countries in the Western Pacific region, and over 460,000 deaths linked to second-hand intake of tobacco smoke. As a result of the scale of the issue and serious consequences, Pacific countries have set up stop smoking campaigns and begun to implement the WHO MPOWER policy guidelines (The Lancet Regional Health–Western Pacific, 2021).

Illicit drugs

Some Pacific countries have long histories of psychoactive drug use. For example, seafarers and labourers brought cannabis or Indian hemp traditions to Fiji, where sugar cane plantations provided fertile ground for cultivation. Favourable cultivation conditions led to a number of Pacific communities increasing production of cannabis, which are consumed mainly by young Pacific men (Puamau et al., 2011). For instance, high rates of teenage substance use have been identified in Tonga and Pohnpei (Smith et al., 2007). Very little robust evidence is known about illicit drugs.

Betel nut

Another substance with the potential to be addictive is betel nut. These are the seed of a type of palm tree. They are chewed after being ground or sliced up. Betel nuts can have stimulant effects similar to caffeine and tobacco. They can also cause vomiting, diarrhoea, gum problems, kidney issues, chest pain, abnormal heartbeat, low blood pressure, shortness of breath, and rapid breathing. Betel nut chewing is a growing concern for the Melanesian Islands groups of Vanuatu, Papua New Guinea, and the Solomon Islands. Research found that people who chew betel nuts often are not aware of the potential harmful impact on their health (Joo et al., 2020).

Strategies targeting alcohol and substance use in the Pacific region

Substance use in the Pacific has many harmful effects, including physical and mental health issues (Leckie & Hughes, 2017). This is particularly concerning because there may not be sufficient services and support for people with problematic use of alcohol and other substances. The World Health Organization explored mental health services in 19 Pacific countries, finding that services were extremely limited, poorly distributed, and underfunded (Government of Samoa, 2006).

The problem is heightened due to a lack of funding. Many Pacific countries and territories depend on aid to support their internal infrastructures, including alcohol and substance use programmes and mental health support. A coordinated regional response may be needed along with more robust research and data about alcohol and drug use in Pacific Island countries (Power et al., 2015).

However, there is some good, targeted work underway. For instance, various alcohol and substance use prevention programmes target young people. Programmes have been found to be effective if they are school or community-centred and focus on increasing cultural pride, character development and connectivity to family and community (Durand, 2016).

Alcohol, tobacco, and other drugs, use for Pacific people in New Zealand

Many Pacific families migrated to New Zealand for better opportunities, particularly from the 1940s onwards. The Pacific community in New Zealand is diverse and colourful but is also beset by health and economic issues. Pacific people in New Zealand have higher mortality rates and lower life expectancies than European and Asian ethnic groups. They also have higher rates of hazardous alcohol consumption, tobacco, and substance use. Some of these issues are likely linked to economic disadvantage and systemic issues. This is compounded by lower rates of accessing health services for support compared to the general New Zealand population (Health Quality & Safety Commission, 2021; Ministry of Health, 2020; Ryan, et al., 2019).

In this section we summarise what is known about alcohol, tobacco, and other drug use in Pacific communities in New Zealand.

Alcohol

It is estimated that 64% of Pacific people aged 15 years and over in New Zealand consume alcohol (Ministry of Health, 2020), 66% of Pacific males and 49% of females. A study found that 49% of all Pacific adults engaged in heavy drinking, with over five drinks consumed on one occasion in the past month compared to 23% of non-Pacific people (Ataera-Minster et al., 2020).

Pacific adults are 1.5 times more likely to be hazardous drinkers than non-Pacific adults in New Zealand (Futures, 2017). Hazardous drinking rates for Pacific people were ranked second to Māori (33.2%), Pacific (26.5%), and European/Other (21.1%) (Ministry of Health, 2021). The Pacific peoples most likely to drink alcohol are New Zealand-born and younger (Nosa et al., 2021).

Harmful effects of hazardous alcohol consumption for Pacific people are similar to other groups, namely physical and mental health issues, death and injury, suicide, violence, high-risk sexual behaviour, family dysfunction, and legal issues. However, there may be a lack of awareness about the consequences among Pacific peoples. A study of Tongan females in New Zealand aged 16–25 years found that they consumed high quantities of alcohol. They reported that their peers, family, and culture all influenced heavy drinking and did not know the dangers (Manuopangai, 2012).

Tobacco

In New Zealand, rates of smoking are decreasing in the population overall, but smoking prevalence remains disproportionately high for Pacific people, particularly in areas of high socioeconomic deprivation. An estimated 59,000 Pacific adults smoke tobacco regularly, which is 22% of the Pacific population (Ministry of Health, 2020). Pacific Island adults are 1.7 times more likely to be current tobacco users than non-Pacific adults. Pacific males had a higher prevalence of tobacco use than females, 26.8% and 18.9%, respectively (Ministry of Health, 2020). Pacific people daily smoking rates were ranked second to Māori (22.3%), Pacific (16.4%), European/Other (8.3%), and Asian (3.9%) (Ministry of Health, 2021).

Pacific-born men are more likely to smoke than New Zealand-born Pacific men. More Pacific children are exposed to second-hand smoke in their households compared to European children (Teevale et al., 2013).

Illicit drugs

Pacific people in New Zealand have higher rates of substance use disorder than the general New Zealand population (Newcombe et al., 2019).

The most common illicit drugs consumed by Pacific people in New Zealand are cannabis, methamphetamine, and synthetic cannabinoids, and use of each of these is increasing (Ministry of Health, 2020). Based on the latest (2019/2020) New Zealand

Health survey, illicit drug use is increasing rapidly among Pacific people compared to the general NZ population. For example, 8% of Pacific people in New Zealand reported using cannabis in 2011/2012 compared to 15% in 2019/2020. Methamphetamine use rose from 0.7% in 2011/2012 to 1.1% in 2019/2020.

Males are more likely to use cannabis than females, but the rates of use of methamphetamine are about the same (Ministry of Health, 2020). One study found that New Zealand-born Pacific people were three times more likely to have used cannabis in the past month than those born overseas (NZ Drug Foundation, 2020).

Since the 2000s, the use of synthetic cannabinoids or alternative 'legal highs' such as 'K2' and 'Spice' has increased significantly in young people. There is evidence that use of these drugs may be higher in Pacific people compared to European people. These drugs have been associated with deaths (Ministry of Health, 2020; Hu et al., 2011).

Gambling

Pacific people are less likely to gamble than the general population in New Zealand, but those Pacific people who do are at high risk of becoming problem gamblers. Women and young people are at higher risk (Urale et al., 2015; Abbott et al., 2014). A survey found that 3% of Pacific students reported spending more than 30 minutes a day gambling compared with just 0.5% of European students (Francis Group, 2009).

Research suggests that most Pacific gamblers use non-casino gaming machines located in lower socioeconomic and deprived communities, though horse racing bets, card games, lotto, and online gaming activities are also used (Fehoko, 2020). Gambling-related harms include financial hardships, health problems, and relationship difficulties (Taufa, 2006).

Kava

In New Zealand, kava is consumed as part of some traditional Pacific practices. It is also sometimes used socially, particularly among New Zealand Tongan communities. However, negative impacts have been reported including effects on family relationships, employment, loss of income, health problems such as sleep deprivation, poor nutrition, and concurrent alcohol use with kava consumption. Outlining the health impact of heavy kava use and the need for family discussions about the overall effect is needed (Taufa, 2014).

Pacific alcohol and other drug services in New Zealand

A number of initiatives and services have been set up in response to the high rates of alcohol, tobacco, and other drug use in New Zealand Pacific communities. Most treatment services are mainstream and intervention-focused programs by district health board providers or non-government organisations (Annadale et al., 2006). In the past two decades, culturally developed interventions have been tested. These need to be embedded in culturally specific services so communities can develop interventions specifically for themselves rather than taking a one size fits all approach.

Some targeted approaches for Pacific communities have been developed including performance dance, theatre, drama, public speaking, and music. These health promotion strategies in schools and church-based interventions have been found to effectively raise awareness of the dangers of alcohol use (Warren et al., 2006).

Research suggests that key elements of effective strategies include being Pacific-led, family-centred, holistic, community-based, and connected (Faleafa, 2020). Services are now trying to use a holistic model of care that includes Pacific values, beliefs, languages, and Pacific models of care (New Zealand Mental Health and Wellbeing Commission, 2021). An example is TUPU (meaning to grow), a service catering explicitly to Pacific people with alcohol, other drug, and gambling issues (Waitemata ADHB website, 2021).

Conclusion

This chapter has shown that alcohol, tobacco, and other drugs use is a concern both in the Pacific Island region and in Pacific communities in New Zealand. This can have significant effects for individuals and families. There are few services specifically targeting these issues for Pacific people, and even where good programmes exist, Pacific people can be reluctant to use them.

In the Pacific region, varying degrees of political stability and finance make the issue particularly difficult to tackle. We know that substance use is a potential problem, but in most cases very little data is available to show the extent. Effective legislation and policy to implement regular data collection and support programmes requires political will and finance.

In New Zealand, there is greater recognition of the issue among health services and policy makers, driven by data that shows that Pacific communities are more at risk and are suffering substantial harm. More work is needed to raise this awareness in communities, with education campaigns that encompass the wider family as well as the individual. Visual images of the physical impact of substance use may work well. These programmes can be incorporated through the Pacific churches and Pacific social media platforms. National policies to reduce substance abuse related harm for Pacific communities are also needed.

Much of the research available about the prevalence of harmful and addictive behaviours is outdated. Relatively little is known about why higher proportions of Pacific people drink and smoke, and particularly why younger Pacific people continue to undertake heavy binge drinking sessions. More Pacific and ethnic specific population research is required to gain a better understating for why these harmful behaviours exists.

For Pacific addiction services there is a need for culturally appropriate services to cater to Pacific people's needs relating to harmful behaviours, alcohol, tobacco, and other drugs use. Research has found that effective programs include stable governance, social accountability, commitment from community leaders, clarity of plan and strategy, strong managerial leadership and support, appropriate staff with Pacific language speakers, holistic flexible interventions, and intra and inter-agency collaboration. There are currently limited alcohol, drug, or gambling services that cater to Pacific people in the Pacific region and New Zealand, but the increasing prevalence of the issue means it should be a priority to develop them.

References

Abbott, M., Bellringer, M., Garret, S., & Mundy-McPherson, S. (2014). *New Zealand 2012 National Gambling Study: Overview and gambling participation (Report No. 1).* Auckland University of Technology, Gambling and Addictions Research Centre. http://niphmhr.aut.ac.nz/research-cetnres/gambling-and-addictions-research-centre/research-reports

Anderson, I., Crengle, S., Kamaka, M.L., Chen, T.H., Palafox, N., & Jackson-Pulver, L. (2006). Indigenous health in Australia, New Zealand, and the Pacific. *The Lancet, 367* (9534), 1775–1785. https://doi.org/10.1016/S0140-6736(06)68773-4.

Annandale, M., Macpherson, C., Richard, T., & Solomona, M. (2006). *A Stocktake of Pacific Alcohol and Drug Services and Interventions.* Alcohol Advisory Council of New Zealand, Health Research Council of New Zealand and Accident Compensation Corporation. https://www.hpa.org.nz/sites/default/files/imported/field_research_publication_file/LeAla_Stocktake_Report.pdf

Aporosa, S. (2015). The new kava user: Diasporic identity formation in reverse. *New Zealand Sociology, 30*(4), 58–77.

Ataera-Minster, J., Guiney, H., & Cook, S. (2020). *Taeao Malama: Alcohol use in Pacific peoples. Results from the New Zealand Health Survey & Attitudes and Behaviour towards Alcohol Survey.* Te Hiringa Hauora/Health Promotion Agency. https://www.hpa.org.nz/sites/default/files/Taeao%20Malama%20-%20Alcohol%20use%20among%20Pacific%20peoples.pdf

Durand, Z., Cook, A., Konishi, M., & Nigg, C. (2016). Alcohol and substance use prevention programs for youth in Hawaii and Pacific Islands: A literature review. *Journal of Ethnicity in Substance Abuse, 15*(3), 240–251. https://doi.org/10.1080/15332640.2015.1024811

Faleafa, M. (2020). *Core Elements of Pacific Primary Mental Health and Addiction Service Provision.* Niu Mindworks Ltd. https://www.health.govt.nz/system/files/documents/pages/core_elements_of_pacific_primary_mental_health_and_addicion_service_provision.pdf

Fehoko, E. S. (2020). *From Games to Gambling: An Exploratory Study of Tongan-born and New Zealand-born Male Perceptions and Experiences of Gambling and Problem Gambling in New Zealand.* [Doctoral Thesis, Auckland University of Technology]. Tuwhera. http://hdl.handle.net/10292/13818

Francis Group. (2009). *Informing the 2009 problem gambling needs assessment: Report for the Ministry of Health.* Ministry of Health. https://www.health.govt.nz/system/files/documents/publications/informing-2009-problem-gambling-needs-assessment-09.pdf

Government of Samoa. (2006). *Samoa mental health policy.* Ministry of Health, Strategic Development and Planning Division. https://catalogue.nla.gov.au/catalog/5017498

Health Quality & Safety Commission. (2021). *Bula Sautu - A window on quality 2021: Pacific health in the year of COVID-19.* Health Quality & Safety Commission. https://www.hqsc.govt.nz/assets/Health-Quality-Evaluation/PR/BulaSautu_WEB.pdf

Hu, X., Primack, B. A., Barnett, T. E., & Cook, R. L. (2011). College students and use of K2: an emerging drug of abuse in young persons. *Substance Abuse Treatment, Prevention, and Policy*, 6, 16. https://doi.org/10.1186/1747-597X-6-16

International Narcotics Control Board (2014). Report of the International Narcotics Control Board for 2013. United Nations. https://www.incb.org/documents/Publications/AnnualReports/AR2013/English/AR_2013_E.pdf

Joo, Y. J., Newcombe, D., Nosa, V., & Bullen, C. (2020). Investigating Betel Nut Use, Antecedents and Consequences: A Review of Literature. *Substance Use & Misuse*, 55(9), 1422–1442. https://doi.org/10.1080/10826084.2019.1666144

Kessaram, T., McKenzie, J., Girin, N., Roth, A., Vivili, P., Williams, G., & Hoy, D. (2015). Tobacco Smoking in Islands of the Pacific Region, 2001–2013. *Preventing Chronic Disease*, 12, E212. https://doi.org/10.5888/pcd12.150155

Leckie, J., & Hughes, F. (2017). Mental Health in the Smaller Pacific States. In: H. Minas & M. Lewis (Eds.), *Mental Health in Asia and the Pacific: Historical and Cultural Perspectives.* (pp. 253–272). International and Cultural Psychology. Springer. http://doi.org/10.1007/978-1-4899-7999-5_17

Linhart, C., Naseri, T., Lin, S., Taylor, R., Morrell, S., McGarvey, S. T., Magliano, D. J., & Zimmet, P. (2017). Tobacco smoking trends in Samoa over four decades: can continued globalization rectify that which it has wrought?. *Globalization and Health*, 13(1), 31. https://doi.org/10.1186/s12992-017-0256-2

Manuopangai, S. (2012). *Exploring alcohol consumption patterns and drinking behaviour of Tongan youth females affiliated to the Tongan Methodist churches of Auckland, New Zealand.* [Unpublished Masters thesis]. University of Auckland.

Marshall, M. (2013). *Drinking Smoke: The Tobacco Syndemic in Oceania.* Honolulu: University of Hawai'i Press. https://doi.org/10.1515/9780824837969

Merikangas, K. R., & McClair, V. L. (2012). Epidemiology of substance use disorders. *Human Genetics*, 131(6), 779–789. https://doi.org/10.1007/s00439-012-1168-0

Ministry of Health. (2020). *Ola Manuia: Pacific Health and Wellbeing Action Plan 2020–2025.* https://www.health.govt.nz/system/files/documents/publications/ola_manuia-phwap-22june.pdf

Ministry of Health. (2021). Annual Data Explorer 2020/21: New Zealand Health Survey. https://minhealthnz.shinyapps.io/nz-health-survey-2020-21-annual-data-explorer/

Newcombe, D., Seini, T., Tanielu, H., & Nosa, V. (2019). Substance misuse stories among Pacific peoples in New Zealand. *Kōtuitui: New Zealand Journal of Social Sciences Online*, 14(1), 68–79. https://doi.org/10.1080/1177083X.2018.1528991

New Zealand Mental Health and Wellbeing Commission (2021). Access and Choice Programme: Report on the first two years – Te

Hōtaka mō Ngā Whai Wāhitanga me Ngā Kōwhiringa: He purongo mo ngā rua tau tuatahi. Wellington: New Zealand. https://www.mhwc.govt.nz/assets/Our-reports/MHWC-Access-and-Choice-report-Final.pdf

Nosa, V., Duffy, S., Singh, D., Lavelio, S., Amber, U., Homasi-Paelate, A., & Alfred, J. (2018). The use of home brew in Pacific Islands countries and territories. *Journal of Ethnicity in Substance Abuse,* 17(1), 7–15. https://doi.org/10.1080/15332640.2017.1362732

Nosa, V., Malungahu, G., Paynter, J., Gentles, D., & Gentles, D. (2021). Pacific peoples and alcohol: a review of the literature. *The New Zealand Medical Journal*, 134(1529), 86–96.

Ofanoa, M., Buetow, S., Ofanoa, S., Huggard, P., Paynter, J., & Nosa, V. (2020). Reasons for and Impacts of Kava Use by Tongan Men in Kava Clubs in Auckland and Tonga. *Social Sciences,* 9(2), 56–60. http://doi.org/10.11648/j.ss.20200902.13

Ofanoa, M., & Ofanoa, S. (2021). Kava Consumption and Family Violence: Fake News by Men no Longer Hidden. *Advances in Social Sciences Research Journal*, 8(9), 303–310. https://doi.org/10.14738/assrj.89.10928

Power, R., Schmich, L., & Nosa, V. (2015). A response for substance and harm reduction in Pacific Island countries and territories. *Harm Reduction Journal*, 12, 48. https://doi.org/10.1186/s12954-015-0080-z

Puamau, E. S., Roberts, G., Schmich, L., & Power, R. (2011). Drug and alcohol use in Fiji: a review. *Pacific Health Dialog,* 17(1), 165–171.

Ryan, D., Grey, C., & Mischewski, B. (2019). *Tofa Saili: A review of evidence about health equity for Pacific Peoples in New Zealand.* Pacific Perspectives Ltd. https://www.pacificperspectives.co.nz/publications/

Smith, B. J., Phongsavan, P., Bauman, A. E., Havea, D., & Chey, T. (2007). Comparison of tobacco, alcohol and illegal drug usage among school students in three Pacific Island societies. *Drug and*

Alcohol Dependence, 88(1), 9–18. https://doi.org/10.1016/j.drugalcdep.2006.08.030

Pasifika Futures. (2017). Pasifika people in New Zealand: How are we doing. Auckland: Pasifika Futures. Pasifika Medical Association.

NZ Drug Foundation. (2020). State of the Nation 2020: A stocktake of how New Zealand is dealing with the issue of drugs. https://www.drugfoundation.org.nz/assets/uploads/State-of-the-Nation-2020-WEB2.pdf

Taufa, A. (2014). Her side of the kava story: Exploring the effects of heavy kava use based on the perspective of Tongan women residing in Auckland, New Zealand. Unpublished Masters in Public Health Thesis, The University of Auckland, Auckland, New Zealand.

Taufa, S. (2006) Gambling and Tongan adolescents. Unpublished Masters in Public Health Dissertation, The University of Auckland, Auckland, New Zealand.

Teevale, T., Denny, S., Percival, T., & Fleming, T. (2013). Pacific secondary school students' access to primary health care in New Zealand. The New Zealand Medical Journal, 126(1375), 58–68.

The Lancet Regional Health- Western Pacific region. (2021). *Tobacco control in the Western Pacific region (Editorial)*. https://doi.org/10.1016/j.lanwpc.2021.100179

Urale, P., Bellringer, M., Landon, J., & Abbott, M. (2015). God, family and money: Pacific people and gambling in New Zealand. International Gambling Studies, Volume 15, 2015- Issue 1. 15:1, 72–87. DOI: 10.1080/14459795.2014.998252

Warren, H. Kirk, R. Lima, L. and Siataga, P. (2006). Alcohol Community Interventions and Services for Pacific Peoples: Literature Review. Wellington: Alcohol Advisory Council of New Zealand, Health Research Council and Accident Compensation Corporation. https://www.hpa.org.nz/sites/default/files/imported/field_research_publication_file/Le_Ala_Lit_Review-Final_May2010.pdf

Waitemata District Health Board (2021). Website ttps://www.waitematadhb.govt.nz/hospitals-clinics/clinics-services/tupu-pacific-alcohol-and-other-drug-and-gambling-service/

Suggested further readings

Gray, J., & Nosa, V. (2009). Tau Fifine Fiafia: the binge drinking behaviours of nine New Zealand born Niuean women living in Auckland. *Pacific Health Dialog, 15*(1), 104–111.

Hale, M., McCool, J., Bullen, C., & Nosa, V. (2012). Views from a small Pacific Island: prospects for tobacco control on Niue. *Health Promotion Practice, 13*(3), 404–411.

Joo, Y. J., Moadsiri, A., Newcombe, D., Nosa, V., & Bullen, C. (2020). E-learning: A Tool to Upgrade the Skills of Health Workers to Address Betel Quid and Areca Nut Chewing. *Substance Use & Misuse, 55*(9), 1525–1527. https://doi.org/10.1080/10826084.2019.1666143

Joo, Y. J., Newcombe, D., Nosa, V., Walker, N., & Bullen, C. (2020). Betel Nut Use in Vanuatu: Investigating Opportunities to Reduce Harms to Health. *Substance Use & Misuse, 55*(9), 1457–1464. https://doi.org/10.1080/10826084.2020.1716803

Newcombe, D., Tanielu-Stowers, H., McDermott, R., Stephen, J., & Nosa, V. (2016). The validation of the Alcohol, Smoking and Substance Involvement Screening Test (ASSIST) amongst Pacific people in New Zealand. *New Zealand Journal of Psychology, 45*(1), 30–39.

Nosa, V., Leau, K., & Walker N. (2018). Cytisine as an alternative smoking cessation product for Pacific smokers in New Zealand. *Pacific Health Dialog, 21*, (2).

Nosa, V., Adams, P., & Hodges, I. (2011). Distinctive alcohol cultural practices amongst Niuean men living in Auckland, New Zealand. *Kotuitui: New Zealand Journal of Social Sciences, 6*(1–2), 62–72.

Nosa, V., Adams, P., & Hodges, I. (2010). A Pacific migrant experience: A case study on the impact of alcohol on migrant

Niuean men to Auckland, New Zealand. In A. Hayes & M. Robert (Eds.), *Migrant Security 2010: Citizenship and Social Inclusion in a Transnational Era* (pp. 166–173). University of Southern Queensland.

Nosa, V., & Ofanoa, M. (2009). The Social, cultural and medicinal use of Kava for twelve Tongan born men living in Auckland, New Zealand. *Pacific Health Dialogue, 15*(1), 96–102.

Fonua Ola: Re-imagining Pacific health promotion for the wellbeing of humanity and the planet

Sione Tu'itahi

Chapter summary

Our common home, Planet Earth, is broken. This global challenge is affecting all beings – plants, animals, and humans, as well as the earth-supporting systems such as air, water, and land. Along with international entities such as states, global organisations, educational institutions, professional associations, the world health promotion community is trying to offer solutions. Addressing global challenges to health is crucial for Pacific peoples[1] because Pacific Island nations, as part of the world community, are already suffering from the consequences of the convergence of the human-induced economic crisis, pandemics, and environmental catastrophes. This chapter posits that through health promotion, Indigenous knowledge from the Moana[2], also known as the Pacific, can contribute solutions. To explore this idea, this chapter discusses the state of the planet, the state of Indigenous peoples, and the on-going development of Pacific health promotion, especially in the Aotearoa New Zealand context. Additionally, it analyses a case study of how indigenous Moana leadership and knowledge were used to elevate health promotion to contribute to addressing the health of the planet and human wellbeing. Importantly also, it examines insights from the case study for the purpose of advancing Pacific health promotion and building the capacity of Pacific peoples and communities. Furthermore, it discusses learnings for communities and institutions, looking into future challenges and opportunities for health promotion.

Introduction

In today's globalised and interdependent world community, global challenges directly affect the national and local contexts, and vice versa. Therefore, understanding the international context and its challenges helps in analysing and finding solutions for all levels, especially the local. But how serious is this environmental challenge? Trying in his State of the Planet address 2020[3] to raise greater awareness and engender international collaboration, United Nations Secretary General Antonio Guterres (2020) pointed out that the planet is broken because humanity was waging war on nature. He warned that:

> *We cannot go back to the old normal of inequality, injustice and heedless dominion over the Earth. Instead we must step towards a safer, more sustainable, and equitable path… Now is the time to transform humankind's relationship with the natural world – and with each other. And we must do so together. Solidarity is humanity. Solidarity is survival.* (Guterres, 2020, n.p.)

Almost a year later at the COP26 climate change summit 2021[4], Guterres further observed that humanity was facing a stark choice; either we stop the crisis – or crisis stops us: 'It's time to say: enough. Enough of brutalizing biodiversity. Enough of killing ourselves with carbon. Enough of treating nature like a toilet… We are digging our own graves…' (Guterres, 2021, n.p.).

Gutterres' (2021) warning sums up succinctly the convergence of the inter-related challenges of a pandemic, an environmental catastrophe, and an economic crisis – that humanity is being confronted with, and what it can do in order to avoid a total collapse of human civilisation. His concern is part of an increasing chorus of disquiet from various professional communities around the world, including the world health promotion community. For example, over 1,000 delegates at the 2019 World Conference on Health Promotion, in New Zealand, unanimously called on the global community to urgently act to promote planetary health and sustainable development for all, now and for the sake of future generations. Issued through the two Legacy Statements of the conference[5], they further called for 'urgent action…because mounting evidence tells us that the current economic and social development paradigm of infinite growth and endless exploitation of limited natural resources is unjust and unsustainable, leading to inequities within and among countries and across generations' (IUHPE, n.d.).

A similar call was made by members of the Planetary Health Alliance, in its São Paulo Declaration[6] (Planetary Health Alliance, n.d.), raising the alarm that:

> *The COVID-19 pandemic is the most recent in a series of distress signals ringing around the world. Climate change, biodiversity loss, and destruction of the quality of air, water, and soil are eroding the fundamental life support systems that we all depend on…Every dimension of human health and well-being is now affected by global environmental change. The planetary health science is clear: we can no longer safeguard human health unless we change course.* (Planetary Health Alliance, 2021, n.p.)

Within health promotion, a commitment to the wellbeing of humanity and the environment was explicitly stated by the World Health Organization (WHO) at its 1986 world conference on health promotion. A stable-eco system was one of nine fundamental conditions and resources for health that the Ottawa Charter called for when it was launched. The other eight and inter-related pre-requisites called for by the WHO-sponsored charter are: peace, shelter, education, food, income, sustainable resources, social justice, and equity (World Health Organization, 1986). However, over the years health promotion has largely been ecologically blind (Hancock, 2019).

Calling to appreciate the environment as a major determinant of health might have been new and novel to many in the world health promotion community, but it resonated, and still does, with Indigenous communities. This is because Indigenous Peoples, including those in the Pacific region, deeply understand health and wellbeing as a state of material and spiritual balance within beings and between all beings, including Mother Nature. They see wellbeing as holistic with several, inter-connected dimensions within the web of life. Naturally then, health promotion is largely understood and practised by Indigenous Peoples, including those in the Pacific region, within their worldview of health and wellbeing. More broadly, Indigenous peoples understand humans as inextricably one with the rest of the environment, a symbiotic, dynamic relationship of an inherent oneness and interdependence.

It is estimated that there are between 370 and 500 million Indigenous Peoples worldwide, in over 90 countries (World Bank, n.d.). While they make up only 5 per cent of the world's population, they account for about 15 per cent of the extreme poor, and their life expectancy is up to 20 years lower, compared to the life expectancy of non-indigenous people worldwide. The bank adds: 'While Indigenous Peoples own, occupy, or use a quarter of the world's surface area, they safeguard 80% of the world's remaining biodiversity. They hold vital ancestral knowledge and expertise on how to adapt, mitigate, and reduce climate and disaster risks.'

Recognising the potentials of Indigenous knowledge to addressing global challenges, especially the ecological crisis, is one of the reasons why national and international institutions and communities are beginning to include Indigenous peoples and their knowledge in the discourse on the environment.

The world now realises that current, dominant political and economic frameworks, with their underpinning values and assumptions, which have served humanity for a few centuries are major contributing factors to our current global challenges of material poverty, inequities within and between countries. But to Indigenous peoples, a major reason for their participation in the planetary discourse is for their survival, their wellbeing, and their rights. Indigenous peoples have been relentless in advocating for their rights to exist, and for the protection of their land and livelihood. Meanwhile, many Pacific people do not readily identify with being Indigenous because most small Pacific nations were freed of colonisation several decades ago. However, there are a handful of states and nations that are still colonial territories, and in some of which, its original inhabitants are still advocating for freedom. Being formerly colonised is often used to define being Indigenous. But as Durie (2011) noted, being the first inhabitants of a place, and a culture that is inherently socio-ecological and inextricably one with the environment is an important identifying factor for the Indigenous peoples of the world, and a foundation for organising their knowledge.

Acknowledging the rights of Indigenous peoples have always been violated and are among the most vulnerable and disadvantaged groups of people in the world, the United Nations (UN, n.d.) noted that special measures are required to protect their rights and maintain their distinct cultures and way of life. One such measure is the UN Declaration on the Rights of Indigenous Peoples, 2007 (UN, n.d.). Further, the United Nations recognises the 500 million Indigenous peoples of the world as:

> *...inheritors and practitioners of unique cultures and ways of relating to people and the environment. They have retained social, cultural, economic and political characteristics that are distinct from those of the dominant societies in which they live. Despite their cultural differences, indigenous peoples from around the world share common problems related to the protection of their rights as distinct peoples.* (UN, n.d. Indigenous Peoples, n.p.)

Regarding Indigenous knowledge as part of the solution, Guterres (2020) observed that because it has been distilled over times of close and straight contact with nature. Although they make up less than 6 per cent of the world's population, Indigenous peoples are stewards of 80 per cent of the world's biodiversity on land. He added: 'Already, we know that nature managed by indigenous peoples is declining less rapidly than elsewhere. With indigenous peoples living on land that is among the most vulnerable to climate change and environmental degradation, it is time to heed their voices, reward their knowledge and respect their rights' (Guterres, 2020, n.p.).

The São Paulo Declaration (2021) calls for health promotion and traditional knowledges led by Indigenous Peoples to be part of the solution of the transition that humanity needs to go through. It also calls for the contribution of all faiths and spiritual leaders, noting that they could lead in the creation of unity and solidarity among all peoples of the world, based on our shared, common home. Further, the declaration calls on faiths and spiritual leaders to 'guide people to reinvest in our relationship within Nature with the reverence and awe that is felt by so many, ... emphasize the moral dimension of protecting all life on Earth' (n.p) and 'Utilize religious and spiritually affiliated institutions for planetary health education, training, engagement, and action' (n.p.) (Planetary Health Alliance, n.d.).

Such deep ecological worldviews and wisdom being called for are embedded in Indigenous knowledge systems, such as the Moana socio-ecological, philosophical concept of fonua, land, in Tongan (Mahina, 1992; Tu'itahi, 2009). Some of its other Pacific cognates are whenua in Māori, vanua in Fijian, fanua in Samoan, and enua in Cook Islands Māori and Tahitian. Simply put, fonua means people and their environment. On a deeper level, it refers to the interdependent and symbiotic relationship between humans and the environment. In Aotearoa New Zealand, Pacific health promotion approaches, frameworks, and practices within the diverse Pacific ethnic groups, share common values and principles that inform health promotion practices, and are based on these socio-ecological concepts and principles (Tu'itahi & Lima, 2015). These core principles and concepts include, but not limited to, humanity being one and organic with Mother Nature, life and wellbeing have a material and spiritual component, wellbeing is a relational state of being healthy within and between beings. In other words, we are all connected to each other and to the environment. Therefore, the wellbeing of the individual is nested within the wellbeing of the collective.

Tu'itahi and Lima (2015) charted the development of Pacific health promotion in Aotearoa, noting that while non-Pacific-specific worldviews, approaches, and frameworks largely shape Pacific health promotion activities over the years, Pacific knowledge and approaches also played a part in the effort by various stakeholders to improve the health of Pacific communities. Most notable is the collective effort of the Pacific institutions, groups, and individuals in the communities, who used Indigenous community development and other health promotion strategies to address the determinants of health that Pacific communities face. While these protagonists might not have framed their plans and action within an academic conception of health promotion, their initiatives contributed to shaping public policies and initiatives that have contributed to the wellbeing of Pacific peoples, dealing with determinants that mostly lie outside the health sector, such as education, housing, employment, and institutional racism.

Faith-based communities such as churches, women's groups, and professional collectives were among the advocates, leading in navigating for Pacific health in the early days of Pacific migration to New Zealand in the 1960s. Responding to emerging needs, social and service providers were established soon after to deal with issues ranging from diseases and housing to education and normalising immigration status of over stayers. There is no scope in this chapter to analyse the history of Pacific health promotion in the country. The reader is invited to refer to the chapter on Pacific health promotion, by Tu'itahi and Lima (2015), listed in the references.

Relevant to this discussion, however, Tu'itahi and Lima (2015) noted that despite the best of intentions, and efforts of public institutions and Pacific communities, the results for Pacific health over the years have been mixed, due to a number of factors, especially the lack of appropriate public policies and adequate resourcing. They also observed that a re-conceptualising of health promotion from a Pacific-centric position could tap more into the strengths of Pacific peoples and their communities which could help them take greater ownership and more meaningful engagement with government-funded initiatives. Additionally, they outlined examples of community-led initiatives that were informed more by Pacific Indigenous principles and concepts. Importantly also, they offered a definition of health promotion from a Pacific perspective, 'the empowering of Pacific peoples and their communities to take control of their holistic health and wellbeing and their future.' (Tu'itahi & Lima, 2015, p. 76).

While the Pacific definition was partly inspired by inspired by the 1988 Ottawa Charter definition that health promotion is the process of enabling people to increase control over, and to improve, their health (World Health Organization, 1986, n.p.) there are Indigenous elements within the Pacific definition that are worth noting. These include the notions of 'holistic health and wellbeing', and 'their future.' Holistic wellbeing depicts the Indigenous conception of health having physical, mental, spiritual, social, cultural, and environmental dimensions. The definition also suggests a health promotion for Pacific peoples that is built on the knowledge of the past, the experience of the present, and the aspiration to have greater control of their future development. Additionally, their definition suggests a process that should be owned and led by Pacific peoples, in collaboration with others, with sharing of knowledge and experience. These dimensions and features of Pacific health promotion are reflected in the two Pacific health models, Fonofale and Fonua that the authors discussed.

Fonofale and Fonua are among several models on the health and education sectors that have been constructed out of Pacific experience in the context of Aotearoa. While these models are relevant to health, Fonua was specifically developed for Pacific health promotion in 2007 and was reconceptualised as Fonua Ola in 2017. As its name depicts, the model reflects two indigenous concepts of fonua and ola. As mentioned earlier, Fonua is the Pacific Indigenous philosophy, based on the natural reality that humanity is inextricably one with the environment. So central is fonua to the life and wellbeing of peoples of the Moana that the human placenta, this physical plane of existence, the grave, and the hereafter are all named fonua or its equivalent cognates in many other Pacific Indigenous languages. Ola refers to holistic wellbeing as also seen in Māori Indigenous concepts such as Wai Ora, healthy water, Whanau Ora, healthy family, and Whenua Ora, or health people, healthy environment. Like its Māori equivalent, Fonua Ola means healthy environment, healthy people. It reflects the natural reality that humans are part of the environment and are inherently organic with it. Without a healthy environment, humanity will be unhealthy and confronted by environmental catastrophes, which we as a global community are currently experiencing.

As an Indigenous health promotion model, six inter-connected dimensions of wellbeing are identified in Fonua Ola: spiritual, mental, physical, socioeconomic, cultural, and environmental. Reflecting the natural life cycle and seasonal phases of Mother Nature, the model also depicts four major circular stages of Kumi, search, langa, build, tauhi – maintenance, and tufunga, re-conceptualisation. At the human level, the Kumi phase is the search for a new space of holistic wellbeing, ola. It implies leading from a space of Fonua Mate, unhealthy, dying stage of a current environment, and, therefore, navigating for a new space of holistic wellbeing, of balanced material and spiritual prosperity, Fonua Ola. The second phase of Langa, refers to building a new life and culture of wellbeing in a new environment, Fonua Ola, found as a result of the process of navigation and search in Kumi. The third phase of Tauhi, maintenance, depicts a period of sustaining and maintaining the new environment for the wellbeing of all. The fourth and final phase of Tufunga Fonua implies that when the environment changes due to internal and external contributing factors which can change both the physical and social realties and conditions, life, and wellbeing should be re-conceptualised, re-imagined, re-constructed, and the life circle begins again with the first phase of Kumi. Another over-arching and related concept is Tufunga Fonua Ola, Good Governance, Leadership, and society-building, refers to the wise and collaborative leadership that is involved in all four phases, a servant-leadership approach that is guided by the leadership framework of Fakapotopoto (Tu'itahi, 2009), the way of the wise and prudent. Fonua Ola and Fakapotopoto[7] are both underpinned by core Indigenous values such as reciprocity, love, justice, equity, serve, and lead for the wellbeing of all. In terms of where it can be applied, five levels are identified in Fonua Ola: the individual, family, local, national, and the global.

A recent application of Fonua Ola and other associated tools, such as Fakapotopototo, to guide and inform the process of introducing indigenous health promotion knowledge to address planetary health and sustainable development, is an example of how Pacific indigenous knowledge can contribute to global challenges. The process is briefly analysed here as a case study, with some lessons that can be replicated in other fields and groups. Noting in the 2000s the potential to contribute indigenous knowledge and leadership, through health promotion, to addressing planetary health, Indigenous leaders, Māori and Pacific, at the Health Promotion Forum of New Zealand (HPF) appraised the series of triennial World Conference on Health Promotion of the International Union for Health Promotion and Education (IUHPE). They saw the conference as a possible strategic platform for a process of advancing and elevating health promotion to the planetary level, in order to contribute to the health of the planet and the wellbeing of humanity, as reflected in the United Nations' sustainable development goals. Being Indigenous, this small team were guided by the knowledge of their mind, and their wisdom in their heart, closely collaborating with high trust and unity. Inspired by reflections and prayers, they agreed that their purpose was to offer Indigenous knowledge to help humanity. Their guiding maxim was: do the right things the right way, with the right spirit, for the right purpose, and the right outcomes will come. They were also supported by a group of eminent leaders and elders in health and leadership, who were invited to provide over-arching guidance. In existence for 70 years, IUHPE is the largest international organisation and professional network that leads the on-going advancement of health promotion, and HPF has been an institutional member for almost 20 years.

Following a successful bid at the 2016 IUHPE conference in Brazil, IUHPE and agreed to HPF's proposal to adopt Te Tiriti o Waitangi as the guiding framework for organising and designing of both form and contents of the 2019 World Conference on Health Promotion, in Rotorua. It was also agreed that the work relationship between IUHPE and HPF will be one of equal partnership. As a result, most components of the conference reflected a partnership and a prominent presence of Indigenous leadership and knowledge. For example, the theme of the conference was 'Waiora: Promoting Planetary Health and Sustainable Development for All.' Including the Indigenous concept 'Waiora' at the front of the theme signals clearly that Indigenous knowledge, co-ownership, co-leadership, and co-designing, inform how the conference is to be planned and organised. Featuring Te Reo Māori as a fourth official language of the conference, along with English, French, and Spanish, was another agreed aspect, and a world first. Moreover, having Indigenous plenary speakers and presenters to share their knowledge, was another significant element. Equally significant, invited Indigenous leaders and elders graced the meeting with their daily presence, opening daily sessions with words of wisdom and karakia and lotu (prayers), ensuring that the socio-cultural milieu of the conference was fused with intellectual and spiritual wisdom and enrichments, and a conducive and dynamic but peaceful learning and networking environment was sustained. A physical and cultural space was also created outside the main plenary room as a global Indigenous elders' hub, adding to the ambiance of unity in diversity the conference was planned to achieve. More than 1,000 delegates from 73 countries participated, the biggest public health conference to be held in New Zealand. Of special significance, two legacy statements, one focusing on general key messages, and the other focusing on Indigenous matters, were unanimously approved at the end of the conference and disseminated throughout the world health promotion community. Papers on the conference and the legacy statements have been published in at least two world health promotion journals. The statements are becoming reference points for health promotion, indigenous knowledge, and planetary health among members of IUHPE. It has inspired some international health promotion initiatives too.

As part of its post-conference strategy, HPF co-founded in 2020 the Global Working Group on Waiora Planetary Health and Human Wellbeing, under IUHPE. The aim is to advance not only the goals of the Legacy Statements within IUHPE, but also to promote them across the world health community. The membership includes Indigenous and non-Indigenous health promotion leaders from across the world and from different cultures (IUHPE, n.d.). In 2021, the strategic goals of the Global Working Group on Waiora, which are based on the legacy statements, were incorporated into the 2021–2026 strategy of IUHPE by its global board. This inclusion is a significant milestone, the inclusion of planetary health and Indigenous knowledge into the centre of thinking and work programme of IUHPE. Earlier in the year, the Waiora Group was invited to organise a workshop on planetary health, indigenous knowledge, and spirituality, at the annual conference of the Planetary Health Alliance (PHA). The presenters were also invited to contribute to the drafting of its Sao Paulo Declaration on planetary health. PHA is the largest network of professionals and institutions that focus their work on planetary health. HPF, the Waiora Working Group and IUHPE are among the signatories to the declaration.

In two other related developments, at the end of 2021, and through IUHPE, the Waiora Working Group was invited to run a workshop on planetary health and indigenous knowledge at the 10th Global Conference on Health Promotion of the World Health Organization. The invitation may be regarded as another measure of the importance and timeliness of HPF and IUHPE's work on planetary health and Indigenous knowledge. Equally important, HPF was approved in June 2021 by IUHPE to be a national accreditation organisation (NAO). This approval made HPF a member of the global accreditation framework established by IUHPE to assess and formally recognise health promoters across the world. The global framework is also to accredit degree-level qualifications in health promotion that universities around the world teach, if they choose to join the voluntary system. A unique feature of the HPF accreditation is that IUHPE has approved that Te Tiriti o Waitangi and the political, socioeconomic, and cultural contexts of New Zealand to be components of the New Zealand accreditation. While it is a world first, in terms of including Indigenous knowledge into the framework, there will also be learning from our New Zealand experience for IUHPE and the world health promotion community, especially for countries with Indigenous peoples.

At least nine learning and insights can be drawn from the case study. First, it demonstrates that Pacific indigenous knowledge can contribute solutions to global health challenges. Second, it shows that Pacific indigenous leadership, health promotion approaches and frameworks such as Fonua Ola can produce outcomes, which is the main thesis of this chapter: that indigenous knowledge can contribute, through health promotion, to address the global challenges the world is facing. Third, it suggests that Pacific health promotion can be more transformative if it aligns more with Pacific Indigenous knowledge. Fourth, for the enhancement of Pacific leadership in health promotion and other fields, the analysis denotes that the value-based, collaborative, and servant-leadership approaches of Indigenous peoples can be effective with results of mutual benefits. Such a strategic and courageous leadership, based on Indigenous intellectual and spiritual wisdom, can be transformational in elevating consciousness from national health promotion to planetary health promotion. Worth noting in discussing leadership is the value of solidarity and collaboration between Māori and Pacific peoples on matters such as human rights, inequities, wellbeing, determinants of health, and planetary health. Not only there is cultural affinity and kinship ties, but they share common challenges.

Fifth, along with good leadership, values and principles must inform and shape institutions and structures that are established to serve for the wellbeing of all. Sixth, also evidential from the narrative there is high degree of commitment expected of personnel who are called to lead and serve in public institutions and the expectations to embody the institutional values and principles, goals, and expected outcomes. Seventh, principles such as reciprocity, humility, justice, love, trustworthiness, and collaboration for the collective wellbeing of all, can contribute to re-conceptualising the dominant socio-political and economic systems, driven by individualism, racism, and materialism, which are major contributing factors to the ecological, economic, and ethical challenges that are breaking the planet and humanity. Eighth, the spiritual dimension of knowledge and wellbeing is not only vital to Pacific peoples but it is an important, dimension the wellbeing of humanity and the planet today. Spiritually provides guiding principles that balance the extremes of materialism and consumerism and can help to promote an outward orientation to serve the collective wellbeing, rather than an inward-looking approach to accumulate resources for individualistic purposes, at the peril of the whole.

Finally, the chapter and the case study, highlight that in our broken and only home, Planet Earth, we urgently need to elevate our consciousness to the level of global citizenship, of planetary thinking and practice. We are diverse, but fellow humans. We live in different locations, but they are connected rooms in our broken planetary home. Some rooms are sinking like the Pacific region, because our home temperature is rising, melting the poles. Some rooms are flooded and razed by monsoons and cyclones. Other rooms are burning while others are in long draughts and famine. Despite knowing that our home is burning, melting, and sinking, and that we are the root-cause, we still focus largely on our individual rooms, as shown at the 2021 COP26 summit. We must raise our thinking to the level of global unity and collaboration in order to recognise the solutions that are latent within inherent interdependence, oneness, and unity in diversity. Born of this new consciousness will be values and principles that will inform and shape policies, institutions, and practices for institutions, communities, and the individual on how to live peacefully and sustainably with each other and with Mother Earth. Our planet is but one island in space and we are all members of one human family. While retaining their Indigenous identity and national loyalty, Pacific peoples are also global islanders. They have the capacity to be part of the solution and co-lead for the wellbeing of Pacific peoples, and all of humanity. We either work together to live, or perish together. The choice is ours.

> *This is a moment of truth for people and planet alike. COVID and climate have brought us to a threshold. We cannot go back to the old normal of inequality, injustice and heedless dominion over the Earth. Instead we must step towards a safer, more sustainable and equitable path…Now is the time to transform humankind's relationship with the natural world – and with each other. And we must do so together. Solidarity is humanity. Solidarity is survival.* (Guterres, 2020)

As a poet, let me conclude this chapter with a poem that was inspired during the Covid-19 pandemic:

Dawn, deep, devotional, beach reflections

Meditating deeply
on the one book of life
helps me to understand
the inner meaning
and inherent oneness
of the many books of revelation
that I have traversed
Listening to the healing songs
of Mother Nature
heals mine own soul,
and helps me to find
my life song and pathway

and to live in peace
and harmony with Her,
and with my fellow,
global islanders

Milford Beach, North Shore, Auckland, Aotearoa New Zealand ©Sione Tu'itahi, October 3, 2021.

References

Durie, M. (2011). *Ngā Tini Whetu: Navigating Māori Futures* (1st ed.). Huia Publishers.

Guterres, A. (2020, December 2). *State of the Planet*. United Nations. https://www.un.org/sg/en/content/sg/speeches/2020-12-02/address-columbia-university-the-state-of-the-planet

Guterres, A. (2021, November 1). *Secretary-General's remarks to the World Leaders Summit - COP 26*. United Nations. https://www.un.org/sg/en/node/260423

Hancock, T. (2019). *Healthy Cities 2.0 Towards One Planet Cities: IUHPE Plenary 2 Rotorua* [PowerPoint slides]. International Union for Health Promotion and Education 2019 World Conference on Health Promotion. https://secure.tcc.co.nz/ei/images/IUHPE19/PDF/IUHPE%202019%20-%20Trevor%20Hancock.pdf

International Union for Health Promotion and Education. (n.d.). *23rd World Conference on Health Promotion and The Legacy Statements.* https://www.iuhpe.org/index.php/en/iuhpe-conferences/1273-23rd-iuhpe-world-conference

Mahina, O. (1992). *The Tongan traditional history Tala-E-Fonua: a vernacular ecology-centred historico-cultural concept.* [Doctoral thesis, The Australian National University]. The Australian National University Open Access Theses. https://openresearch-repository.anu.edu.au/handle/1885/114566

Planetary Health Alliance. (n.d.). *The São Paulo Declaration on Planetary Health.* https://www.planetaryhealthalliance.org/sao-paulo-declaration

Tu'itahi, S., & Lima, I. (2015). Pacific Health Promotion. In M. Ratima & L. Signal (Eds.), *Promoting Health in Aotearoa New Zealand* (1st ed., pp. 64–81). Otago University Press.

Tu'itahi, S. (2009). *Langa fonua: In Search of Success - How a Tongan Kainga Strived to be Socially and Economically Successful in New Zealand.* [Master's thesis, Massey University]. Massey University. https://mro.massey.ac.nz/items/dc4d6037-157d-45e2-90cd-6c8f67322828

United Nations. (n.d.). *Indigenous Peoples at the United Nations.* https://www.un.org/development/desa/indigenouspeoples/about-us.html

United Nations. (n.d.). *United Nations Declaration On The Rights Of Indigenous Peoples.* https://www.un.org/development/desa/indigenouspeoples/declaration-on-the-rights-of-indigenous-peoples.html

World Bank. (n.d). *Indigenous Peoples.* https://www.worldbank.org/en/topic/indigenouspeoples#1

World Health Organization. (1986). *The Ottawa Charter.* https://www.who.int/westernpacific/about/how-we-work/programmes/health-promotion

Pacific health data in Aotearoa New Zealand: Users, sources, and important considerations

Corina Grey

Chapter summary

Accurate, reliable, and timely data is crucial for monitoring Pacific health outcomes and developing plans to achieve Pacific health equity. The aim of this chapter is to highlight some of the key considerations for people using and interpreting data about Pacific peoples that has been collected by government agencies or elsewhere within the health system. It discusses the uses of Pacific health data and the definitions and classification of ethnicity, which form a robust foundation for monitoring Pacific health over time. The three major ethnicity outputs (prioritisation, total response, and single/combination) are also described, along with their advantages and limitations with respect to the analysis of Pacific data. Two major sources of population health data (the Census and Integrated Data Infrastructure) are also described, as well as the implications for Pacific peoples of the move to a 'digital-first' approach for the 2018 Census. The chapter then finishes with a brief description of the emerging issue of Pacific data sovereignty.

Introduction

Moana Research and the Pacific Data Sovereignty Network aptly define Pacific data as 'data produced by Pacific or that is about Pacific and the environments we have relationships with' (Moana Research, 2021, p. 14). They differentiate 'data *from* Pacific' (e.g., traditional cultural information, oral literature, Pacific epistemology) from 'data *about* Pacific' (e.g., information collated by government and non-governmental organisations).

This chapter deals with considerations about the latter (data *about* Pacific), but strongly encourages readers to think about how the former (data *from* Pacific) can be more carefully nurtured and systematically integrated within the health system. Furthermore, data *about* Pacific can only be useful when it is framed within an appropriate Pacific context, taking into account Pacific world-views and interpreted by Pacific peoples and experts.

Accurate and timely data is critical for the monitoring, evaluation, and achievement of Pacific health equity. As health planners, funders, and practitioners, it is important that our knowledge about the populations we serve is sufficiently detailed to: develop and continuously tailor services to meet the diverse needs of different populations, train, and recruit a workforce that is fit-for-purpose, and advocate for wider public policies and programmes that enable Pacific peoples to achieve and maintain optimal health and well-being.

Over the last two decades, a number of national Pacific health strategies and action plans have been published, all unified by a goal to improve Pacific health outcomes and achieve equity in health for Pacific peoples in Aotearoa New Zealand (NZ) (Minister of Health, 2002; Minister of Health & Minister of Pacific Island Affairs, 2010; Ministry of Health, 2014; Ministry of Health, 2020). Up-to-date data has formed the basis of these various plans, highlighting priority areas and providing a strong rationale for focusing on Pacific health due to well-documented, long-standing, and persistent inequities in health outcomes for Pacific peoples.

In 2021, the Health Quality & Safety Commission (HQSC) published *Bula Sautu – A window on quality: Pacific health in the year of COVID-19*. *Bula Sautu* brings together health system indicators from various sources to provide an up-to-date snapshot of how well the NZ health system is performing for Pacific peoples at various stages of life (Health Quality & Safety Commission, 2021). Unfortunately, almost 20 years on from the publication of the first *Pacific Health and Disability Action Plan* (Minister of Health, 2002), *Bula Sautu* demonstrates that the health system continues to under-perform, failing to meet the needs of Pacific populations in many areas. However, it also clearly demonstrates that there is much that can (and should) be done, including specific actions within and across services, to rectify and lift the performance of the health system for Pacific peoples and populations (Health Quality & Safety Commission, 2021).

To accelerate progress in Pacific health, a concerted effort, across health and related sectors, will be necessary. A cornerstone of this concerted effort will include the collection, regular reporting, and ongoing monitoring of Pacific health data.

While the health system currently collects and reports a great deal of data, much of this information is not reported by ethnicity. Even where ethnicity is regularly reported, these analyses are often only presented by Māori/non-Māori. The analysis of data for Māori, as *tangata whenua*, is of utmost importance and in line with the government's obligations under *Te Tiriti o Waitangi*. However, given the well-known and longstanding nature of Pacific health inequities, good practice also demands that, where appropriate, health data should also be specifically reported for Pacific peoples (not least because, in most cases, not doing so will underestimate the magnitude of inequities between Māori and non-Māori non-Pacific populations).

Further, given that 'Pacific peoples' is an umbrella term encompassing a number of different ethnic groups, data would ideally be presented to Level 4 ethnicity (see *Ethnicity Classification* below), and include Pacific-specific ethnic groups.

Regular reporting of Pacific health data, tied to specific actions, and accountability mechanisms (outlining what will be done if measures do not show improvement), is crucial to determining what works (and therefore should be supported and scaled up) and what hinders progress in Pacific health (and therefore should be stopped or changed).

The following sections will outline some of the important uses of Pacific health data, the main methods of reporting and output of ethnicity data and its implications for Pacific people, and the major sources of population data. It will also briefly describe the emerging issue of Pacific data sovereignty.

Uses of Pacific health data

Data is fundamental to *informed action* within health and other sectors. Without a good understanding of what is happening now, what has happened previously, and what is projected to happen in the future, we are essentially 'flying blind'. Good data, with appropriate framing and interpretation, enables us to take control and measure the impact of different actions on Pacific health equity.

Common uses of Pacific health and population data include:

- Monitoring the changing ethnic diversity, language, and social needs of the population at national, regional, and local levels so that services can be appropriately tailored and targeted.
- Monitoring health outcomes, over time and in different regions.
- Measuring access to, utilisation, timeliness, and uptake of various services and interventions (e.g., primary care access, immunisation rates, screening uptake).
- Assessing quality of care received (e.g., diabetes care, surgical infections, cardiovascular risk management).
- Examining patient and whānau/aiga experience of care.
- Planning health services and programmes.
- Prioritising limited health resources and allocating funding.

- Evaluating the implementation, acceptability and impact of services, programmes, and other interventions.

Ethnicity data: Definitions and methods of output

To ensure that the health of Pacific peoples can be reliably compared (to that of other groups, as well as over time), clear and consistent definitions of ethnicity are crucial. NZ is recognised as a world leader in its ability to analyse health data by ethnicity due to a long-term and ongoing focus on capturing high-quality ethnicity data (Ministry of Health, 2017). This has been enabled through a standard definition of ethnicity and the development of ethnicity data protocols for the health and disability sector.

Definition of ethnicity

Statistics New Zealand (Stats NZ) is responsible for the definition of ethnicity across all-of-government, including health. Ethnicity is defined as 'the ethnic group or groups that people identify with or feel they belong to. It is a measure of cultural affiliation, as opposed to race, ancestry, nationality or citizenship' (Stats NZ, 2005). There are three important elements to the definition of ethnicity: (1) it is self-perceived and therefore must be self-identified, (2) people may identify with multiple ethnic groups, and (3) ethnicity may change over time (termed 'ethnic mobility') (Ministry of Health, 2017).

In 2004 the Ministry of Health published *Ethnicity Data Protocols for the Health and Disability Sector* to develop a standardised process for the collection, recording, and output of ethnicity data for the health sector (Ministry of Health, 2004). These protocols were revised and updated in 2009 and again in 2017, to include the following recommendations: (i) collect ethnicity data with a standard question (the 2018 Census ethnicity question) at least once every 3 years, (ii) record all ethnicity data to Level 4 (the most detailed level of ethnicity classification), and (iii) use information systems capable of recording up to six ethnic group responses (Ministry of Health, 2017).

Ethnicity classification

Ethnicity categories are organised into a hierarchical structure with 4 different levels of detail. Levels 1, 2, and 3 have 6, 21, and 36 ethnic categories respectively. Level 4 includes 233 different ethnic groups.

Ethnicity data must be recorded at Level 4 (Ministry of Health, 2017). Ethnicity information is typically output at either Level 1 or Level 2 in official statistics (Stats NZ, 2005).

The six categories at Level 1 include: Māori, Pacific Peoples, Asian, Middle Eastern/Latin American/African (MELAA), Other, and European.

At Levels 2 and 3, there are eight Pacific ethnic group categories: Samoan, Cook Islands Māori, Tongan, Niuean, Tokelauan, Fijian, Other Pacific Peoples, and Pacific Peoples Not Further Defined (NFD).

At Level 4, there are 19 Pacific ethnic group categories: Samoan, Cook Islands Māori, Tongan, Niuean, Tokelauan, Fijian, Indigenous Australian, Hawaiian, Kiribati, Nauruan, Papua New Guinean, Pitcairn Islander, Rotuman, Tahitian, Solomon Islander, Tuvaluan, Ni Vanuatu, Pacific Peoples NFD, and Pacific Peoples Not Elsewhere Classified (Ministry of Health, 2017).

The 2017 update of the ethnicity data protocols also specifically noted data quality issues associated with the collection, classification, and recording of the 'Fijian Indian' ethnic group. The Ethnicity NZ Standard Classification categorises 'Fijian Indian' as Level 4 code 43112 (which aggregates at Level 1 output to 'Asian') (Ministry of Health, 2017). However, it has been noted that in many instances, instead of using the appropriate Level 4 code, some respondents and providers have instead chosen to select 'Fijian' (which aggregates to Level 1 'Pacific Peoples') and 'Indian' (Level 1 'Asian') separately. This combination would result in a Level 1 prioritised output (see *'Ethnicity Data Outputs'* below) of 'Pacific Peoples', when in most cases it should actually be 'Asian'.

These inconsistencies in the coding of Fijian Indians have implications for resource allocation and health status monitoring for both Pacific and Asian populations. Most recently, the issue was observed when reporting of COVID-19 vaccination rates showed an unusually high number and proportion of Fijians getting vaccinated very early on in the vaccination programme (substantially higher than any of the other Pacific ethnic groups), leading experts to conclude that there was a mismatch in the numerator and denominator of the Fijian ethnic group.

It is important that respondents identifying as 'Fijian Indian' be coded correctly (Ministry of Health, 2017). Previous research into cardiovascular disease risk profiles of different Pacific ethnic groups has also previously noted discrepancies in health statistics reported for the Fijian ethnic group, suggesting that a number of Fijian Indians are being inadvertently counted in the indigenous Fijian group (Grey et al., 2010). This is an area that requires caution and further exploration.

Ethnicity data outputs

Ethnicity data protocols are clear that respondents who report multiple ethnicities must not be asked to choose a principal or primary ethnicity (Ministry of Health, 2004; Ministry of Health, 2017). However, reporting data about people with multiple ethnicities can present a challenge, due to overlapping denominators and groups that are not mutually exclusive. This is particularly an issue for the Pacific population, which has a high proportion of people who identify with two or more ethnic groups (41% according to 2018 Census data, compared to 13% of the total population) (Stats NZ, 2021).

There are three standard forms of output of ethnicity data: prioritised, total response, and single/combination (Stats NZ, 2005; Ministry of Health, 2017).

1. Prioritised output

Prioritised ethnicity is the most commonly used ethnicity output in health. Prioritisation is a method where individuals are classified into one ethnic group, in a hierarchical order (at Level 1) as follows; Māori, Pacific Peoples, Asian, MELAA, Other, European (Ministry of Health, 2017). This means that anyone who identifies as Māori and any other ethnic group (including Pacific) will always be categorised as Māori. Similarly, a Pacific person who also identifies with a non-Pacific ethnicity, except Māori, will be categorised as Pacific.

The aim of prioritisation is to ensure that, in instances where people must be assigned to a single ethnic group, ethnic groups of policy importance, or of small size, are not swamped by the NZ European ethnic group (Ministry of Health, 2004). Prioritisation is a reduction process for output purposes and does not assume that this is the ethnic group that a respondent identifies most strongly with (Ministry of Health, 2017).

One of the main advantages of prioritisation is the focus on the Māori population, as it is at the top of the prioritisation hierarchy. Prioritised categorisation reflects the importance of accurate counts for documenting Māori health inequities and enabling a *Te Tiriti o Waitangi* lens on health outcomes (Cormack & Robson, 2010). Another advantage is that each respondent is classified into a single mutually exclusive group, which means data is easier to work on because individuals only appear once in the data (Ministry of Health, 2017).

However, the prioritised output method has a number of limitations, and is the only standard form that is *not* recommended by Stats NZ. Stats NZ largely discontinued this type of output following the 2004 Review of the Measurement of Ethnicity, because it conceals diversity within and overlapping between ethnic groups (Stats NZ, 2004). Another disadvantage is a misalignment with the concept of self-identification (as respondents are not given the opportunity to self-identify the single ethnic group into which they are placed) (Cormack & Robson, 2010; Leather, 2009), which is therefore inconsistent with the conceptual foundations and definition of ethnicity outlined by Stats NZ (Kukutai & Stats NZ, 2008).

Over many years, the Pacific ethnic group has been shown to be the group most affected by the prioritisation method, resulting in significant under-counts and age-based selection bias for Pacific peoples (Boven et al., 2019; Didham & Callister, 2012; Kukutai &

Callister, 2009; Reid et al., 2016). These undercounts are primarily due to the large proportion of Pacific people who identify with more than one ethnic group (41% reporting two or more ethnic groups, compared to 16% of NZ Europeans and 10% of Asians at the 2018 Census) (Stats NZ, 2021).

A 2012 study that examined the effect of prioritisation on 2006 Census data reported that the Pacific population was 15% larger than the prioritised data would suggest (Didham & Callister, 2012). This reduction in number due to prioritisation was seen across all age groups for Pacific peoples, but was particularly marked in the youngest age groups, due to the increasing number of children and young people reporting multiple ethnicities, particularly Māori and Pacific in combination (Didham & Callister, 2012).

Similarly, a 2019 study that examined the impact of different ethnicity output methods on smoking prevalence in adults aged 15 and older reported a 10% difference in the Pacific population as defined by the total response and prioritisation methods (Boven et al., 2019). This study concluded that prioritisation 'may be inappropriate for use by government agencies and for policy-relevant research principally concerned with children, young people, Māori or Pacific Peoples' (Boven et al., 2019).

Total response and single/combination data are considered the best means of outputting ethnicity data (Kukutai & Stats NZ, 2008), but there has been surprisingly little focus on how this should be done from a Pacific perspective.

2. Total response output

Total response is the preferred output method according to Stats NZ. The Ministry for Social Development also changed all its reporting from prioritised ethnicity to total response from December 2021 (Ministry for Social Development, 2021).

The total response output captures up to six ethnic groups for each respondent, utilising more information about an individual's ethnic identity than prioritisation (Cormack & Robson, 2010). People who indicate more than one ethnic group are counted more than once (in each of the ethnic groups with which they identify), so the sum of the ethnic group populations will exceed the total population. This means that the total response output does not lead to undercounting of any ethnic categories (Cormack, 2010), which is an important consideration for the Pacific ethnic group. However, it does make analyses more difficult, as groups are not mutually exclusive (Cormack & Robson, 2010).

Given that total response is the preferred method of output for Stats NZ, it is perplexing that there is very little information on how to use total response categorisation appropriately in statistical modelling (Boven et al., 2019). It is likely that this is primary reason that prioritisation continues to be the favoured method for regression models (Ministry of Health, 2017; Boven et al., 2019).

3. Single/combination output

The single/combination output counts people in mutually exclusive categories. Individuals who report two or more ethnic groups are counted once in the relevant 'combination' group. This means that the total number of responses equals the total number of people who stated their ethnicity, making it straightforward to use in statistical models (Cormack & Robson, 2010; Didham, 2005; Hobbs et al., 2018).

This method allows a more nuanced depiction of the overlap between ethnic groups (Boven et al., 2019). Different characteristics and outcomes associated with combination ethnic groups (e.g., Māori/Pacific peoples) and single ethnic groups (e.g., Pacific Peoples only) may be missed with other methods (Didham, 2005).

In 2018 a *Growing Up in New Zealand* study examined the impact of different ethnicity outputs on risk estimates for hospitalisation with infectious disease in the first 5 years of life (Hobbs et al., 2018). This study found the highest hospitalisation rates among Pacific children, and significantly higher risk estimates among individuals who identified with the 'single Pacific' ethnic group, compared to those who identified as Pacific-NZ European, Pacific-Māori, and prioritised Pacific. The authors of this study concluded that 'single-combined ethnicity revealed diversity of risk within the broader Māori and Pacific groups and for this reason, and with mixed ethnicity becoming increasingly common, the single-combined method should be preferred where sample size and data structure allow it' (Hobbs et al., 2018).

A limitation of the single/combination output, however, is that there are a large number of possible combinations of ethnicity, and some will have very small numbers (Cormack & Robson, 2010), therefore this method is not appropriate for smaller datasets (Didham, 2005).

It should be noted that these output methods are mostly based on reporting of ethnicity to Level 1, which aggregates Pacific ethnic groups into one (as 'Pacific Peoples'), but a more nuanced understanding of Pacific health demands reporting of ethnicity to at least Level 2, and preferably higher (i.e., Level 4). There is currently a dearth of information on the impact of output methods for different Pacific ethnic groups.

Data sources

There are many different sources of Pacific health data. This chapter will focus on two major sources: the Census and the Integrated Data Infrastructure (IDI).

Census

The Census is an important part of the ecosystem for health and other data, providing the basis for population health estimates and projections. The collection of ethnicity information in the Census of population and dwellings is a legislative requirement under the Statistics Act 1975, and the census is an important source of ethnicity data for small areas and small ethnic groups (Reid et al., 2016).

Usually undertaken every 5 years, the 2018 Census represented a significant change from its predecessor in 2013, with Stats NZ opting to follow countries such as Australia and Canada by taking a 'digital-first' approach. Letters were posted to all households containing an internet access code for online completion of census questionnaires. Paper questionnaires (the mainstay of previous Censuses) were made available primarily as a back-up and generally only upon request (2018 Census External Data Quality Panel, 2019a).

Unfortunately, Stats NZ significantly overestimated the uptake of the online Census and underestimated the need for community engagement and availability of paper questionnaires. Total response rates in the 2018 Census (87.5%) were significantly worse than in 2013 (93.2%). Māori (74.3%) and Pacific peoples (73.5%) and those aged 15–29 (81.1%) were disproportionately missed – a notable change from 2006 when there was a 90% response rate for each of these groups (2018 Census External Data Quality Panel, 2019a).

In order to bridge the gap created by disproportionately low response rates and to achieve coverage of the population comparable to 2006 and 2013, Stats NZ initiated a large-scale census mitigation project that involved the extensive use of alternative government data (primarily through the IDI). However, this represented a *significant* change from previous Censuses, and the 2018 Census was the first for which the usual resident population count included a count of those who did not complete a Census questionnaire – and a disproportionate proportion of these people were Māori, Pacific, and/or aged 15–29 years (2018 Census External Data Quality Panel, 2019a).

An External Data Quality Assurance Panel was convened by the Government Statistician in August 2018. The panel provided ongoing advice and guidance to Stats NZ with regard to their mitigation methods and considered the quality of the population statistics that resulted from that work (2018 Census External Data Quality Panel, 2019a; 2019b; 2020). The Panel consisted of esteemed experts in geography, demography, Māori health, statistics, biostatistics, and social research. Unfortunately, despite Pacific peoples having the lowest response rates of the 2018 Census and the highest proportion of data from administrative datasets, there were no Pacific experts on the Panel.

The Panel developed three detailed reports (an initial report, an assessment of variables, and a final report) (2018 Census External Data Quality Panel, 2019a; 2019b; 2020). These reports seem comprehensive but are not simple to follow. Therefore, it is difficult to assess the exact nature and magnitude of the impact on Pacific population statistics that the changes in the 2018 Census have had.

Key findings from the three documents released by the Panel in relation to Pacific data include:

- Data quality ratings for Pacific ethnic groups range from moderate to high (in comparison to NZ European, Chinese, and Indian groups, which are rated very high). Most Pacific groups at Level 2 are rated high, although Niuean, Tokelauan, and Cook Islands Māori are close to the moderate threshold. The Fijian group has only a moderate quality rating, due to a low percentage of data sourced from Census 2018 and poor consistency between ethnicity responses on the received forms and the 2013 Census and administrative data.
- Because of the changes in the way Census data was collected in 2018, the Panel's view was that Census 2018 should be treated as a break in the time series, and that comparisons with ethnicity data prior to 2018 should be undertaken with extreme caution, particularly for Māori and Pacific ethnic groups.
- The quality of data at the small area level varies widely, due to large variation in response rates across different areas of the country. Some small areas were particularly affected by low response rates, and as such have lower quality data across many variables (including, for example, relationship

status, occupation, usual residence 1 year ago). There were 24 small area units (1% of the total) with less than 60% census responses. 15 of the 24 areas were in the Auckland region, with 12 in the South Auckland local boards of Otara-Papatoetoe (6), Manurewa (4), and Mangere-Otahuhu (2), all areas with very high Pacific populations. This means that detailed data about Pacific people may not be possible in the areas in which many reside.

- There is great variation in the assessment of the quality of different variables. Those intending to use 2018 Census data should start with the 2018 Census Review Panel's document *Assessment of Variables* (2018 Census External Data Quality Panel, 2019b).

To allow users of Pacific health data in the 2018 Census to appropriately analyse, interpret, and frame data, Stats NZ (or another interested group) should consider developing an easy-to-follow document or 'how-to' manual outlining the key considerations, potential pitfalls, and implications of using Pacific data from the 2018 Census.

Integrated data infrastructure

Many analyses across government and in academia are now utilising Stats NZ's IDI. The IDI is a collection of NZ whole-population administrative data sources from government agencies, the 2013 Census and several questionnaire-based social and socioeconomic surveys from samples of the population (Stats NZ, 2020). The IDI allows whole-population and longitudinal analysis across different sectors of government (e.g., health, social services, education) (Milne et al., 2019).

The IDI provides one place to securely link the various data sources for 'research for public good' (Atkinson & Blakely, 2017). Before data is made available to approved researchers, all personal identifiers have been either removed or encrypted (replaced with another number) to ensure the data records are not associated with named individuals.

There are eight broad categories of data in the IDI:

1. Health, e.g., hospitalisations, cancer registrations, mortality, B4 school checks.
2. Education and training.
3. Benefits and social services, e.g., youth services, ACC injury claims, family start.
4. Justice – data from the Ministry of Justice and police.
5. People and communities – e.g., data from Auckland City mission, transportation (driver's licences and motor vehicle registrations), government surveys.
6. Population – e.g., visa applications, births, deaths, marriages, and civil unions.
7. Income and work – e.g., tax and income, household economics.
8. Housing – e.g., tenancy and social housing information.

There are many advantages of using the IDI, including the fact that health data can be linked to other administrative data (e.g., tax, education, migration), it facilitates collaboration between agencies from different sectors, and it allows for repeated measures and longitudinal data analysis (Atkinson & Blakely, 2017).

Currently, there are nationally-standardised processes for ensuring that 'only responsible and capable researchers with appropriate research questions have access to the relevant anonymised data' (Atkinson & Blakely, 2017). However, there is currently no oversight over what Pacific data is being used, who is doing the research and how it is being interpreted. Good governance over the data to ensure Pacific data is being framed appropriately, is crucial.

Growing concerns over safeguards for Pacific data in the IDI and other data sources, as well fallout from the 2018 Census, have resulted in the emergence of the issue of Pacific data sovereignty and the establishment of a Pacific Data Sovereignty Network (PDSN) (Moana Research, 2021).

Pacific data sovereignty

Indigenous data sovereignty is an important issue that has emerged in recent years as a result of the increased use of 'open data' globally. Indigenous data sovereignty refers to the right of Indigenous peoples to control data from and about their communities and lands, articulating both individual and collective rights to data access and to privacy (Rainie et al., 2019). In NZ, *Te Mana Raraunga,* the Māori Data Sovereignty Network, was established in 2015, with the purpose of asserting Māori rights and interests in relation to data and ensuring data for and about Māori can be safeguarded and protected (Te Mana Raraunga, 2021).

Pacific peoples are not indigenous to NZ, but are a unique population with a rich history and special ties to NZ and its *tangata whenua.* Health research and data on Pacific peoples is often framed through a deficit framework with 'outsider' perspectives (Tualaulelei & McFall-McCaffery, 2019), highlighting the importance of Pacific data sovereignty (Moana Research, 2021). With support from *Te Mana Raraunga,* the PDSN, hosted by Moana Research, was established in 2019.

The PDSN describes Pacific data sovereignty as 'understanding our ancestral heritage while upholding the ethos that "nothing is about us – Pacific Peoples – without us – Pacific Peoples". This ensures that the lineage of Pacific data paves its paths and linkages back to Pacific ancestors and the generations following to present-day Pacific peoples.' (Moana Research, 2021, p15).

Pacific data sovereignty is focused on:

- Rights and responsibilities to determine the means of collection, access, analysis, management, and dissemination of Pacific data.
- Producing information from and/or about Pacific peoples that is driven by Pacific cultural values, worldviews, epistemologies, and traditional knowledge systems.
- Pacific stewardship of data, through supporting and enhancing Pacific peoples' understanding of data, its sources, access pathways, management, and current and future use.
- Ensuring that data is curated and cared for by Pacific peoples (Moana Research, 2021).

As it is still in its infancy, the area of Pacific data sovereignty will continue to evolve and mature, but is a significant step forward in ensuring there is good stewardship of Pacific health (and other) data.

References

2018 Census External Data Quality Panel. (2019a). *Initial Report of the 2018 Census External Data Quality Panel*. https://www.stats.govt.nz/reports/initial-report-of-the-2018-census-external-data-quality-panel

2018 Census External Data Quality Panel. (2019b). *Assessment of variables*. Stats NZ. https://www.stats.govt.nz/assets/Uploads/Reports/2018-Census-External-Data-Quality-Panel-Assessment-of-Variables/Download-data/2018-census-external-data-quality-panel-assessment-of-variables.pdf

2018 Census External Data Quality Panel. (2020). *Final report of the 2018 Census External Data Quality Panel*. Stats NZ. https://www.stats.govt.nz/reports/final-report-of-the-2018-census-external-data-quality-panel

Atkinson, J., & Blakely, T. (2017). New Zealand's Integrated Data Infrastructure (IDI): Value to date and future opportunities. *International Journal of Population Data Science*, 1(1), 124. https://doi.org/10.23889/ijpds.v1i1.124

Boven, N., Exeter, D., Sporle, A., & Shackleton, N. (2019). The implications of different ethnicity categorisation methods for understanding outcomes and developing policy in New Zealand. *Kōtuitui: New Zealand Journal of Social Sciences Online*, 15(1), 123–139. https://doi.org/10.1080/1177083X.2019.1657912

Cormack, D. (2010). *The politics and practices of counting: ethnicity in official statistics in Aotearoa/New Zealand*. Te Rōpū Rangahau Hauora a Eru Pōmare. https://www.otago.ac.nz/wellington/otago600095.pdf

Cormack, D., & Robson, C. 2010. *Classification and output of multiple ethnicities: considerations for monitoring Māori health*. Te Rōpū Rangahau Hauora a Eru Pōmare. https://www.health.govt.nz/publication/classification-and-output-multiple-ethnicities-considerations-monitoring-maori-health

Didham, R. (2005). *Understanding and Working with Ethnicity Data*. Stats NZ. https://www.researchgate.net/publication/289801509_Understanding_and_working_with_ethnicity_data_a_technical_paper

Didham, R., & Callister, P. (2012). The effect of ethnic prioritisation on ethnic health analysis: a research note. *The New Zealand Medical Journal*, 125(1359), 58–66.

Grey, C., Wells, S., Riddell, T., Pylypchuk, R., Marshall, R., Drury, P., Elley, R., Ameratunga, S., Gentles, D., Erick-Peleti, S., Bell, F., Kerr, A., & Jackson, R. (2010). A comparative analysis of cardiovascular disease risk profiles of five Pacific ethnic groups assessed in New Zealand primary care practice: PREDICT CVD-13. *New Zealand Medical Journal*, 123(1325),41–52.

Health Quality & Safety Commission. (2021). *Bula Sautu – A window on quality 2021: Pacific health in the year of COVID-19*. Health Quality & Safety Commission. https://www.hqsc.govt.nz/assets/Health-Quality-Evaluation/PR/BulaSautu_WEB.pdf

Hobbs, M. R., Atatoa Carr, P., Fa'alili-Fidow, J., Pillai, A., Morton, S. M. B., & Grant, C. C. (2018). How differing methods of ascribing ethnicity and socio-economic status affect risk estimates for hospitalisation with infectious disease. *Epidemiology and Infection, 147*, e40. https://doi.org/10.1017/S0950268818002935

Kukutai, T. (Tahatū Consulting) & Stats NZ. (2008). *Ethnic Self-prioritisation of Dual and Multi-ethnic Youth in New Zealand*. Stats NZ. https://ndhadeliver.natlib.govt.nz/delivery/DeliveryManagerServlet?dps_pid=IE1632044

Kukutai, T., & Callister, P. (2009). A "Main" Ethnic Group?: Ethnic Self-Prioritisation among New Zealand Youth. *Social Policy Journal of New Zealand, 36*, 16–31.

Leather, F. (2009). Prioritising ethnic data from schools: Who are we missing? A research note. *Social Policy Journal of New Zealand, 36*, 82–87.

Milne, B. J., Atkinson, J., Blakely, T., Day, H., Douwes, J., Gibb, S., Nicolson, M., Shackleton, N., Sporle, A., & Teng, A. (2019). Data Resource Profile: The New Zealand Integrated Data Infrastructure (IDI). *International Journal of Epidemiology, 48*(3), 677–677e. https://doi.org/10.1093/ije/dyz014

Minister of Health. (2002). The Pacific Health and Disability Action Plan. https://www.health.govt.nz/system/files/documents/publications/pacific_health.pdf

Minister of Health & Minister of Pacific Island Affairs. (2010). *'Ala Mo'ui: Pathways to Pacific Health and Wellbeing 2010–2014.* Ministry of Health. https://www.health.govt.nz/publication/ala-moui-pathways-pacific-health-and-wellbeing-2010-2014

Ministry of Health. (2004). *Ethnicity Data Protocols for the Health and Disability Sector.* https://www.fmhs.auckland.ac.nz/assets/fmhs/faculty/tkhm/tumuaki/docs/ethnicity-data-protocols.pdf

Ministry of Health. (2014). *'Ala Mo'ui: Pathways to Pacific Health and Wellbeing 2014–2018.* https://www.health.govt.nz/publication/ala-moui-pathways-pacific-health-and-wellbeing-2014-2018

Ministry of Health. (2017). *HISO 10001:2017 Ethnicity Data Protocols.* https://www.health.govt.nz/publication/hiso-100012017-ethnicity-data-protocols

Ministry of Health. (2020). *Ola Manuia: Pacific Health and Wellbeing Action Plan 2020–2025.* https://www.health.govt.nz/publication/ola-manuia-pacific-health-and-wellbeing-action-plan-2020-2025

Ministry of Social Development. (2021). *Improving how we report ethnicity.* https://www.msd.govt.nz/about-msd-and-our-work/tools/how-we-report-ethnicity.html

Moana Research. (2021). *Pacific Data Sovereignty Network, Consultation Document.* https://www.moanaresearch.co.nz/wp-content/uploads/2021/03/PDS-consultation-document.pdf

Rainie, S.C., Kukutai, T., Walter, M., Figueroa-Rodríguez, O.L., Walker, J., & Axelsson, P. (2019). Indigenous data sovereignty. In T. Davies, S. Walker, M. Rubinstein, & F. Perini (Eds.), *The state of open data: Histories and horizons* (1st ed., pp. 300–319). African Minds and International Development Research Centre.

Reid, G., Bycroft, C., & Gleisner, F. (2016). *Comparison of ethnicity information in administrative data and the census.* Stats NZ. https://www.stats.govt.nz/assets/Research/Comparison-of-ethnicity-information-in-administrative-data-and-the-census/comparison-of-ethnicity-information-in-administrative-data-and-the-census.pdf

Stats NZ. (2004). *Report of the Review of the Measurement of Ethnicity: June 2004.* https://statsnz.contentdm.oclc.org/digital/collection/p20045coll1/id/1460/

Stats NZ. (2005). *Ethnicity New Zealand Standard Classification 2005V2.0.0.* http://aria.stats.govt.nz/aria/?_ga=2.254044168.1822128773.1641531104-1485014763.1575591675#ClassificationView:uri=http://stats.govt.nz/cms/ClassificationVersion/l36xYpbxsRh7IW1p

Stats NZ. (2020). *Integrated Data Infrastructure.* https://www.stats.govt.nz/integrated-data/integrated-data-infrastructure/

Stats NZ. (2021). *2018 Census ethnic group summaries.* https://www.stats.govt.nz/tools/2018-census-ethnic-group-summaries

Te Mana Raraunga. (2021). *Our Data, Our Sovereignty, Our Future.* https://www.temanararaunga.maori.nz/

Tualaulelei, E., & McFall-McCaffery, J. (2019). The Pacific Research Paradigm: Opportunities and challenges. *MAI Journal: A New Zealand Journal of Indigenous Scholarship*, *8*(2), 188–204. https://doi.org/10.20507/maijournal.2019.8.2.7.

Healthcare horizons: Scanning the data to navigate the barriers and enablers for Pacific communities

Roannie Ng Shiu

Asetoa Sam Pilisi

Chapter summary

This chapter presents some of the key health data and research to highlight some of the disparities on the health care needs of Pacific people in response to their health burden. Pacific communities' health burden as a result of higher prevalence rates of long-term conditions (LTCs) is an issue for all New Zealanders as it impacts on resources. In addition, many presentations to hospital could easily be treated and managed in primary health services if access to these services was greatly improved. Data and research from the last several decades demonstrate that while access to health care and health inequities are worsening despite research identifying the various barriers and new innovations and advances in medicine that could assist in improving access.

Introduction

Barriers to accessing adequate healthcare and unmet health needs have remained a challenge for Pacific communities for several decades in Aotearoa New Zealand. Consequently, these challenges contribute to persistent health inequalities between Pacific and Māori communities in comparison to other ethnic groups such as Pākehā and Asian New Zealanders. Despite this being a persistent, well-known feature of health outcomes for many years, the gap between Pacific people's outcomes and other New Zealanders continues to grow despite modest nominal improvements in certain areas. Some barriers to accessing health care include cultural, social, economic, and systemic issues, which require a multifaceted approach to ensure favourable and equitable health outcomes for Pacific communities and all New Zealanders.

Another area of concern regarding Pacific health outcomes is the challenge of 'good data.' Reliable and quality Pacific health data and research are important to assist with targeted interventions and identify gaps and needs to improve health outcomes. However, there are significant gaps in data on Pacific health outcomes and population health needs. Ethnic-specific public health data is often not available or is out of date. Additionally, issues with sampling and undercounting of Pacific peoples limit the validity and reliability of quantitative analysis data, as was witnessed during the 2018 Census. Despite these challenges, there are some useful datasets that can provide a snapshot of health service access and use and health needs of Pacific communities.

This chapter begins by reviewing some of the current data on health outcomes and long-term conditions (LTCs), unmet needs, and access to healthcare and medicine for Pacific communities before discussing some of the key socioeconomic, cultural, and systemic issues affecting access to healthcare. This chapter draws on some of the identified barriers and enablers of access to health care identified in *Tofa Saili: A review of evidence about health equity for Pacific Peoples in New Zealand* (Ryan et al., 2019) as well as drawing on the Pacific response to COVID-19 in Aotearoa New Zealand. Pacific leadership during the COVID-19 pandemic in Aotearoa New Zealand provides a unique opportunity to highlight the strengths and resilience of Pacific communities in responding to their own health needs and demonstrates the potential and possibilities that Pacific-led health interventions present for better Pacific health outcomes.

Long-term conditions

LTCs are a range of long-term or recurring illnesses and health conditions that require health services for a range of prevention, management, and treatment that can have a significant impact on people's lives. Often, these conditions have many of the same underlying causes, which are sometimes described as modifiable risk factors and include hypertension, also known as high blood pressure, infectious diseases, tobacco, diet, obesity, and alcohol (Meredith et al., 2012).

Pacific data on modifiable risk factors from the New Zealand Health Survey 2022/2023 (Ministry of Health, 2023a) results showed that:

- Pacific adults have the highest prevalence rates for hypertension. They were 1.4 times more likely to be diagnosed with hypertension and currently taking medication.
- Rates of obesity for Pacific adults (67.3%) and children (27.8%) are disproportionately higher compared to the total New Zealand population. Children (13.5%).
- Smoking rates have declined over the last decade but smoking rates still remain higher compared to other population groups except for Māori. After adjusting for age and gender Pacific people were 1.3 times as likely to be current smokers compared to their non-Māori and non-Pacific counterparts.
- Hazardous alcohol consumption for Pacific adults was 21.5% compared to 16% for the total New Zealand population.

Pacific adults are more likely to develop one or more LTCs over their lifetime, leading to multimorbidity, that is, the diagnosis of two or more LTCs. They are also more likely to develop LTCs at a younger age compared with other ethnic groups. The most prevalent conditions are obesity, anxiety or depression, hypertension, asthma or chronic obstructive pulmonary disease, gout, diabetes, cardiovascular disease, and osteoarthritis (Stokes et al., 2018).

The current healthcare system is complex and difficult to navigate and tends to specialise and focus on one disease or disease system. Therefore, multimorbidity patients present a challenge to the healthcare system and workforce, as they require intense clinical management of LTCs. As a result, Pacific communities find the health system fragmented, confusing, and difficult to navigate (Ministry of Health, 2023b). Multimorbidity is also associated with increasing age and with socioeconomic deprivation, which has impacts on access to adequate healthcare to ensure health needs are being met.

Access to healthcare

Primary care provides a pivotal role in screening, diagnosing, and managing LTCs. New Zealand data indicate that primary care is less accessible to Pacific people in Aotearoa New Zealand compared to the wider population. Data from annual New Zealand Health Surveys[1] provide data on key indicators of unmet need due to cost and transport. The results below show that the Pacific adult population have lower rates of visits to GP despite data showing Pacific people have higher rates of illness and disease.

The table above highlights cost and transport as barriers to accessing health care. In addition, the data also supports research which has shown that Pacific people are less likely to report referrals and tests and scans ordered (Ryan et al., 2019)

Snapshot of access to healthcare:

- **Tagata saili malo – Pacific peoples with disabilities in New Zealand**:
    - There is limited data to describe the access and quality of care and support for Pacific peoples with disabilities in New Zealand. This includes comprehensive data on the delivery of support services, funding, equipment, and the barriers to access for disabled Pacific peoples in New Zealand.

Table 1: New Zealand Health Survey data on barriers to healthcare.

	2020/21 Pacific	**Total population**	**2022/23**	**Total population**
Visits to GP in the past 12 moths	68.0	73.9	64.6	73.2
Unmet need for primary care in the past 12 months due to cost	15.2	10.2	17.6	12.9
Unfilled prescription due to cost in the past 12 months	6.6	3.1	8.5	4.0
Unmet need for dental care in the past 12 months due to cost	44.4	39.8	58	44
Unmet need for GP due to transport	4.8	2.4	3.4	2.2
Visited ED at least once in the past 12 months	14.8	14.2	20.1	17.9
Was referred to a specialist			34.5	50.9

- **Pacific children:**
  - o Data from the New Zealand Health Survey 2021/22 found Pacific children aged 0 to 14 years were twice as likely to experience unmet need for a GP due to cost and transport and have an unfilled prescription due to cost.
  - o Pacific children also have lower rates of health and developmental screening at the Before School Checks at age four compared with the total population (Ministry of Health, 2022).
  - o Research has shown that at each age barriers to primary health care for Pacific children were more prevalent compared to New Zealand European children (Jeffreys et al., 2022).
- **Pacific adults**:
  - o Pacific adults with a mental health condition, were twice as likely as other ethnic groups to report the cost of prescriptions as a barrier to treatment.
  - o Research has shown that Pacific peoples have lower rates of specialist mental health service use than non-Māori, non-Pacific peoples despite higher rates of psychological distress (Ataera-Minster & Trowland, 2018).

Ambulatory sensitive hospitalisations

Ambulatory sensitive hospitalisations (ASH) are acute admissions that are considered avoidable through preventative or therapeutic interventions deliverable in primary care (Ryan et al., 2019). Lower ASH rates are associated with access to quality primary care, continuity of care and having a regular source of care. Therefore, ASH rates and emergency department visits are often used as proxies to determine unmet primary health care needs.

Current data on ASH rates highlight the significant disparities between Pacific populations and the total New Zealand population. The ASH rates for 0- to 4-year-olds show that while there have been slight improvements for the total population between 2016 and 2022, the rates for Pacific children have worsened. Conversely, the rates for Pacific adults have improved over the same time period but a large gap between the total New Zealand population remains.

The following table provides the rates of the top ten conditions of avoidable hospital admissions. In most of these instances the disparities are remarkable and considerable.

Table 2: Standardised ASH rate per 100,000 to December 2022.

	2016 Pacific		**2022 Pacific**	
Ambulatory sensitive hospitalisations per 100,000 0–4 years	12,079	6,690	14,083	6,475
Ambulatory sensitive hospitalisations, per 100,000 per 45–64 years	8,787	3,789	7,219	3,835

High ASH rates come at a considerable cost to the government and have an adverse effect on the capacity of hospital services and emergency departments. Improvements in access to quality primary health care and medicines should ease the pressure on secondary health services.

Medicine access equity and polypharmacy

In Aotearoa New Zealand, medicine access equity refers to everyone having a fair opportunity to access funded medicines to attain their full health potential, and that no one should be disadvantaged from achieving this potential. In this context, unequal inputs are required to attain a fair opportunity to access funded

Table 3: Top ten condition for standardised ASH rate per 100,000 for 45–64 age group to December 2022 (Ministry of Health, 2023c).

	Pacific	**Total New Zealand population**
Angina and chest pain	1,893	1,085
Myocardial infarction	451	32
Cellulitis	722	310
Gastroenteritis/dehydration	355	281
Chronic inflammatory lung disease	293	217
Pneumonia	502	211
Kidney/urine infection	336	181
Congestive heart failure	478	160
Stroke	344	158
Diabetes	277	137

medicines (PHARMAC, 2019). Access to medicines includes issues broader than the cost of prescriptions and medicines but includes ensuring there is an adequate supply of publicly funded medicines, that all New Zealanders have access to and optimally use available medicines and that these medicines lead to effective health outcomes.

Access to medicines is vitally important in the management and treatment of health conditions. Common diseases where there are significant Pacific health disparities, such as asthma, diabetes, gout, hypertension, and primary and secondary prevention of a cardiovascular event, respond well to established scientific medicines. Research has shown that Pacific and Māori people are often under-prescribed these medicines, which, in addition to prescription costs, are barriers to accessing effective medication (Ofanoa et al., 2023). Reasons for underprescribing medicines also highlight issues of discrimination and racism in the health care system.

Management and treatment of multimorbidity include the need for multiple medical prescriptions or polypharmacy. Polypharmacy is where multiple medications are concurrently prescribed to one individual. High rates of polypharmacy are a concern, as it is also associated with poor health outcomes, including increased admissions to hospitals and death. Pacific adults have the highest rate of polypharmacy, and rates were significantly higher in younger Pacific and Māori adults compared to other ethnic groups. This is consistent with national rates of multimorbidity by ethnic group (Health Quality & Safety Commission, 2021b). Polypharmacy comes at a significant cost to patients and health services, and Pacific adults are twice as likely to have unfilled prescriptions due to cost compared to the total population (see Table 1).

Appropriate polypharmacy can be beneficial, while problematic polypharmacy is harmful. The 'triple whammy' treatment is an example of problematic polypharmacy, which is the combination:

1. angiotensin converting enzyme (ACE) inhibitor/angiotensin receptor blocker (ARB)
2. a diuretic
3. non-steroidal anti-inflammatory drug (NSAID)

This combination should be avoided to prevent the increased risk of acute kidney injury. However, Pacific adults between the ages of 65 and 74 years are more likely to be prescribed the triple whammy compared to any other ethnic group (Health Quality & Safety Commission, 2021b). While the overall, rate of long-term medicine use has reduced since 2012, the rates continue to be high for Pacific peoples. Addressing multimorbidity in Pacific populations will assist in reducing rates of polypharmacy and improve health outcomes generally.

COVID-19: Pacific health service delivery leadership and opportunities

Aotearoa New Zealand's response to the COVID-19 pandemic was to follow an elimination strategy in order to achieve health and economic outcomes. Consideration was given to the impact on population health outcomes and health services, impacts on inequities, control of new variant spread, and time to allow New Zealand to better prepare for outbreaks, administer vaccines, and gather better data and intelligence from the international health community.

Since the global outbreak of the COVID-19 pandemic Aotearoa New Zealand experienced three distinct clusters resulting in 29.3% of cases among Pacific peoples. Hospitalisation rates were higher for Pacific peoples compared to NZ European/Pākehā communities – approximately 10% and 4%, respectively (Ministry of Health, 2022). One of the clusters, also known as the Auckland August 2020 outbreak, significantly affected Pacific communities in South Auckland (Colmar Brunton, 2021; Tukuitonga, 2021), resulting in 59% of confirmed cases among Pacific peoples.

In response to this particular cluster, Pacific communities were encouraged and supported to lead a localised Pacific response to limit the spread of the virus and improve vaccination rates. Churches became the focal points for testing and distribution sites for essential goods such as food parcels, medications and sanitation prevention packs, and social support. Church leaders and Pacific media became vital health communicators providing critical information that was translated and interpreted for the seven main Pacific community groups (Samoan, Tongan, Cook Islands, Niuean, Fijian, Tokelauan, and Tuvaluan).

The ability for a range of Pacific leaders to collaborate and respond effectively and efficiently to COVID-19 meant that testing rates were the highest among Pacific populations and the spread of COVID-19 was limited and contained. This response highlights the opportunities that Pacific leadership has on improving health outcomes through effective health communication and messaging, how to better deliver health services and care, and how to increase engagement with the health sector in a community that has typically been disengaged with the health sector as a consequence of being underserved by mainstream health services. Lessons learnt include flexible and rapid deployment of funding and resources, cross sectoral and interagency collaboration and appropriately enhancing the trusted relationships of Pacific providers with Pacific communities in delivering holistic models of care that integrate approaches to address health, social, and education needs (Health Quality & Safety Commission, 2021a).

Stigma and discrimination

Research has shown that Pacific individuals and families experience racism across all areas of the health system. Experiences of discrimination are associated with poorer health outcomes, particularly in mental health, lower rates of life satisfaction, and poorer self-rated health. Researchers investigating stigma and discrimination in New Zealand found that Māori, Pacific, and Asian populations were more likely to experience racial discrimination one area in which research on stigma and discrimination has been researched is in mental health. A recent study on caregiver experiences of racism and child mental health outcomes noted a higher prevalence of vicarious racism for Pacific children compared to European/Other children (Juang et al., 2023). A qualitative study explored the barriers and supports for Pacific communities accessing and using mental health services. The researchers found that Pacific clients were more likely to seek help from a Pacific practitioner compared to non-Pacific practitioners due to previous experiences of stigmatisation and a lack of trust and knowledge of services (Fa'alogo-Lilo & Cartwright, 2021).

Treatment differences, such as underprescribing medicines between ethnic groups, also point to discrimination and racism (Ofanoa et al., 2023). These challenges have long been echoed by Pacific community members, who want to have a health system that is fair and equitable to all New Zealanders. Negative experiences of racism and discrimination lead to intergenerational disengagement with the health system, which will further exacerbate current health challenges for Pacific peoples. These studies acknowledge that while there are efforts to help address stigma and discrimination, culture changes, and shifts remain slow highlighting the need for ongoing cultural training for health service providers.

Cultural competence

Critically, patients and families have experienced challenges when health professionals aren't equipped with the necessary tools to understand Pacific worldviews and cultural values. A one size fits all approach to healthcare does not work for Pacific patients and Pacific cultural competency in healthcare is the ability to understand and appropriately apply cultural values and practices that are essential to Pacific peoples' worldviews of health and wellbeing (Tiatia-Seath, 2018). One such way of acknowledging Pacific cultural values is to understand and place greater emphasis on building and sustaining relationships. For most Pacific peoples protecting relationships are imperative and is conveyed through the Samoan phrase *teu le va* (Wendt, 1996). Thus, health professionals and the spaces in which healthcare is delivered can value and protect relationships that align with Pacific worldviews as an active commitment to reducing inequities in a population where health disparities and injustices have been rife.

Healthcare providers are encouraged to undergo cultural competence training to better understand and respond to the cultural needs of Pacific patients. Efforts are made to create a culturally sensitive healthcare environment to make Pacific people feel more comfortable and respected. By Pacific, for Pacific services are more than just having Pacific peoples at the frontline to work with their own. By Pacific, for Pacific services means that the model of care reflects the values and philosophies of Pacific. One such successful model of care is the Pacific Whānau Ora model which is a family-centric, culturally responsive, and strength-based, co-created solution to ensure better wellbeing outcomes for Pacific whānau to thrive in Aotearoa (Pasifika Futures, 2023). By employing a strengths-based approach to healthcare, Pacific patients and their families are able to feel respected while navigating various health challenges.

Language and communication

Ensuring that there is good communication between health professionals and patients and their families is a key facet to delivering high-quality health services (Mohammed et al., 2014). A recent review on health literacy and culture among Pacific peoples in New Zealand found that Pacific female adults and older adults in low socioeconomic areas had lower levels of health literacy. Pacific adults with compromised health also struggled with health literacy which has implications for their management of illness and disease. For example, those with diabetes reported difficulties in understanding what normal blood sugar levels and blood pressure ranges complicated their management of hypoglycaemia (Lilo et al., 2020)

In-depth analyses of the experiences of Māori and Pacific whanau with children treated for cancer at Starship Hospital (Auckland, New Zealand) and of families with children hospitalised with unintentional injury have highlighted mismatches in the cultural values of whanau and the system in which their children were being treated (Arlidge et al., 2009; Brown, 2018). In both studies, families spoke of communication barriers, a clash in cultural worldviews and, at times, discriminatory and racist behaviour.

According to current literature, barriers to effective communication for Pacific communities include discriminatory and racist behaviour, lack of clear communication of relevant health information, and challenges with translating and interpreting a complex health system and medical jargon. To ensure effective communication to improve health outcomes for Pacific communities' health services and professionals require culture competence training to provide them with the skills to communicate relevant health information in an effective and timely manner. While having Pacific language translators and interpreters who are skilled in relaying complex medical jargon and information is the most preferred option, they are not always available particularly in small communities and rural areas. Therefore, it is important that all health workers have some form of cultural competence training as part of their health training. Furthermore, time spent to explain how the health system works and who people can reach out to for further information provides Pacific communities with the knowledge and tools to manage their health and access healthcare more effectively in a timely manner and therefore is more likely to have an impact in reducing prevalence rates of ASH.

Pacific health services

More and more, digital technologies are used to manage health issues and are often touted as providing easy access to individual health information. However, inequities in accessing technology for Pacific communities means they are often at a disadvantage. Pacific providers understand these issues and prioritise more face-to-face engagement at their services (Ministry of Health, 2023b).

Pacific people are more likely to attend very low-cost clinics that operate walk-in only services but critically are in areas with high Pacific populations for example, South Auckland, West Auckland, Porirua with appropriate opening hours to accommodate patients who find it difficult to get time off for appointments (Ryan et al., 2019). Pacific Primary Health Organisations (PHO's) provide critical services which address some of the above barriers particularly in response to cultural competence and language and communication. However, these services are overloaded and under-resourced (Barthow et al., 2023).

Research has suggested that targeted investment in Pacific primary health community care commission is needed to provide adequate health care for Pacific patients with multimorbidity (Sheridan et al., 2023). As presented above Pacific people are disproportionately affected by multiple health issues, therefore a targeted approach would provide healthcare that addresses the full picture rather than siloed approaches to individual health issues. This encourages efficient health service delivery and declutters the confusing multiple touch points for Pacific patients and their families.

Pacific workforce

A representative Pacific health workforce is critical to addressing unmet need. Increased numbers of Pacific health workers across the country provides choice for Pacific peoples and supports a culturally safe environment to respond to Pacific health needs (MOH, 2023). Contributing to a representative Pacific workforce include initiatives and policies such as Mirror on Society and POPO (University of Otago), MAPAS (University of Auckland), and FOU Health Science Academies (Counties Manukau Health/ Te Whatu Ora). Incremental increases to the Pacific regulated health care graduates entering the workforce continue to provide impact in Pacific communities, however longer strides are needed to have a workforce that is reflective of Aotearoa New Zealand's diverse population. The current Pacific health workforce and forecasts for the future demonstrate the need for intensive support required to meet the burden of care needed for Pacific communities given the growing disparities in health prevalence rates (See Table 4).

Training a clinical workforce that is commensurate with the Pacific population in New Zealand will take time and intensive resourcing. To aid in improving health outcomes and access to health services for Pacific communities requires a multi-faceted and multidisciplinary approach to also address some of the critical social determinants of health like poverty and inadequate

Table 4: Pacific Health Workforce – regulated health care workers (Ministry of Health, 2023c).

	Pacific	**2032 Forecast**
Doctor	2.3	2.7
GP	2.2%	4.1
Nurse	3.9	4.1
Midwife	3.0%	4.1
Pharmacist	2.3	2.9
Clinical psychologist	1.9%	No forecast available
Dentist	1.2%	
Dental hygienist	1.6%	
Dietician	1.5%	
Occupational therapist	2%	
Oral health/dental therapist	5.9%	
Optician	1.5%	
Paramedic	2.1%	
Podiatrist	3.6%	
Psychologist	2.1%	

housing. Non-regulated health care workers including community health workers and leaders may play a role in disseminating health information, assisting in systemic issues related to social determinants of health and encouraging preventive care within Pacific communities. Information on these health workers is limited highlighting the need for more research into the links between community health workers and improved access to healthcare. A recent study into primary health services among Pacific adults with Type 2 Diabetes mellitus (T2DM) in South Auckland investigated the growing Pacific community-based, non-clinical workforce to support Pacific people living with T2DM to achieve better outcomes. This workforce was able to work well with clinical counterparts to undertake a multidisciplinary approach to improve diabetes outcomes for Pacific adults in their service (Mullane et al., 2022).

Conclusion

Improvements in Pacific outcomes for a more equitable, just and healthy New Zealand necessitates the removal of barriers to care across the entire health sector. These barriers have been identified as access to essential medicines, particularly for the treatment and management of LTCs, ensuring health services address stigma and discrimination, and ensuring health professionals and services communicate effectively and efficiently important health information and understand the complex health system to enable Pacific patients to better manage their illnesses.

The compounding effects of social determinants of health on Pacific health outcomes requires innovation in health service delivery and health equity. A multifaceted approach to address socioeconomic issues as well as investment into access to adequate and high-quality health care and medicine remains a priority to address persistent, pervasive, and preventable health outcomes for Pacific people. The COVID-19 Pacific response has shown the benefits and effectiveness of investment in Pacific led responses. There are already established models of care and service delivery in primary health care that can be scaled up to increase the capacity of Pacific health providers and increase Pacific health workforce capacity and capability.

References

Arlidge, B., Abel, S., Asiasiga, L., Milne, S. L., Crengle, S., & Ameratunga, S. N. (2009). Experiences of whānau/families when injured children are admitted to hospital: a multi-ethnic qualitative study from Aotearoa/New Zealand. Ethnicity & Health, 14(2), 169–183. https://doi.org/10.1080/13557850802307791

Ataera-Minster, J., & Trowland, H. (2018). *Te Kaveinga: Mental health and wellbeing of Pacific peoples. Results from the New Zealand Mental Health Monitor & Health and Lifestyles Survey.* Health Promotion Agency. https://www.hpa.org.nz/sites/default/files/FinalReport-TeKaveinga-Mental%20health%20and%20wellbeing%20of%20Pacific%20peoples-Jun2018.pdf

Barthow, C., Krebs, J., & McKinlay, E. (2023). A multiple case study of pre-diabetes care undertaken by general practice in Aotearoa/New Zealand: de-incentivised and de-prioritised work. BMC Primary Care, 24(1), 109.

Brown, R. (2018). Surviving the System: Māori and Pacific Whānau Coping Strategies to Overcome Health System Barriers. [Doctoral thesis, Auckland University of Technology]. Tuwhera. https://openrepository.aut.ac.nz/items/403a5513-569a-4ab6-8c77-5a88fcf7799e

Colmar Brunton. (2021). *Impact of COVID-19 on Pacific peoples living in South Auckland. Ministry of Health.* https://www.health.govt.nz/system/files/documents/pages/impact_of_covid-19_on_pacific_peoples_living_in_south_auckland.pdf

Fa'alogo-Lilo, C., & Cartwright, C. (2021). Barriers and supports experienced by Pacific peoples in Aotearoa New Zealand's mental health services. Journal of Cross-cultural psychology, 52(8–9), 752–770.

Health Quality & Safety Commission. (2021a). *Bula Sautu – A window on quality 2021: Pacific health in the year of COVID-19.* Wellington: Health Quality & Safety Commission. https://www.hqsc.govt.nz/resources/resource-library/bula-sautu-a-window-on-quality-2021-pacific-health-in-the-year-of-covid-19-bula-sautu-he-mata-kounga-2021-hauora-pasifika-i-te-tau-covid-19/

Health Quality & Safety Commission. (2021b). *Polypharmacy in people aged 65 and over.* https://www.hqsc.govt.nz/our-data/atlas-of-healthcare-variation/polypharmacy-in-people-aged-65-and-over/

Jeffreys, M., Smiler, K., Ellison Loschmann, L., Pledger, M., Kennedy, J., & Cumming, J. (2022). Consequences of barriers to primary health care for children in Aotearoa New Zealand. *SSM - Population Health*, *17*(101044). https://doi.org/10.1016/j.ssmph.2022.101044

Juang, R., Li, C., Harris, R. B., & Paine, S. J. (2023). Caregiver experiences of racism and child mental health outcomes: cross-sectional analysis from Aotearoa New Zealand. New Zealand Medical Journal, *136*, 28–43.

Lilo, L. S. U., Tautolo, E. S., & Smith, M. (2020). Health literacy, culture and Pacific peoples in Aotearoa-New Zealand: A review. Pacific Health, 3.

Meredith, I., Sarfati, D., Ikeda, T., & Blakely, T. (2012). Cancer in Pacific people in New Zealand. *Cancer Causes & Control*, *23*(7), 1173–1184. https://doi.org/10.1007/s10552-012-9986-x

Ministry of Health. (2022). Annual Data Explorer 2021/22: New Zealand Health Survey. https://minhealthnz.shinyapps.io/nz-health-survey-2020-21-annual-data-explorer/

Ministry of Health. (2023a). Annual Data Explorer 2022/23: New Zealand Health Survey. https://minhealthnz.shinyapps.io/nz-health-survey-2020-21-annual-data-explorer/

Ministry of Health. (2023b). *Te Mana Ola: The Pacific Health Strategy.* https://www.health.govt.nz/publication/te-mana-ola-pacific-health-strategy

Ministry of Health. (2023c). *Ambulatory sensitive (avoidable) hospital admissions.* https://www.health.govt.nz/new-zealand-health-system/accountability-and-funding/planning-and-performance-data/ambulatory-sensitive-avoidable-hospital-admissions

Mohammed, K., Nolan, M.B., Rajjo, T., Shah, N.D., Prokop, L.J., Varkey, P., & Murad, M.H. (2014). Creating a Patient-Centered Health Care Delivery System: A Systematic Review of Health Care Quality From the Patient Perspective: A Systematic Review of Health Care Quality From the Patient Perspective. *American Journal of Medical Quality*, 31(1), 12–21. https://doi.org/10.1177/1062860614545124

Ofanoa, S., Ofanoa, M., Tu'akoi, S., Lutui, H., Heather, M., Jansen, RM., Dalbeth, N., Grey, C., & Goodyear-Smith, F. (2023). Interventions designed to improve uptake of allopurinol for gout treatment in Aotearoa New Zealand: a scoping review. *Journal of Primary Health Care, 15*(1), 48–58. http://doi.org/10.1071/HC22094

Ofanoa, S., Ofanoa, M., Tu'akoi, S., Lutui, H., Heather, M., Jansen, RM., Dalbeth, N., Grey, C., & Goodyear-Smith, F. (2023). Interventions designed to improve uptake of allopurinol for gout treatment in Aotearoa New Zealand: a scoping review. *Journal of Primary Health Care, 15*(1), 48–58. http://doi.org/10.1071/HC22094

Pasifika Futures Limited (2023, March 23–24). *Pasifika Futures Limited Whanau Ora Model.* [Paper presentation], PFL Whanau Ora Conference 2023: Navigating New Waters, Auckland, New Zealand.

PHARMAC. (2019). *Achieving medicine access equity in Aotearoa New Zealand: towards a theory of change.* https://pharmac.govt.nz/about/access-equity/achieving-medicine-access-equity-in-aotearoa-new-zealand-towards-a-theory-of-change

Ryan, D., Grey, C., & Mischewski, B. (2019). *Tofa Saili: A review of evidence about health equity for Pacific Peoples in New Zealand.* Pacific Perspectives Ltd. https://www.pacificperspectives.co.nz/publications/

Sheridan, N., Love, T., & Kenealy, T. (2023). Is there equity of patient health outcomes across models of general practice in Aotearoa New Zealand? A national cross-sectional study. *International Journal for Equity in Health, 22*(1), 79.

Stokes, T., Azam, M., & Doolan Noble, F. (2018). Multimorbidity in Māori and Pacific patients: cross-sectional study in a Dunedin general practice. *Journal of Primary Health Care, 10*(1), 39–43. https://doi.org/10.1071/HC17046

Tiatia-Seath, J. (2018). The importance of Pacific cultural competency in healthcare. Pacific Health Dialog, 21(1), 8–9. https://doi.org/10.26635/phd.2018.909

Tukuitonga, C. (2021). COVID-19 in Pacific Islands People of Aotearoa/New Zealand: Communities Taking Control. Y Campbell & J Connell. (Eds.) *COVID in the Islands: A comparative perspective on the Caribbean and the Pacific*, 55–69.

Longitudinal and life course research: Pacific birth cohort study

El-Shadan Tautolo

Leon Iusitini

Chapter summary

This chapter focuses on longitudinal and lifecourse research in Aotearoa New Zealand. Our brief unpacking of the Pacific Islands Families Study as a longitudinal and lifecourse research takes into consideration today's context. A longitudinal lifecourse approach recognises the significant developmental factors across childhood, adolescence, and adulthood that affect Pacific health and wellbeing outcomes. The Pacific Islands Families Study utilises this understanding to support Pacific families to be successful and lead fulfilling and productive lives in Aotearoa New Zealand.

Introduction

Background context

Pacific peoples are an integral part of Aotearoa New Zealand (NZ) society with approximately 443,000 people of Pacific ethnicity residing in NZ (9% of the total population) (Stats NZ, 2025). Auckland has the largest population of Pacific people in NZ and is home to one of the largest Pacific populations in the world. Comprising at least 17 different Pacific ethnic groups, this ethnic diversity is manifested in differing cultures, languages, strength of acculturation, and corresponding access to (and utilisation of) health and social services. This young and growing Pacific population has a median age of 24.9 years, 13 years younger than the NZ population overall (Stats NZ, 2025).

Pacific peoples are woven intricately into the fabric of NZ society, and are a dynamic and diverse group that make a strong contribution to the community, the arts, religion, academic, sports, politics, and education. However, compared with the population as a whole, there is a lot of potential for Pacific people that remains under-utilised within the workforce and educational settings, which must be addressed and supported (Ministry of Pacific Peoples, 2021). The influence of Pacific peoples will only continue to increase in New Zealand as the future of this young population continues to materialise.

To understand and address the inequities experienced by Pacific families in NZ, it is necessary to examine the underlying drivers of health and wellbeing for Pacific families, as well as identify the barriers and support mechanisms necessary to improve these. In addition, strong cultural links and relationships with peers, family, and the wider community may also be instrumental in improving resilience in the face of adversity, and cultivating the potential for successful outcomes. Examining these facets of health and development using a longitudinal lifecourse approach is essential to recognising the important drivers for Pacific wellbeing, and utilising this understanding to support Pacific families to be successful and lead fulfilling and productive lives.

The PIF Study: A Pacific birth cohort study

The scarcity of robust culturally specific data, upon which to base appropriate health and wellbeing policies for Pacific families, led to the initiation of the Pacific Islands Families (PIF) birth cohort study. The PIF Study is a unique longitudinal study of Pacific children born in Middlemore Hospital, Auckland, in the year 2000, and includes their mothers and fathers as participants, something that has been rarely undertaken in previous longitudinal studies of this nature (Paterson et al., 2008).

The PIF Study team is based within the AUT Pacific Health Research Centre at the Auckland University of Technology (AUT). The PIF Study is specifically focused on exploring the health and wellbeing of Pacific children and their mothers, fathers, and the cultural nuances that impact on family wellbeing. The PIF Study also provides a platform for developing Pacific researchers and postgraduate scholarship within the research programme, and provides a valuable resource for Pacific stakeholders and policy-makers.

The specific aims of the PIF Study are to:

1. identify and characterise those individuals and families experiencing both positive and negative health and well-being outcomes
2. understand the mechanisms and processes shaping the pathways to those outcomes
3. make empirically-based strategic and tactical recommendations to improve the wellbeing of Pacific children and families, and thereby benefit New Zealand society as a whole.

Study design

Participants

The PIF Study team recruited 1,376 mothers of a cohort of 1,398 Pacific infants (22 pairs of twins) born at Middlemore Hospital (a large tertiary hospital) in South Auckland between 15 March and 19 December 2000. An infant was deemed eligible for the study if at least one of their parents identified themselves as being of a Pacific ethnicity and was a permanent resident of New Zealand. The cohort was recruited from Middlemore Hospital because its maternity division has the largest number of Pacific births in New Zealand.

A high response rate of 93% was achieved upon confirmation of eligibility criteria and since then regular contact has been maintained with a majority of the cohort.

While the composition of individual families has changed over time, adult participation in the study has always been determined by who the child's main caregivers are at any given phase (their mother or primary caregiver and father or secondary caregiver), as it is these adults who typically have the greatest influence on the child's development, health, and wellbeing. Attempts to contact all families are conducted at every phase, resulting in a fluctuating response rate, with most losses to follow-up occurring due to families moving outside the Auckland region. Information gathered at each phase confirms the current family structure and documents any changes that have taken place between phases.

Theoretical framework

The PIF Study draws from a life-course approach to understand the biological, behavioural, and psychosocial pathways to wellbeing and health among Pacific families within the New Zealand context (Ben-Shlomo & Kuh, 2002). Physical and social exposures over time are measured within a socio-ecological context (Bronfenbrenner, 1992). This integrated approach provides a broad, yet culturally appropriate, modelling structure to understand the way external factors impact on the wellbeing, health, and development of Pacific families. Specifically, this approach provides insights into the central role of parents, the supporting roles performed by family and peers during childhood and adolescence and the influence of institutions such as schools and health services on the health and development of the family.

Documenting the timing, duration, and context of exposures to advantage and disadvantage is important for designing optimal interventions that promote healthy outcomes. Implicit to this approach is the notion of the clustering of risks (Graham, 2002). Accumulated success or disadvantage across time predicts a range of interpersonal circumstances and health and wellbeing outcomes throughout life (Poulton et al., 2002). These models recognise that development is not simply a process of progressively building on what has gone before, with changes in individual trajectories being important for identifying the pathways and the markers that predict outcomes. Such transition points are regarded as the key time for effective policy intervention (Sanders, 1995). The longitudinal research methodology of the PIF Study enables the research team to leverage the extensive data already obtained, in order to model pathways to successful adaptation.

Data collection

The PIF Study primarily collects self-reported data through structured interviews with mothers (*maternal interview*) and fathers (*paternal interview*) in their homes, and with teachers (*teacher questionnaire*) and children (*child assessment*) in their schools or homes depending on their age at the time of survey. Children and their families have been visited when the children were aged 6 weeks, and 1, 2, 4, 6, 9, 11, 14, 17, 22 and most recently at 25 years of age (Figure 1), providing valuable data at key transition points (for example, the transition to school, and from childhood to adolescence).

Maternal and child measures of psychosocial and physical health outcomes have comprised the core measures completed at every time point (for example, general health; child behaviour; growth and development; peer, family, and community relationships; acculturation; physical health), while paternal and teacher assessments have occurred at specific stages throughout the lifecourse.

The longitudinal nature of the data provides the ability to look at stability and changes in these phenomena throughout the

Figure 1: PIF Study data collection phases and participant involvement at each timepoint.

Teacher questionnaire					✓	✓	✓		
Child assessment	✓	✓	✓	✓	✓	✓	✓	✓	✓
Paternal interview		✓	✓		✓		✓	✓	✓
Maternal interview	✓	✓	✓	✓	✓	✓	✓	✓	✓
	6 weeks	1 year	2 years	4 years	6 years	9 years	11 years	14 years	18 years
				Different timepoints of data collection					

lifecourse development of the participants. The specific dimensions and instruments employed in the main PIF Study have been described elsewhere (Paterson et al., 2008).

The importance of the family has been described as the basis for individual and social wellbeing (Bogenschneider & Corbett, 2010). Individuals benefit from the emotional and financial support of their family, and families fulfil a range of functions that benefit society. The role of caring for children and providing education and socialisation for the next generation represents the cornerstone of a society in which individuals flourish (Coleman & Ganong, 2004). However, family wellbeing is impacted by a complicated range of factors.

The following section focuses on selected case study examples that examine particular facets of family wellbeing, physical growth, metabolic risk, and cultural resilience.

Case study: Physical growth, metabolic risk, and potential lifecourse outcomes

The trajectories of growth and weight gain from early childhood to adolescence and potential risk for metabolic disease are not well understood (Plank et al., 2019). An important objective of the PIF Study has been to examine the trajectories for bodyweight and physical growth among Pacific children from 2 to 14 years of age, as well as identifying potential metabolic risk factors in the later years.

Statistical analysis of PIF Study data on the weight of each cohort member (expressed as z scores relative to the mean) was calculated at a range of ages (2, 4, 6, 9, 11, and 14 years). Growth trajectories or curves were then constructed by estimating the linear trend of z scores across age for each child. The results indicated a higher bodyweight in early childhood (compared to the World Health Organization reference child) with relatively rapid weight gain over subsequent years. This rapid growth was associated with a number of risk factors for metabolic disease, including insulin resistance, blood pressure, vitamin D, and urate levels.

A more intensive suite of testing was undertaken with a subgroup of 204 PIF cohort members at age 14/15, using blood samples to measure biomarkers of metabolic risk and comparing them with the growth trajectories previously constructed. These comparisons indicated that more rapid growth was associated with higher concentrations of insulin, leptin, urate, and markers of liver function, insulin resistance, and inflammation. Both rapid weight gain and a higher body weight in early childhood were associated with higher risk for metabolic disease. Monitoring growth trajectories and understanding the underlying patterns and associations with metabolic risks may supports the development of targeted interventions to optimise nutrition and growth for Pacific children. In addition, these trajectory patterns linking rapid growth with metabolic risk are only possible because of the longitudinal design of the study, highlighting the value of this kind of data.

Case study: Role of cultural alignment and identity in maintaining wellbeing

Pivotal research findings throughout several waves of the PIF Study suggest the retention of strong cultural links to Pacific cultures is likely to have positive health and wellbeing benefits for Pacific families (Borrows et al., 2011; Tautolo, 2011; Tautolo et al., 2009, 2011).

The PIF Study has explored this phenomenon of acculturation or cultural alignment across several different waves of the PIF Study. The concept of acculturation describes the process or changes that groups and individuals undergo when they come into continuous contact with another culture (Berry, 2006, 2010).

Maternal acculturation and its association with infant and maternal health risk indicators, was investigated among the PIF Study cohort. Results revealed that mothers with strong alignment to Pacific culture had better infant and maternal outcomes than those with weak cultural alignment (Borrows et al., 2011). The children of mothers who possess a strong link to their Pacific culture are also significantly less likely to experience clinical-range internalising and externalising behavioural problems across early childhood compared to children of mothers with weaker links to their Pacific culture, suggesting a protective effect of retention of Pacific cultural practices.

Further research found significantly different patterns of acculturation between immigrant and New Zealand-born Pacific mothers (Schluter et al., 2011). The length of time resident in New Zealand was positively associated with increased alignment to New Zealand mainstream culture. Moreover, foreign-born Pacific mothers generally maintain their strong Pacific cultural alignment for approximately 12 years after arriving in New Zealand, after which time the strength of this alignment decreases and approaches the level observed by mothers who have lived their lives entirely in New Zealand (Schluter et al., 2011). This pattern is consistent with international findings (Berry, 2010), and could suggest that the positive influence of strong cultural alignment may need to be maintained or strengthened once migrants have been resident within NZ society for an extended period. Nonetheless, these findings demonstrate the benefits of PIF Study's longitudinal study design, and the possibilities for this kind of information to support beneficial outcomes for Pacific peoples.

Knowledge translation and impact

Findings have been utilised by numerous government agencies such as the Ministry of Pacific Peoples (inform policy advice to Government), Ministry of Social Development (domestic violence), the Ministry of Health (Food and Nutrition Guidelines, Food security), and other stakeholders such as Counties Manukau District Health Board (Let's Beat Diabetes project, Otitis media screening), and the National Heart Foundation (Pacific Heartbeat Certificate in Pacific Nutrition programme).

In addition, generalisability of PIF Study research to migrant populations in other countries continues to make important contributions to dissemination and international research impact in Pacific health and related areas.

Current and future research with the PIF Study

The PIF Study provides extensive quantitative and qualitative data on the risk and protective factors that affect individual and family wellbeing for Pacific people. However, the cohort has transitioned from childhood to adolescence and now, 20 years later, into early adulthood. This has necessitated a focus on exploring issues and priorities for young Pacific adults, such as mental wellbeing, economic status and employment, and cultural resiliency and identity. The context in which such issues and priorities for young Pacific adults occur has been affected by the health and societal impacts linked to COVID-19. Many of these current themes were the focus of an upcoming data collection with the cohort at 22 and 25 years of age.

In addition, with the global increase in older aged people within the population, including for Pacific communities, it is crucial to understand how best to support and meet the needs and aspirations of our older Pacific population. The PIF research team has been undertaking research as part of the Ageing Well New Zealand National Science Challenge to explore healthy ageing among older Pacific people, and utilising older parents and grandparents of the PIF birth cohort as participants. Alongside stakeholder partnerships with Vaka Tautua and other Pacific agencies, the findings have been beneficial in identifying priority focus areas for the health of older Pacific people, and ensuring research findings can be directly implemented for the benefit of our Pacific families and communities.

The PIF Study continues to be an integral part of both national and international research collaborations, particularly involving lifecourse development and the impact of early life exposures across the lifecourse. Funding continues to be an important consideration in continuing this essential work, however the continued support from the Health Research Council, Royal Society of New Zealand, and other funding bodies throughout the last 20 years, is gratefully acknowledged and recognised.

Conclusion

Findings from the PIF Study highlight the importance of longitudinal research in understanding the impact of family environments and interactions upon child development. Healthy and well-functioning families contribute to healthy children and support better long-term outcomes across the lifecourse. The PIF team will continue to work more closely with key stakeholder agencies to improve our overall understanding of the wellbeing of Pacific families. This collaborative approach will ensure that PIF findings will continue to bring Pacific issues to the fore, and equip Pacific groups with the tools to improve their own outcomes. It also enables agencies to lobby for policy and organisational change while providing them with robust pragmatic knowledge to promote family health and wellbeing for Pacific peoples in New Zealand.

References

Ben-Shlomo, Y., & Kuh, D. (2002). A life course approach to chronic disease epidemiology: conceptual models, empirical challenges and interdisciplinary perspectives. *International Journal of Epidemiology*, *31*(2), 285–293.

Berry, J. (2006). Contexts of Acculturation. In D. L. Sam & J. W. Berry (Eds.), *Cambridge Handbook of Acculturation Psychology* (1st ed., pp. 27–42). Cambridge University Press. https://doi.org/10.1017/CBO9780511489891

Berry, J. (2010). Intercultural Relations and Acculturation in the Pacific Region. *Journal of Pacific Rim Psychology, 4*(2), 95–102. http://doi.org/10.1375/prp.4.2.95

Bogenschneider, K., & Corbett, T. J. (2010). Family policy: Becoming a field of inquiry and subfield of social policy. *Journal of Marriage and Family, 72*(3), 783–803. https://doi.org/10.1111/j.1741-3737.2010.00730.x

Borrows, J., Williams, M., Schluter, P., Paterson, J., & Langitoto Helu, S. (2011). Pacific Islands Families Study: The Association of Infant Health Risk Indicators and Acculturation of Pacific Island Mothers Living in New Zealand. *Journal of Cross-Cultural Psychology, 42*(5), 699–724. https://doi.org/10.1177/0022022110362750

Bronfenbrenner, U. (1992). Ecological systems theory. In R. Vasta (Ed.), *Six theories of child development: Revised formulations and current issues* (1st ed., pp. 285–296). Jessica Kingsley Publishers.

Coleman, M., & Ganong, L. (2004). *Handbook of Contemporary Families: Considering the Past, Contemplating the Future.* Sage.

Graham H. (2002). Building an inter-disciplinary science of health inequalities: the example of lifecourse research. *Social Science and Medicine, 55*(11), 2005–2016. https://doi.org/10.1016/s0277-9536(01)00343-4

Ministry for Pacific Peoples. (2021). *Pacific Economy Research Report on Unpaid Work and Volunteering in Aotearoa.*

Paterson, J., Percival, T., Schluter, P., Sundborn, G., Abbott, M., Carter, S., Cowley-Malcolm, E., Borrows, J., Gao, W., & PIF Study Group (2008). Cohort profile: The Pacific Islands Families (PIF) Study. *International Journal of Epidemiology, 37*(2), 273–279. https://doi.org/10.1093/ije/dym171

Plank, L. D., Obolonkin, V., Smith, M., Savila, F., Jalili-Moghaddam, S., Tautolo, E. S., & Rush, E. C. (2019). Pacific Islands Families Study: Physical growth to age 14 and metabolic risk. *Pediatric Obesity, 14*(5), e12497. https://doi.org/10.1111/ijpo.12497

Poulton, R., Caspi, A., Milne, B. J., Thomson, W. M., Taylor, A., Sears, M. R., & Moffitt, T. E. (2002). Association between children's experience of socioeconomic disadvantage and adult health: a life-course study. *The Lancet, 360*(9346), 1640–1645. https://doi.org/10.1016/S0140-6736(02)11602-3

Sanders, M. (1995). *Healthy Families, Healthy Nation: Strategies for Promoting Family Mental Health in Australia.* Australian Academic Press.

Schluter, P. J., Tautolo, E., & Paterson, J. (2011). Acculturation of Pacific mothers in New Zealand over time: findings from the Pacific Islands Families study. *BMC Public Health, 11*, 307. https://doi.org/10.1186/1471-2458-11-307

Stats NZ. (2025). *Pacific Peoples ethnicities in Aotearoa New Zealand.* https://www.stats.govt.nz/infographics/detailed-ethnicity-infographics-from-2023-census/pacific-peoples-ethnicities-in-aotearoa-new-zealand/

Tautolo, E., Schluter, P. J., & Sundborn, G. (2009). Mental health well-being amongst fathers within the Pacific Island Families Study. *Pacific Health Dialog, 15*(1), 69–78.

Tautolo, E. (2011). *Pacific fathers cultivating the future: The health of Pacific fathers and their influence upon and involvement with their children.* [Doctoral Thesis, Auckland University of Technology]. Tuwhera. https://openrepository.aut.ac.nz/items/f7329e73-0ca7-4f2c-9d43-a55657f8da37

Tautolo, E., Schluter, P. J., Paterson, J., & McRobbie, H. (2011). Acculturation status has a modest effect on smoking prevalence among a cohort of Pacific fathers in New Zealand. *Australian and New Zealand Journal of Public Health, 35*(6), 509–516. https://doi.org/10.1111/j.1753-6405.2011.00774.x

Prosperous Pacific families through Whānau Ora

Debbie Sorensen

John Huakau

Chapter summary

This chapter focuses on advancing Pacific peoples wellbeing through Whānau Ora and the work of Pasifika Futures, the first and former Pacific Whānau Ora Commissioning Agency in Aotearoa New Zealand. This chapter begins with a short section on the background to the origins of the New Zealand government's Whānau Ora initiative (called Whānau Ora) and how Pasifika Futures defines Whānau Ora for Pacific peoples in Aotearoa. Throughout this chapter the nomenclature uses lower case when referring to the concept of Whānau Ora and upper case when referring to the Whānau Ora policy (as used in Moore (2014) and in Boulton, Gifford, Allport and White (2018)). This chapter's focus is on Pasifika Futures the Pacific Whānau Ora commissioning agency and its commissioning for outcomes approach and how it has progressed the Vision of 'Prosperity for Pacific Peoples' through 'Supporting Pacific Families to Shape a better Future'.

Introduction

Whanau Ora began as a government initiative in 2009 when the Taskforce on Whānau Centred Initiatives was established to develop an evidence-based framework to strengthen Whānau capabilities and support families to become self-determining. The Whānau Ora framework drew on extensive evidence, hui Māori and consultation of what works to build whānau capabilities and outcomes. Pacific families are resilient, dynamic, and experience the worst social, economic, and health outcomes in New Zealand with persistent inequities despite decades of government interventions. To transform our future, we created the Pacific Commissioning Agency, Pasifika Futures, deeply anchored in our cultural contexts. We developed a shared outcomes framework co-designed with communities and commissioned Pacific partner organisations to improve outcomes with Pacific families. To harness our collective power, we have a relational commissioning model that invests in growing the capacity and capability of our organisation and our partners to measure and achieve outcomes.

Background to Whānau Ora

Whānau Ora, the government initiative, began in 2009 with the development of an evidence-based framework to strengthen Whānau capabilities and self-determination (Taskforce for Whānau Centred Initiatives, 2010). In 2013, the government expanded Whānau Ora to include Pacific families, while also establishing three Non-Governmental Commissioning Agencies. Pasifika futures, a Pacific owned (owned wholly by the Pasifika Medical Association) and led organisation was appointed as the Pacific Commissioning Agency for Pacific Families in Aotearoa.

The concept of whānau ora and origins of the Whānau Ora Initiative

In 2009, Dame Tariana Turia, Minister for the Community and Voluntary Sector under the 2008 National-led government, convened the Taskforce on Whānau-Centred Initiatives with the main objective of the Taskforce to be to construct an evidence-based framework that will lead to:

- Strengthened Whānau capabilities
- An integrated approach to Whānau wellbeing
- Collaborative relationships between state agencies in relation to Whānau services
- Relationships between government and community agencies that are broader than contractual, and
- Improved cost-effectiveness and value for money.

Dame Turia stated that the main goal of the Taskforce on Whānau-Centred Initiatives was to develop a policy framework for 'a new method of government interaction with Māori service providers to meet the needs of whānau' Moore (2014).

He Korowai Oranga stated that:

'The outcomes sought for whānau included:

- Whānau experience physical, spiritual, mental, and emotional health and have control over their own destinies
- Whānau members live longer and enjoy a better quality of life
- Whānau members (including those with disabilities) participate in te ao Māori and wider New Zealand society.

And that these outcomes are more likely where:

- Whānau are cohesive, nurturing, and safe
- Whānau are able to give and receive support
- Whānau have a secure identity, high self-esteem, confidence, and pride
- Whānau have the necessary physical, social, and economic means to participate fully and to provide for their own needs, and
- Whānau live, work, and play in safe and supportive environments

(Source: Ministry of Health, 2002).

Sir Mason Durie stated that the Taskforce on Whānau-Centred Initiatives further expanded the meaning of Whānau Ora to reflect outcomes across social, cultural, and economic dimensions, and used the Whānau Ora philosophy that is based on Māori cultural foundations of a communal approach to wellbeing, group capacities for self-determination, intergenerational transfers of knowledge and values, and full participation within society. Whānau Ora's aim was to shift attention from individuals to collectives, from sectoral interventions to intersectoral collaboration, from crisis intervention to capability building, and from process indicators to measures of outcomes for Whānau (Ministry of Health, 2011).

The Taskforce on Whānau-Centred Initiatives in their 2010 Report entitled Whānau Ora laid the framework for Phase one and Phase two of Whānau Ora.

In a summary of the Taskforce on Whānau-Centred Initiatives Framework the Auditor General noted that the Taskforce recommended that:

- Providers should work with Whānau instead of focusing on the specific needs of one or two people within a Whānau.
- That funders, government and non-government providers, and whānau – would need to change from a 'deficit approach' to a 'strengths-based approach' to achieve best outcomes for Māori, and that funders, providers, and Whānau would also need to start, working together.
- Providers working within a Whānau Ora framework should have more flexibility in how they meet Whānau needs. Contracts should focus on the improvements achieved by Whānau rather than outputs.
- Providers (as well as government agencies and community organisations) should have networks or alliances to ensure smooth referrals and co-ordinated services for Whānau.
- An independent trust should be formed to govern, co-ordinate, and implement Whānau Ora, and report to a Minister for Whānau Ora; a specific Whānau Ora appropriation be established for the trust to manage;
- Whānau ora services should be integrated and comprehensive, and focused on measurable outcomes that will help to empower whānau; Whānau Ora services should be shaped by te ao Māori; all government agencies with responsibilities for any aspect of Whānau well-being commit to Whānau Ora principles and support Whānau Ora initiatives; and the trust establish regional groups to ensure that Whānau Ora contributes in positive and realistic ways in local communities.

The Taskforce on Whānau-Centred Initiatives recommendations laid the foundation for commissioning for outcomes and the establishment of the three independent Whānau Ora Commissioning Agencies that have existed since 2014. Based on the recommendations a paper to cabinet charged Te Puni Kōkiri (TPK) with the responsibility to establish the Whānau Ora initiative for both Māori and Pacific peoples. Governance and accountability arrangements were put in place, TPK under Vote Māori Development would be the Crown Agency responsible for Whānau Ora and would report directly to the Minister for Whānau Ora.

In July 2013, Cabinet decided to set up three Whānau Ora Commissioning Agencies, whose purpose was described as funding support for building the capability of Whānau (Auditor General's 2015 Report). With the main idea being that more Whānau Ora funding would be distributed by TPK to the Whānau Ora Commissioning Agencies who were independent trusts that were at arm's length from TPK and who would be better able to commission the funding to Whānau Ora Partners in the community who were closest to whānau and families.

Commissioning can be defined as a set of inter-related tasks that need to be undertaken to turn policy objectives into effective social services. Effective commissioning is fundamental to well-functioning social services (The Productivity Commission, 2015).

This led to the establishment of the sole Whānau Ora commissioning agency for all Pacific peoples in Aotearoa called Pasifika Futures Ltd (Pasifika Futures).

In the next section we focus on Pasifika Futures; the Pacific Whānau Ora Commissioning Agency and its commissioning for outcomes approach.

Pasifika Futures

At Pasifika Futures the concept of Whānau Ora is defined as a multifaceted approach to supporting family wellbeing, which is family-centred, culturally anchored, evidenced based, supports self-determination, and is unique to each family's circumstance, realities, goals, and aspirations.

Pasifika Futures was the sole Whānau Ora Commissioning Agency for Pacific people across Aotearoa and is an independent trust fully owned by the Pasifika Medical Association. The Pasifika Medical Association was awarded the Whānau Ora Commissioning Agency for Pacific peoples after a 12-month long tender process. Pasifika Futures was established and was funded through TPK to initially commission support to over 2,000 families with its first annual budget of $5 million (in financial year FY2014/15). Fast-forward to FY2023/24 and Pasifika Futures commissions over $45 million of Whānau Ora funding to support over 7,000 families per annum and has a provider network of 78 Whānau Ora partners (including 27 short-term community and emergency response partners). In addition to Whānau Ora funding Pasifika Futures also commissions around $25 million of health and mental health funding. Pasifika Futures since its inception has grown to become the largest non-governmental Pacific organisation in Aotearoa and the Pacific in terms of both revenue and reach, and in the number of wellbeing outcomes achieved with Pacific families.

Commissioning for outcomes is a new and innovative approach that Pasifika Futures has been using since 2014. Pasifika Futures' Whānau Ora commissioning approach is an integrated and inter-generational program that works with the whole family. It includes provider capability and capacity enhancement which was critical in the development of the Whānau Ora partner network. The approach worked with Whānau Ora partners to change how they traditionally operated with families moving away from the transactional approach to a relational approach with families. This required partners (providers) to reimagine the relationship with families, to see themselves as facilitators and supporters rather than experts in aspects of Pacific people's lives. It required a renewed focus with families at the centre, rather than the traditional provider driven services. The approach also supports partners to enhance their knowledge and skills around Whānau Ora with training opportunities for the workforce to become skilled and trained in the navigational model.

The Commissioning for outcomes model is culturally anchored, evidence based, and contracts Whānau Ora Partners on high-trust integrated service contracts for periods of 3–4 years. The contracts are relational and based on achieving outcomes for families and asks partners to describe the impact they are making with families and to provide evidence of progress and how they made a difference to the lives of families. Through this process families are able to chart their own progress.

Vision and purpose

Pasifika Futures vision is 'Prosperous Pacific families' and its purpose is to 'Support Pacific families to shape a better future'. Its values are family, service, integrity, diversity, relationships, leadership, and being strength-based.

From the very beginning, Pasifika Futures positioned families to lead the vision and purpose of the organisation and determine the priorities for focus. Healthy, educated, undertaking vocational work that makes them happy and brings them joy, strengthening cultural understanding, and making sure they were on a pathway to economic and financial prosperity are the pillars that guide the agency.

Leadership and governance

Pasifika Futures Ltd has a Chief Operating Officer (CEO) and board of directors who reflect the shared values and interests of the Pacific communities and have proven leadership and governance skills, as well as experience in operating within cultural frameworks. They have extensive networks throughout Aotearoa and the region built on family, village, kinship, professional, sporting, church, cultural, education, business, and community relationships. As individuals who have dedicated their lives to serving Pacific communities, the relationships are deep and multi-faceted. They have strong credibility and integrity and are recognised community leaders.

Board of directors

Chair Dr Tearikivao (Kiki) Maoate ONZM, FRACS (Cook Islands Māori) is a Paediatric Surgeon and Urologist based in Christchurch. Dr Maoate is the Chair of Pasifika Futures Ltd and President and Chair of the Pasifika Medical Association Group. He is a leader in the Cook Islands community and in the health and education sector in both Aotearoa and internationally. He is Associate Dean, Pacific Health, University of Otago based in Christchurch.

Dr Francis Agnew MNZM, FRANZCP, FACHAM (Cook Islands Māori) is a pioneer in the development of Pacific mental health services in Aotearoa and the Pacific region. He is a leader in Pacific mental health and addiction services in Aotearoa and has served on many government reviews, committees, and task forces. Dr Agnew is a Director of Pasifika Medical Association Group.

Dr Siniva Sinclair FAFPHM, MPH (Samoan) was born and raised in Papua New Guinea. Siniva is a fellow of the Australasian Faculty of Public Health Medicine and has completed a Master's in Public Health.

La'auli Sir Michael Jones KMHZ, MNZH (Samoan) has a wealth of experience having worked in tertiary education and Pacific economic development. La'auli is passionate about economic and social development for Pacific people in Aotearoa and in New Zealand.

Mrs Soana Akolotu Pamaka BA, Auck Dip Tchg ACE (Tongan) is an educational leader, serving the community of Glen Innes for the past 30 years. Soana is passionate about enabling the community through educational opportunities and success and supporting educational innovation. Mrs Pamaka is the Principal at Tamaki College.

Chief Operating Officer

Mrs Debbie Sorensen ONZM, CCT, CMInstD, MNZIOD (Tongan) Debbie Sorensen is the CEO of Pasifika Futures Ltd and the Pasifika Medical Association Group of charitable companies.

Debbie has been instrumental in the development of Pacific health services in Aotearoa and the region over the past 30 years. She has held leadership roles in the Ministry of Health, District Health Boards and International Consultancy firms. She has led the development of the Pasifika Medical Association group over the past 20 years, transforming it into the largest Non-Governmental Pacific organisation in the region.

Pasifika Futures strategy and outcomes framework

Pasifika Futures supports Pacific families to achieve well-being outcomes across the five aspirational outcome domains (see outcomes framework) through its strategy shown below. The strategy highlights its principles, how it delivers programmes, and provides organisational support which is foundational in achieving these aspirational outcomes.

Our Strategy

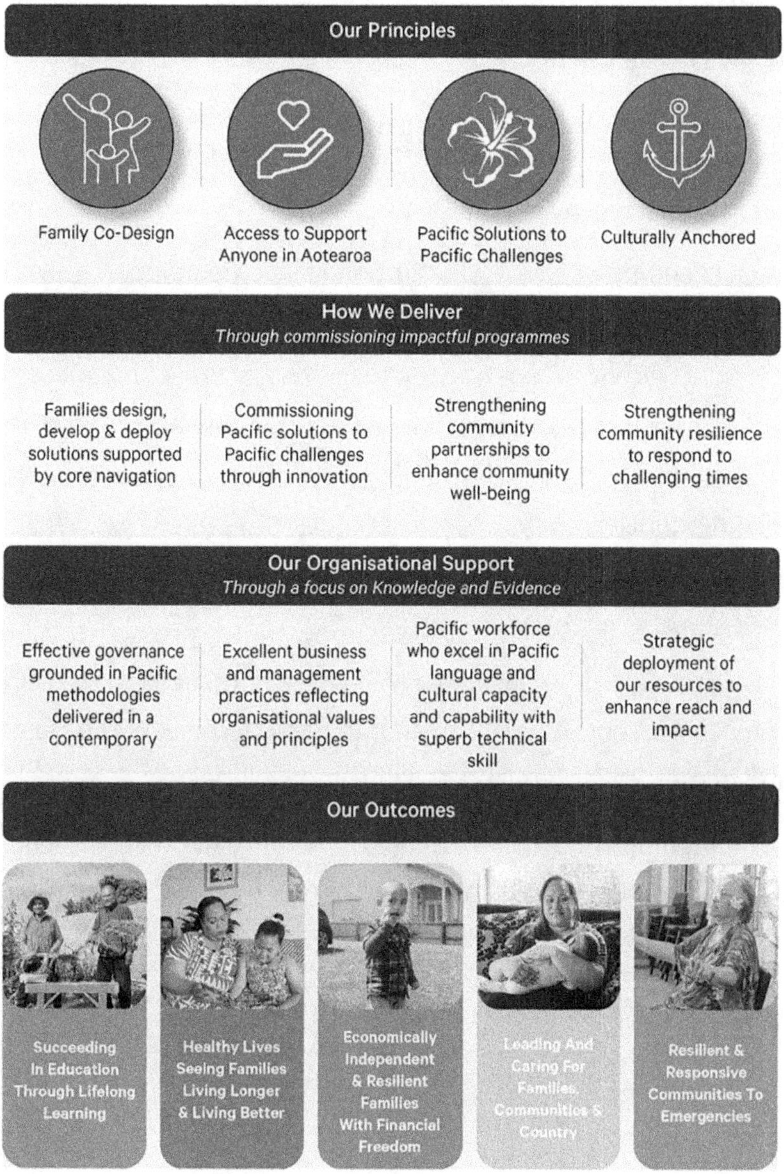
Our Principles
Family Co-Design
Access to Support Anyone in Aotearoa
Pacific Solutions to Pacific Challenges
Culturally Anchored
How We Deliver
Through commissioning impactful programmes
Families design, develop & deploy solutions supported by core navigation
Commissioning Pacific solutions to Pacific challenges through innovation
Strengthening community partnerships to enhance community well-being
Strengthening community resilience to respond to challenging times
Our Organisational Support
Through a focus on Knowledge and Evidence
Effective governance grounded in Pacific methodologies delivered in a contemporary
Excellent business and management practices reflecting organisational values and principles
Pacific workforce who excel in Pacific language and cultural capacity and capability with superb technical skill
Strategic deployment of our resources to enhance reach and impact
Our Outcomes
Succeeding In Education Through Lifelong Learning
Healthy Lives Seeing Families Living Longer & Living Better
Economically Independent & Resilient Families With Financial Freedom
Leading And Caring For Families, Communities & Country
Resilient & Responsive Communities To Emergencies

Pasifika Futures outcomes framework

From several years of Talanoa with over 1,000 Pacific families the high-level outcome domains Pasifika Futures supports Pacific families to achieve are:

- Succeeding in education through lifelong learning
- Healthy lives: Seeing families living longer and living better
- Economically independent and finanically resilient families
- Leading and caring for families, communities, and country
- Resilient and responsive families and communities (to emergencies).

Pasifika futures has developed and utilised a culturally anchored and evidence based outcomes framework that is focussed on a holistic set of Pacific family well-being outcomes (Jensen, Sorensen & Jensen, 2019). The outcomes framework measures and frames Pacific family prosperity and well-being.

The outcomes framework contains short-, medium-, and long-term outcome we expect to see within each of the five outcome domains and is shown below.

OUTCOMES FRAMEWORK

	Short Term Participation (1-4 years)	**Medium Term** Engagement (5-9 years)	**Long Term** Achievement (10+ years)
Succeeding in Education Through Lifelong Learning	**Pacific families are:** ▸ Well prepared for schooling ▸ Identifying their educational pathways ▸ Understanding how to support and nurture educational success	**Pacific families are:** ▸ Achieving educational success ▸ Supporting and nurturing educational success ▸ Technically literate	**Lifelong Learning** ▸ Pacific families are achieving success across all educational pathways.
Healthy Lives: Seeing Families Living Longer and Living Better	**Pacific families are:** ▸ Embarking on the journey to live a smoke-free and healthy lifestyle ▸ Partnering with health professionals in the management of their health ▸ Fully immunized ▸ Progressing towards achieving their aspirations for those living with disabilities	**Pacific families are:** ▸ Smoke free ▸ Physically active and making healthy eating choices ▸ Managing their health in partnership with health professionals ▸ Actively participating in national screening programmes ▸ Able to manage their mental health & well-being needs	**Living longer, living better** ▸ Pacific families experience wellbeing and a high quality of life.
Economically Independent and Resilient With Financial Freedom	**Pacific families are:** ▸ Becoming economically independent ▸ Engaging with support to reduce their debt ▸ Engaged in a range of pathways that provide successful employment and business opportunities	**Pacific families are:** ▸ Economically independent and resilient ▸ Reducing their indebtedness ▸ Owning and operating their own businesses ▸ On a pathway to home ownership	**Financial freedom** ▸ Pacific families are economically independent and resilient.
Community Connections: Leading and Caring For Our Families, Communities and Country	**Pacific families are:** ▸ Taking leadership in providing healthy and safe environments for their families ▸ Strong in their cultural capital and sense of belonging ▸ Understanding the diversity of our communities ▸ Actively participating in their communities	**Pacific families are:** ▸ Living in healthy, safe & violence-free environments ▸ Strong leaders, influential, foster resilience and empower each other to improve their lives ▸ Accept and advocate for the inclusion of our diversity ▸ Involved and influential in their civic duties ▸ Prepared & resilient to face emergencies	**Community Connection** ▸ Pacific families are leading and connected to their families, communities and country.
Resilient And Responsive Families And Communities	**Pacific families are:** ▸ Knowledgeable about how to protect and prepere their families ▸ Have access to resources to support themselves ▸ Are able to stay safe and access support when they need it ▸ Are connected to Whānau Ora support across the country	**Pacific families are:** ▸ Technically literate and support and nurture educational success ▸ are engaged in a range of pathways to employment and business opportunities ▸ are fully immunised and managing their health in partnership with health professionals ▸ are prepared, connected and engaged to face emergencies	**Resilient and Responsive Pacific communities to emergencies:** ▸ Pacific families and leaders are adaptive, connected and prepared

The following graphic highlights what Pasifika Futures does through its regionally based partners to support Pacific families to achieve their aspirations within each of these five outcome domains.

What We Do

Pasifika Futures is a Whānau Ora Commissioning Agency. We work with regionally based partners to build the capability and capacity of Pacific families. Pasifika Futures supports Pacific families to achieve their aspirations in health, housing, education, training and economic development.

Succeeding in Education
We build lifelong learning with Pacific families, through enrolling in early childhood education, achieving at school, helping families support their children's development, supporting school leavers into education, employment or training, and gaining tertiary education qualifications.

Healthy Lives
We work alongside Pacific families to live longer and better lives through supporting Pacific families in healthy eating and exercise, immunisation and screening, healthy homes, primary care access, stopping smoking, managing long-term health conditions, and supporting people with disabilities to achieve their aspirations and access services.

Economically Independent and Resilient
We work with Pacific families to build a pathway to financial freedom, through reducing debt, increasing income and savings, gaining and strengthening employment and owning their own homes.

Leadership, Culture and Community Connections
We build on the strengths of Pacific communities to live in safe and supported environments, through fostering Pacific languages, strengthening community connections and participation, resolving conflict non-violently, and ensuring elderly people are safe and connected.

Resilient & Responsive Communities to Emergencies
Pacific families and leaders are adaptive, connected and prepared.

The basis of what we do is reflected in our values which underpin the Pasifika Futures commissioning approach. This includes:

- All activities and interventions are driven by families.
- Self-determination and empowerment of families.
- The model is relationship based not transactional.

- A skilled navigation workforce that are culturally anchored, hold Pacific language proficiency, and are technically expert.

A key framework and methodology that is used by Pasifika Futures to inform their activities and processes is the Talanoa methodology (Vaioleti, 2016; Jensen et al., 2019). Talanoa provides Pasifika Futures with a culturally embedded and congruent approach to Whānau Ora Commissioning. Talanoa is a term shared by different Pacific ethnicities (Tongan, Samoan, Fijian) and is a concept that is familiar to other nations. Jensen et al. (2019) describe the methodology and its application within Pasifika Futures as more than a method of good empathetic conversation. It is a transformative space that enables 'self-determination for Pacific families and communities' where Pacific social and cultural contexts are considered and integrated. The methodology enables and engages Pacific families, staff, community organisations to identify issues, and co-create knowledge solutions and relationships to support the achievement of outcomes.

Based on the Talanoa methodology a framework called the Knowledge, Engagement, Enablement and Performance (KEEP) Framework that ensures Pasifika Futures processes are evidence based, dialogue and actions focussed, and accountable to improve family outcomes (Jensen et al., 2019). The utilisation of the Talanoa methodology by Whānau Ora programmes has created a strength based culture that is culturally anchored and supports the capability and capacity of navigation staff and organisations to achieve results with families (Jensen et al., 2019).

Whānau Ora services that are offered by Pasifika Futures are based on addressing the social and economic hardships that Pacific families face. The multidimensional approach allows for customisation of each program to suit the needs and aspirations of individual families.

Commissioning programmes

Pasifika Futures commissioning for outcomes approach has four commissioning workstreams. As described below:

- **Commissioning for Core Navigation:** Core commissioning involves working with partners to support Pacific families across Aotearoa to achieve their dreams and aspirations by improving family outcomes.
- **Commissioning for Innovative Pacific Solutions:** Innovation programmes involve working with partners to support families to achieve their aspirations in one or more outcome areas.
- **Commissioning to Strengthen Community Partnerships:** Commissioning for communities enables small community organisations who work with largely volunteer groups to support Pacific families.
- **Commissioning for Responsive and Resilient Communities**: Commissioning a network of community partners who respond when Pacific families are in need due to a disaster, crisis, or public health emergency.

The family journey

The family journey illustrated below describes activities taken as a family advances towards achieving their goals and aspirations. While family strengths, needs, and support are customised to the unique family context, processes for data collection and monitoring are standardised and used to evaluate families between cohorts. The Pasifika Futures Measurement Assessment Scoring Tool (MAST) measures family's strengths and challenges allowing the family to develop their vision and goals. Navigators play a crucial role in ensuring families can achieve their aspirations improving health and wellbeing outcomes. The report by Koloto and Misa (2018) indicate the success of strengthening the role of navigators in Whānau Ora programmes as they play an important part as family advisors, encouragers, guides, connectors, and much more. The skills qualities and characteristics that are possessed by navigators include (Koloto and Misa 2018):

- Empathy towards families.
- Knowledge of the New Zealand health, social, and welfare systems and services.
- Good problem solver.
- Skilled facilitator.
- Culturally competent.

The integration of cultural models and practices into the development of the navigation workforce has been effective in improving the wellbeing outcomes of Pacific families. The 'Our Way' customised training for all navigators has improved engagement of navigators with families. An additional intervention to ensure a well-trained workforce has been the establishment of the micro credentialling course (HLTHSCI 7001MC) at the University of Auckland which has enrolled its first cohort of 40 people.

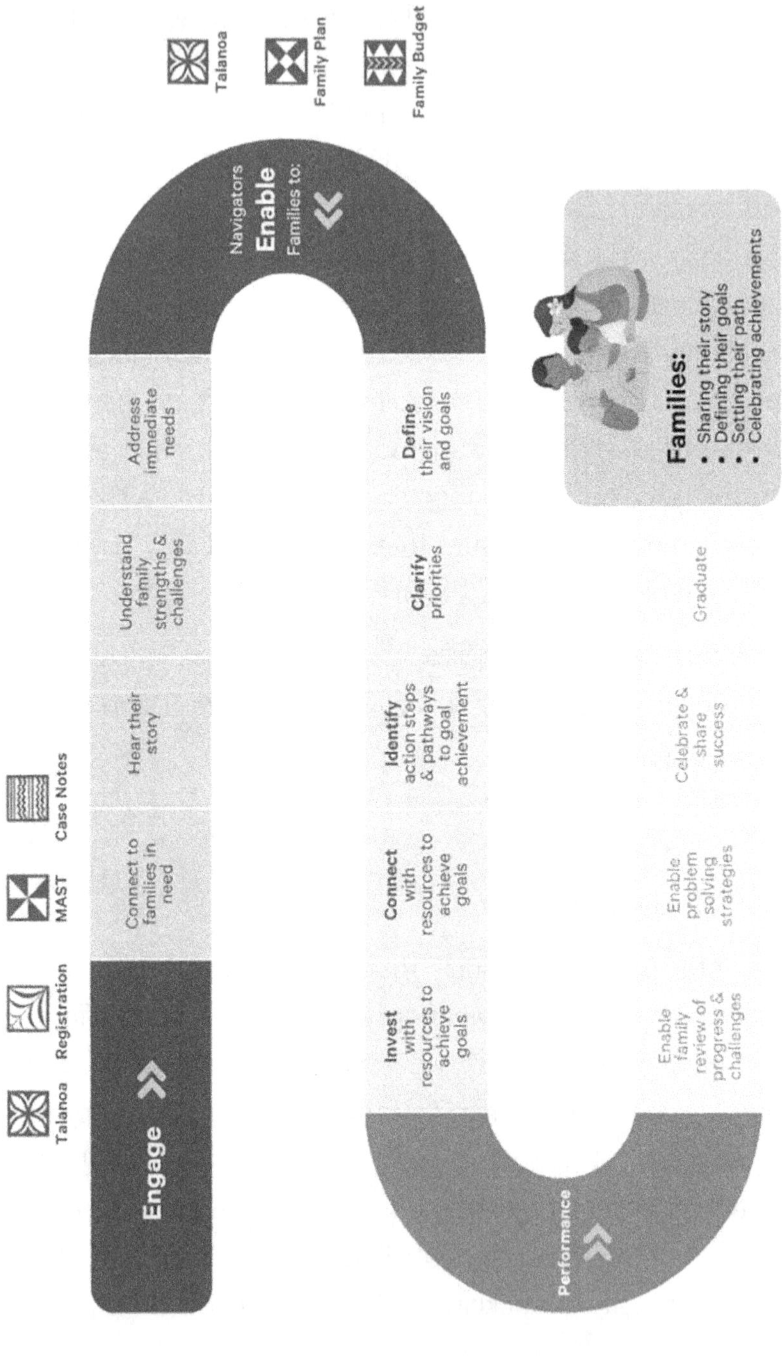
Talanoa
Registration
MAST
Case Notes
Engage
Connect to families in need
Hear their story
Understand family strengths & challenges
Address immediate needs
Talanoa
Family Plan
Family Budget
Navigators
Enable
Families to:
Define their vision and goals
Clarify priorities
Identify action steps & pathways to goal achievement
Connect with resources to achieve goals
Invest with resources to achieve goals
Performance
Enable family review of progress & challenges
Enable problem solving strategies
Celebrate & share success
Graduate
Families:
Sharing their story
Defining their goals
Setting their path
Celebrating achievements

Pasifika Futures results

Pasifika Futures has commissioned Pacific family well-being outcomes, including health and mental health outcomes through the work of its 78 Whānau Ora partners across the country enabling it to grow and reach approximately 84% of Pacific peoples throughout Aotearoa.

The snapshot of success below shows that over the period from July 2014 to March 2024, Pasifika Futures has commissioned support to 79,169 families (or 395,555 individuals) resulting in the achievement of 185,775 well-being outcomes (Pasifika Futures, 2024).

Over the past 4 years, its network of community responsiveness and resilience partners have also distributed 132,847 packages of support to families in emergencies such as the COVID-19 pandemic, the Auckland floods, and Cyclone Gabrielle (Pasifika Futures, 2024).

Pasifika Futures has also responded to growing demand for the mental health services from the Pacific community by commissioning Pacific Primary Mental Health and Addiction Services (Ngalu Fānifo). This has supported the delivery of mental health services to 8,141 individuals conducted by health coaches, health improvement practitioners, mental health nurses, and other mental health professionals in Waitematā, Counties Manukau, and Canterbury (Pasifika Futures, 2024).

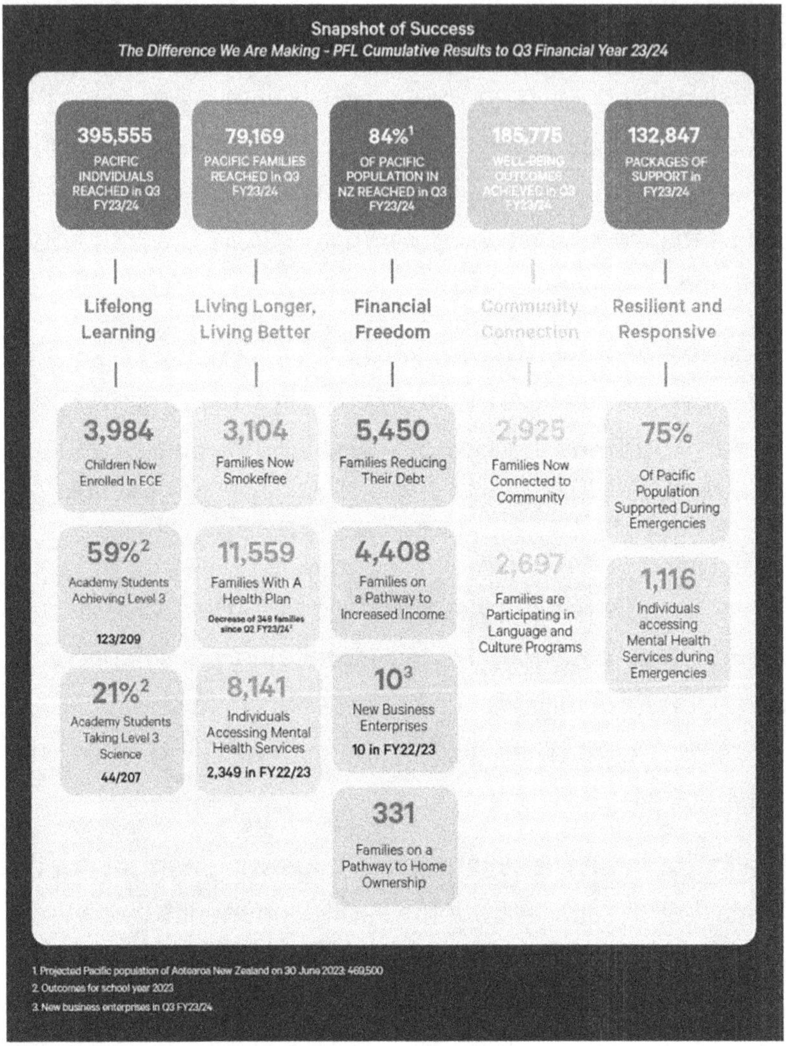

Pasifika Futures limited commissioning case study series

To conclude this chapter, we present a set of mini case studies that detail the impact that Whānau Ora has had on the health and wellbeing of Pacific families. These case studies are shared with the permission of the individuals and organisations involved.

Core navigation case study

Navigating towards financial stability: The Fonua family's success story with Pasifika Futures' Whānau Ora partner Aotearoa Tongan health workers association

Family challenges

The Fonua family, consisting of Siaosi and Tania and their four children, faced significant challenges living on a single income. Siaosi worked part-time and struggled to make ends meet. Their children's health suffered due to the cold and damp living conditions at home, leading to frequent illnesses and intermittent school attendance.

Family goals

When Pasifika Futures' Whānau Ora partner Aotearoa Tongan Health Workers Association (ATHWA) and their navigator met the family to assess their challenges and strengths, they set several goals for the Fonua family to pursue and monitor including:

- paying off debt
- increasing family income
- purchasing furniture for the family to support healthy living
- supporting children's studies and provide needed stationery, and
- strengthening personal health and wellbeing.

Whānau Ora intervention and impact

The ATHWA navigator provided support to the Fonua family through regular engagement. Siaosi was assisted into securing full-time employment, with the outcome of increasing the family's total income by $350 per week. They also devised a debt repayment plan for the Fonua family and facilitated access to financial support entitlements from Work and Income New Zealand. The navigator also ensured the family received proper healthcare by registering them with a local GP.

With the ATHWA navigator's support, the Fonua family experienced a significant transformation in their situation. Financial strain decreased, leading to improved family dynamics and stability. The children's health improved as they received timely medical care. The family's income boost allowed them to address immediate needs like purchasing furniture and supporting their children's education through purchasing stationery and uniforms for school.

The Fonua family's journey from financial hardship, lack of healthcare, and lack of children's educational resources to a state of stability highlights the effectiveness of targeted intervention and support through Whānau Ora that has addressed their underlying challenges enabling them to live more successful and prosperous lives. This case study demonstrates the positive impact of Whānau Ora through the provision of integrated support in the domains of Financial Freedom, Living Healthy Lives, and Succeeding in Education that was delivered in a culturally appropriate way making a significant difference to families' lives.

Commissioning for innovation case study

Navigating academic success: Josefa's Whānau Ora educational journey at Otahuhu College

Student challenges

Josefa, a Year 13 student at Otahuhu College, faced the challenge of balancing his studies with cultural engagements and financial hardship. Despite his potential, he needed support to navigate the complexities of his final year at secondary school and transition to university.

Whānau Ora support

With the support of Otahuhu College's Science, Technology, Engineering and Mathematics (STEM) programme (funded through Pasifika Futures' Whānau Ora Commissioning for Innovation), Josefa received targeted assistance including guidance from a STEM Navigator who provided mentorship and resources to help him excel academically and engage actively in cultural activities. Josefa also benefited from workshops and support sessions tailored to his needs, while ensuring he received support that allowed academic and personal growth.

Impact of Whānau Ora

As a result of the Whānau Ora support he received, Josefa made remarkable progress in his academic journey. He achieved outstanding results in his internal assessments, earning multiple awards including Dux, Head Boy, and Top in Year 13

Chemistry, Drama, and English. He also received scholarships from Victoria University, Auckland University of Technology, and Otago University. Josefa's active participation in cultural activities not only enriched his cultural connectedness but also contributed to his personal development and sense of identity. Josefa also secured a part-time job while studying to help ease financial pressures on his family. Due to the STEM programme support, he was still able to maintain outstanding results in his studies.

Josefa's journey highlights the impact of Whānau Ora and the STEM programme on students. By providing tailored assistance, mentorship, and resources, Josefa excelled academically, participated in cultural activities, preparing him for a bright future. This support not only fostered his overall well-being and resilience but also allowed him to realise his full potential.

Commissioning for communities case study

Empowering cultural connection: Maria's journey with Pasifika Futures' Whānau Ora partner Tupumaiaga A Niue Trust

Need for community connectedness

Maria, a mother of five children, wanted to learn her Niuean language and culture and nurture positive relationships within her community. Seeking opportunities to learn her Niuean language and culture, by attending cultural heritage workshops held by Tupumaiaga A Niue Trust in Auckland.

Whānau Ora support

Maria's journey began with her attendance at workshops and Niue playgroups facilitated by the trust. Despite her introverted nature, Maria eagerly participated in setting up food, games, and books at the playgroups, contributing to a welcoming environment for other families. With her newborn baby in tow, Maria joined these gatherings, supported by her mother-in-law who helped care for the children.

During the workshops, Maria immersed herself in traditional Niuean crafting techniques, particularly the art of making Niuean bedsheets for her newborn. With the guidance of the trust, Maria honed her skills and experienced the joy of crafting a bedsheet for her youngest child.

Impact of Whānau Ora

Through her involvement with Tupumaiaga A Niue Trust, Maria experienced a profound transformation. She not only learned valuable traditional skills but also forged meaningful connections with other Niuean families. Maria's journey exemplified the Trust's commitment to empowering young mothers like her to embrace their cultural heritage and participate actively in their community. Moreover, Maria's husband also found a connection with the Niuean community through her involvement in these workshops.

Maria's journey highlights the impact of Whānau Ora commissioning for smaller community groups. By facilitating spaces for families to connect, engage with their language and culture, and actively participate in their communities, organisations like

Tupumaiaga A Niue Trust play a vital role in nurturing cultural identity and fostering a sense of belonging and identity for Pacific families living in New Zealand.

Commissioning for community resilience case study

Overcoming overcrowded living conditions and financial strain during COVID-19: Pasifika Futures' Whānau Ora and community responsiveness and resilience partner: K'aute Pasifika

Family challenges

The Too family are a family of 11 with 9 children living in Hamilton. The Too family faced significant challenges including overcrowded living conditions, financial hardship, health issues exacerbated by the COVID-19 pandemic, high power usage, and poor housing conditions. With limited resources and a large family to support, the Too's were looking for assistance to improve their quality of life.

Whānau Ora Support

K'aute Pasifika navigators supported the family with vaccinations and immunisations, housing, respiratory health and financial assistance, and saving on energy. The K'aute Pasifika navigator referred the Too family to well child nurses to get the family up to date with their vaccinations, especially COVID-19, to protect against respiratory illnesses. They also referred the family to Whare Ora to provide support for bedding and car seats, addressing overcrowding issues as most of the family were sleeping on the floor, and ensure safety for the children.

The K'aute Pasifika navigators also helped install smooth sensors to address moisture-related respiratory issues, improving the overall health and wellbeing of the children. They also referred the family to a budgeting advisor and a mortgage broker to develop a financial plan and explore options for homeownership. This alleviated financial strain and provided long-term stability for the family. The navigator negotiated with a cheaper power provider, reducing power related expenses, and making it more affordable for the family, easing the financial burden they face.

Impact of Whānau Ora

With the vaccinations and improved housing conditions, the Too family experienced improved health outcomes, resulting in fewer hospital admissions and reduced stress on the parents. The Too family developed a comprehensive financial plan, reduced power expenses, and made progress towards homeownership. This resulted in increased financial stability and reduced stress for the family. Despite challenges posed by the pandemic and associated financial constraints, the children were able to continue their education with minimal interruptions. With the support received, the family managed to secure better housing, addressing overcrowding issues, and creating a healthier environment for all family members.

The interventions provided through Whānau Ora support have contributed to enhancing the quality of life, resilience, and successful future prospects of the Too family. These outcomes demonstrate the effectiveness of Whānau Ora in providing prompt and impactful responses to national emergencies such as COVID-19 pandemic and other natural disasters, and the critical role it plays in supporting families during times of crisis.

References

Boulton, A., Gifford, H., Allport, T., and White, H. (2018). Delivering on diversity: The challenges of commissioning for Whānau Ora. Journal of Indigenous Wellbeing. Te Mauri-Pimatisiwin, Volume 3, Issue 1, Article 4. Retrieved from Journalindigenouswellbeing.co.nz/media/2022/01/111.121.Delivering-on-diversity-The-challenges-of-commissioning-for-Whānau-Ora.pdf

Pasifika Futures. (2024). Celebrating Ten Years of Pasifika Futures. June 2024. Pasifika Futures Limited, Auckland Retrieved from https://s3-ap-southeast 2.amazonaws.com/media.pasifikafutures.co.nz/production/1636/pfl000002-10-year-report_f6-(1).pdf

Jensen, S., Sorensen, D., and Jensen, W. (2019). Whānau Ora and Talanoa: Generating and using knowledge to achieve Pacific family wellbeing and prosperity outcomes. Pacific Health Dialog, 21(4). https://doi.org/10.26635/phd .2019 WOS.621

Koloto, H., A., & Misa, A. (2018). Whānau Ora Tongan Families Evaluation. Unpublished report. Pasifika Futures Limited, Auckland.

Moore, C. (2014). A whakapapa of Whānau Ora. Master of Arts thesis, University of Auckland, Auckland. Retrieved from https://researchspace.auckland.ac.nz/bitstream/handle/2292/22594/whole.pdf?sequence=2&isAllowed=y.

Ministry of Health. (2002). Māori Health Strategy, He Korowai Oranga. Wellington: Ministry of Health. Retrieved from https://www.health.govt.nz/system/files/documents/publications/mhs-english.pdf.

Ministry of Health. (2011). Whānau Ora: Transforming our futures. Wellington: Ministry of Health. Retrieved from https://www.health.govt.nz/system/files/documents/publications/whanau-ora-transforming-futures-v2.pdf.

Office of the Auditor-General. (2015). *Whānau Ora: The first four years*. Retrieved from: https://oag.parliament.nz/2015/whanau-ora/docs/whanau-ora.pdf.

Taskforce on Whānau Centred Initiatives. (2010). Whānau Ora: Report of the Taskforce on Whānau Centred Initiatives. Retrieved from https://www.msd.govt.nz/documents/about-msd-and-our-work/publications-resources/planning-strategy/whanau-ora/whanau-ora-taskforce-report.pdf

The New Zealand Productivity Commission – Te Kōmihana Whai Hua o Aotearoa. (2015). More Effective Social Services. Final Report, August 2015. Retrieved from https://www.productivity.govt.nz/assets/Documents/8981330814/Final-report-v2.pdf

Vaioleti, T. M. (2016). Talanoa Research Methodology: A Developing Position on Pacific Research. Waikato Journal of Education, 12(1). https://doi.org/10.15663/wje.v12i1.296

Mana-mai-le-lagi: Storying the importance of lived experience and community connection in health research with Pacific Rainbow+ communities

Malaeulu Seuta'afili Patrick Thomsen

Allyssa Verner-Pula

Phylesha Brown-Acton

Chapter summary

This chapter provides insights into community research with Pacific peoples using the Manalagi Project as a case study. The Manalagi project marks a significant milestone as the first ever Pacific Rainbow+ health and wellbeing project supported by the Health Research Council (HRC). In this chapter we present a storytelling-focused chapter that details Manalagi's holistic approach to community research, placing emphasis on community co-creation and collaboration. The project's approach to community engagement centres core values of service, or tautua (espoused in Samoan), genealogy, reciprocity, holism, and respect. Incorporating and operationalising Pacific Indigenous knowledge and the lived experiences of Pacific Rainbow+ communities as the foundation for community research in the Pacific context.

Introduction

The Manalagi: Aotearoa Pacific Rainbow/Queer/(L)esbian (G)ay (B)isexual (T)ransgender (Q)ueer (I)ntersex (A)sexual/gender+ (M)āhū (V)akasalewalewa (P)alopa (F)akafifine (A)kavaine (F)akaleiti/Leiti (F)a'afafine+ health and wellbeing project (Manalagi Project) is funded by the Health Research Council of New Zealand (HRC). It is the first project of its kind to be supported by HRC as a Pacific health research project. The arrival of Manalagi marks a special time in Pacific health research in Aotearoa-New Zealand. In acknowledging the internal diversities that exist within Pacific communities, HRC has signalled that it is prepared to support projects with a sound intersectional basis, capable of generating good data to better serve this (Pacific and Rainbow+)

multiply marginalised group. Led by Pacific Rainbow+ researchers Malaeulu Seuta'afili Dr Patrick Thomsen in partnership with F'INE Pasifika Aotearoa Executive Director Phylesha Brown-Acton, Manalagi engages a Pacific research praxis that is uniquely Rainbow+ and community embedded.

The aim of this chapter is to narrate/illustrate through personal experience, how Manalagi's holistic approach to health and wellbeing research can provide insights into how health research with Pacific people can be carried out in an innovative, ethical, and culturally appropriate way. One that centres on lived-experience, community co-creation, co-design, and collaboration. We offer this chapter through talanoa and storytelling to journey through the genesis of the project tied to lived experiences and connections, and to provoke new ideas and discussions around community consultation and our engagement model. This model engagement has helped Manalagi bridge the gap between research and community praxis in exciting ways. We hope this can help us think further about broadening the way we understand the role of research in engaging innovatively with Pacific communities in our country today. A review on the health of Pacific Rainbow+ communities is offered earlier in this textbook. This chapter, by contrast, will focus on storytelling and offers a reflective review of phase 1 of Manalagi: the community consultation processes, which represents phase one of the project. The chapter will have two main narrator voices, the first is from lead researcher Seuta'afili Dr Patrick Thomsen, with the second being short reflections from the project's research assistant Allyssa Verner-Pula. Phylesha Brown-Acton, who is our third named author is referenced across the article as the pivotal unifying force between community and academia, and as such she is honoured in the chapter through our recollections.

In this chapter we demonstrate how values that are expressed in the HRC of New Zealand's Pacific Health Research Guidelines can be practiced in a real-life setting, with a specific Pacific community/communities. In particular, Manalagi's approach to research is derived from Pacific ways of knowing and doing, articulated by HRC as valuing communal relationships, centring reciprocity, holism, and respect from the beginning to the end of the process. This chapter shows how these values are embedded not just in the way the research is carried out, but also how valuing Indigenous knowledges of the Pacific embedded within Pacific communities in New Zealand, also speaks to the value of lived experiences that pre-date and exist outside of research contexts.

Genesis: Lived experience

The story of Manalagi began long before the submission of a funding application to the HRC. It began with me and my history as a Samoan, queer, fa'afafine man, born in Middlemore hospital, raised in South Auckland. Being raised by a solo mum, it was a formative cultural and class inflected experience growing up on the benefit in a state house. Samoan was the first language at home, and as part of a Samoan Catholic family, I attended St Anne's Primary School in Manurewa and completed most of my secondary schooling at De La Salle College in Māngere up until the year 2000.

In my lifetime, I have seen discrimination not just from Aotearoa-New Zealand society, but from within Pacific communities as well (Thomsen, 2022). In addition to this, I have also borne witness to the innovative ways many of the fa'afafine I knew crafted to survive. Some worked unsafe carceral streets, others low-paid factory jobs, and as fa'afafine we experienced ridicule and exclusion from all sides of society. Drug and alcohol misuse was common as a coping mechanism for some, and career prospects were few for many that came directly from Sāmoa or the Pacific. These early experiences tangibly demonstrated to me the barriers that existed in our community from being able to achieve security and safety in Aotearoa-New Zealand (Thomsen, 2020a).

However, I was also a witness to huge acts of service, kindness, and contributions to Pacific communities, churches, families, and organisations from Pacific Rainbow+ people that are rarely acknowledged (Thomsen, 2020b). This was apparent when I attended Church or Samoan community events – where ministers and men delivered heteronormative speeches using heterosexist language, while the women sat at the back or were in the kitchen. Fa'afafine would be further back still, providing service to all. I would join many of them, spending hours preparing before the main event, cooking, cleaning, decorating, and styling. Speaking with many fa'afafine from Sāmoa, their stories of struggle, and their aspirations for their families would sometimes spill out. It perturbed me how I never once saw anyone in Church youth groups and community gatherings show interest in uplifting fa'afafine and their stories. All I heard were demands for their time, labour, and service, and I began to wonder what it would take for our community to stop treating them as invisible.

Connections: The foundation of the project

Manalagi would not have been possible without the people I have in my life and shared bonds. The connection between myself and associate investigator Phylesha Brown-Acton (affectionately known as Auntie Phee in our community) being particularly pivotal. Although I am embedded within Pacific, more specifically, Samoan Rainbow+ communities, I had been living overseas for a substantial period before 2019 pursuing further study and career opportunities. During my absence, Phylesha continued to serve Pacific communities through her work with F'INE and many other initiatives she was crucial in developing. Her mana within Pacific communities and community-facing work is more than substantial, it is revered ('Queen's Birthday Honours, 2019,' 2019; The Governor-General of New Zealand, n.d.)

Phylesha's connection to me is through my mother initially, developed further by shared cross-life events. Despite our modest means, my siblings and I were brought up to understand the importance of tautua (service), a bedrock value in Samoan culture, tied to intentional generosity and care. In the spirit of tautua my mother built around us, our home and family were always a safe space for fa'afafine and queer folk in the Samoan and wider Pacific community to congregate. Amidst the raucous parties filled with roaring laughter and spectacular disagreements, our garage was home to incredible flair and creativity. There, costumes for beauty pageants would be produced, glorious Samoan attire were constructed; many a dream was spoken, few achieved and important connections were made. Auntie

Phee, was part of my mother's community-connected story as they'd cross paths at community events and Auckland's vibrant Samoan night club scene in the '90s.

To this day, many in the fa'afafine community of the elder generation know me and are caring toward me because of my mother. Many see me as an extension of her generosity and care. My bond with the fa'afafine community stems from these rich and intimate relationships. When I hosted my mother's 65th birthday in August 2021, her special guests aside from my family were her fa'afafine friends. When I spoke about Manalagi to one of them at my mum's birthday, the notorious and well-loved character in the Samoan community Jennifer O'Brien (or Jenny as she is more commonly known), stated that she wanted to participate to support me as my mother's child. Anything I needed her help with, she said, she would show up for to honour all the love and care mum had always shown her and other fa'afafine. Though I had no idea that it would be our last, I am grateful for this memory of the conversation we had. Jenny passed away suddenly in October 2021 as Auckland shifted into its longest lockdown of the pandemic. At Jenny's funeral, Auntie Phee and her team were there to tautua.

I also connected with Auntie Phee through the beauty pageant scene. In the '90s and early 2000s, fa'afafine beauty pageants were a key source of community entertainment, which created mini creative and circulative economies of their own. Auntie Phee won many pageants during this time, while I served on multiple organising committees for pageants. She was also seen providing tautua to many in the community through her work with the New Zealand AIDS Foundation, the Love Life Fono. She even won world championships in netball. As an advocate for our communities, she had been doing crucial work in fighting for more resourcing to support Pacific Rainbow+ peoples. When I returned to New Zealand, I spoke to Auntie Phee about where our communities were in terms of data. She told me that one of the biggest issues she had faced, was being able to get Pacific-specific, and targeted data together, capable of speaking the data-language of policymakers to advocate for more resourcing for our communities.

Conceptualising: In search of a research project and name

In 2019, I returned to Aotearoa-New Zealand following graduate and doctoral studies in South Korea and the United States. I also came home in many ways, to rejoin the Aotearoa Pacific Rainbow+ community. Despite physical separation, for over a decade, I had maintained contact with many of the practitioners and community workers I knew through the digital sphere. Following my appointment to a postdoctoral position at the University of Auckland in the Centre for Pacific Studies, I was eager to begin developing my research programme and knew that my ability to stay within the academy would be dependent on my ability to leverage this position in tautua of my communities.

When I began to immerse myself in the existing research on our communities, I found pockets of information extracted from larger surveys that had small amounts of Pacific specific information, however, our Pacific Rainbow+ communities were still being treated as peripheral and as an afterthought to many projects

(Thomsen et al., 2021b; Thomsen, 2022). Likewise, community practitioners working at the coalface of social support and health service and the research community lacks recognition. This contrasts with the hypervisibility through successful queer artists, entertainers, and performers of Pacific heritage who have made major inroads for Pacific Rainbow+/queer representation of late (see Prior, 2017; Ryan, 2021; TheCoconetTV, 2014).

The complexity of the issue around this erasure is further compounded by deficit ways we are referred to in existing scholarship I came across. Though it is acknowledged that there are many ways we are excluded, the language and framing used were not culturally grounded, nor reflective of our multifaceted realities. While I understood language was necessary to highlight systemic faults, it ran the risk of re-marginalisation. Highlighting, and spotlighting our differences as a deficit and perpetuates the idea that we were at risk, misused/abused, under-served, excluded, discriminated against, experiencing homophobia, transphobia – that we were problematic. Many community members I spoke to worried that this portrayal could reinforce an unreflexive position suggesting to health practitioners that *we* needed to be fixed, rather than the system. This type of framing is clearly counterproductive and treated our communities as people with no mana. Committed to remedying this, I turned to health and wellbeing models like the Fonofale Model (Crawley et al., 1995) and Whare Tapa Wha (Durie, 1994), which provided a holistic understanding of health and hauora, and incorporates the pivotal role of culture in understanding impactful health interventions (Manuela & Sibley, 2014; Ponton, 2018; Ryan et al., 2019). These models helped me find a basis to advance the Manalagi approach, incorporating the role of liminality or gender/sex and sexuality to the complex factors that are tied to culture and identity.

Many meetings pre-COVID days, and conversations using the viber application between Phylesha and I and with other community members were also pivotal to the conceptualisation of the project. When I settled on proposing a project idea to the HRC's call for proposals around an Emerging Researcher First Grant targeted for Pacific researchers, I turned to senior Pacific research colleagues and my connections within the community for advice and to get a stronger idea of what would make sense for a project like this. Despite a lack of health research background, there were glaring gaps in research and quantitative data in almost every area that impacted health and wellbeing outcomes for Pacific Rainbow+ communities. After carrying out a scoping literature review, it was found that there was no baseline data on Pacific Rainbow+ communities in New Zealand, few studies that centred our community's intersectional experiences, and very little was known about what was working well for our communities in the health system specifically (Thomsen et al., 2021b). Following this, I crafted the proposal which included a summary of my conversations with Phylesha and other community members to go with the corpus of existing research I was able to gather in time before the submission deadline. Phylesha's thoughts as a community practitioner and her lived experience was invaluable as so little published research existed by Pacific Rainbow+ researchers in the health space, and I specifically incorporated her input, presenting them to the assessing panel as an integral form of data to be considered. Indeed, community voices would prove essential to the Manalagi project.

The initial proposal was submitted in late August of 2019 under the name 'Nuanua: Aotearoa Pacific Rainbow/Queer LGBTQIA+ MVPFAFF+ Health and Wellbeing Project.' Nuanua translates to Rainbow in my native Samoan. Specifically, the proposed aims of the project were articulated as: to create a safe cultural space for members of Pacific Rainbow+ communities to communicate their unique and specific health and wellbeing needs. There are four specified goals: 1. Collect accurate baseline data regarding the presence and make-up of Pacific Rainbow Communities; 2. Document the experiences of Pacific Rainbow+ communities within New Zealand's healthcare service provision; 3. Provide recommendations to policymakers through the establishment of a Pacific Rainbow+ Health and Wellbeing framework to better support our communities' specific health needs; and 4. Apply an intersectional framework in producing scholarship that allows for knowledge generation that is culturally sensitive and accessible to our communities in creating a research architecture that can be used here and abroad by researchers in health and wellbeing research that impacts intersectional and marginalised groups. Progressing through three phases, the first phase of the project was concluded at the end of 2021, the community talanoa/consultations, which this chapter focuses on. Furthermore, the research team prepared a survey instrument based on feedback from these community talanoa, which was taken to community in 2022. This survey focused on collecting baseline data and information regarding our communities' physical and mental health, wellbeing in relation to family, religion, culture, and spirituality. We reached 482 Pacific Rainbow+ respondents nationwide, with community consultations leading to the establishment of a friends and allies survey taking total responses to 750. This was complemented with individual talanoa across New Zealand of 62 Pacific Rainbow+ individuals.

By the time we had passed the peer-review process and confirmed to receive funding, the project name had long changed. We announced ourselves in May 2020 as the Manalagi Project. The term Manalagi is a compound word that combines two mostly pan-Polynesian words/terms: 'mana' – innate spiritual/authority, with 'lagi' the Samoan spelling for the shared Polynesian term (langi/rangi) for the heavens and the sky, which I took from the full statement of 'mai le lagi' to be from the skies/heavens. These concepts meet to denote the innate essence and authority of all peoples, including Rainbow+, who are embedded within, (not outside) our cultures, communities, and families; highlighting an essence imbued from our conception and formation among, and as a continuation of, our ancestors.

Process: Community consultations, protocol, and the power of inclusive collaboration

The Manalagi Project adopts a culturally appropriate mixed methods research design that combines Pacific approaches to knowledge generation, while acknowledging the need for reliable statistics and baseline data to be able to measure health and wellbeing outcomes for our communities. What has been distinctive about the Manalagi approach is our commitment to the community being realised in material, not just discursive ways. The first year of the Manalagi project focused on preparing the survey instrument following a community-driven ethos. Manalagi has been extremely successful in doing this, and although the process has been gruelling in many respects, it has been empowering and led to incredibly important collaborations that will expand the impact and dissemination of research results beyond conventional means.

Even prior to the consultations, it was clear that our communities wanted a platform to be able to tell their stories, to resist, to speak back, to write back to re-establish the acknowledgement of their mana within the process of research, and the Manalagi project was aware of this from its very conception. I have always had an uneasy relationship with academia, holding strong suspicions and critiques of its colonising tendencies (Thomsen et al., 2021a; Leenen-Young et al., 2021). Especially as research communities are dominated by mostly non-Pacific, non-Indigenous, who have tended to undermine and exclude Indigenous and Pacific knowledges from the academy (Smith, 1999; Thaman, 2003; Thomsen et al., 2021a; Leenen-Young et al., 2021). The task of reclamation as a decolonial praxis is pivotal to Manalagi.

The name Manalagi is also a play at reframing the words in the Book of Exodus in the Bible, where manna, or bread is promised to the Israelites as falling from the heavens while they sought out freedom from bondage (English Standard Version Bible, 2001, Ex. 16:1-36). My specific use of the terms mana and lagi, is therefore a political statement that urges for space to be made, and an imperative to acknowledge that we, as Pacific Rainbow+ people, are genealogically tied to the same heavens as the lagi from which all Pacific people's mana derive through their ancestors

(Thomsen & Brown-Acton, 2021). As such, Manalagi, is also tied to the potential space made for our realities when we embrace notions of decoloniality around spirituality. Making space for us, diminishes no one's mana, but enhances the mana of all of us.

Decentring the main centres in community consultations

My initial idea was to take Manalagi to fono to be held in Auckland, Wellington, and Christchurch. However, it was Phylesha whom I took my lead from when we designed our community-engagement strategy for the consultation. She suggested that we try to branch out beyond the main centres, into what Auntie Phee calls the 'hearty-centres' of Whangarei, Gisborne, Tokoroa, and Hamilton. This is because Auckland and our urban interests tend to dominate representation and conversations related to Pacific communities. Thus, the first Manalagi community talanoa took place in Ōtepoti-Dunedin at the beginning of April 2021 to de-centre Aukilani as the locus of all that is Pacific in our country. I remember Auntie Phee saying quite clearly that if we started with Auckland, it would likely dominate and potentially taint the way we were able to receive the rest of the consultations. I am grateful I took her advice, as it really helped to centre the community consultations in communities beyond our own comfort zone.

Aside from this, as a research team, much of our community engagement strategy came from things Phylesha and I intuitively knew through the process of working with community in the past. Protocol played a crucial role in building meaningful relationships with our participants. We engaged in many pre-meetings, months before we hoped to have consultations. Here again, I rested on the connections that Auntie Phee had to complement mine. She set up meetings with providers in the hearty centres and allowed us to build proper relationships with these providers before we embarked on any attempts to consult and draw in communities. In these meetings, full introductions/mihis were given in our own languages, meaningful connections and reconnections were established before business was ever discussed. After whakawhanaungatanga (establishing relationships, relating well to others), we presented a short presentation to the community members present, explaining the entire history of the project, the naming practice, and the message the branding was aiming to deliver. Following this, we broke for refreshments and further talanoa, leading into breakout sessions where members of the research team led groups in talanoa around the areas we had identified as priority areas for the survey.

The importance of meaningfully connecting with community providers meant our engagement strategy took off at a grassroots level that flew mostly under the radar of the high-vis optics of mainstream Rainbow+ representation. In these talanoa, we never engaged in any potentially parochial debates, nor did we attempt to disrupt or underscore reactively to the violences our communities face. Rather, it is more accurate to say that we kept our trauma in-house to be unpacked by our own before we allowed it to be cherry picked and used as trauma voyeurism for mainstream Rainbow+ movements, media, and those seduced by the allure of representational politics. In this way, Manalagi's engagement strategy stayed true to its ethos of seeking ways to enhance mana for all our communities. But also acknowledging that for many within our communities, this means keeping intact as far as we could, the mana of our families and the wider community.

Due to the very real risk of the country being plunged into another lockdown if COVID-19 broke out again, we compressed the consultation session into a 5-week period across the months of April and May. We held 11 separate talanoa across 8 centres in Aotearoa within this period. During this time, we criss-crossed the country, book ending Friday and weekend sessions (doubled) in Christchurch and Wellington, while using weekdays as opportunity to visit our hearty centres (Whangarei, Gisborne, Tokoroa, Hamilton) in honouring the contributions of our providers outside Auckland, Wellington, and Christchurch (Godfrey, 2021). The constant travel was incredibly testing as I was still teaching at the same time, and the core of our team, myself, Phylesha Brown-Acton, and our research assistant Allyssa Verner-Pula, were at all 11 sessions. Our other associate investigators (Professor Jemaima Tiatia-Siau, Dr Sam Manuela, Dr Lara Greaves) joined us at different sessions on different weeks.

In the talanoa, discussing the themes allowed us to see if what we had identified as themes to collect data on from the literature would be useful to our community members and the work they were wanting to do to uplift their own Rainbow+ whanau. We took reams and reams of notes, held long, sometimes trauma-filled conversations, and struggled through difficult topics. In the end, the process became more than just a consultation in many places. It also became a space of connecting Pacific Rainbow+ whanau with each other. The learnings we took as a research team ensured that what we would deliver as a survey instrument were priority areas that community members needed data around (baseline data, physical and mental health, wellbeing in relation to culture, family, identity, and spirituality). The survey needed to be a length palatable to our communities, and we understood our participants do not always connect with surveys to tell their stories, so we committed to allowing community members to suggest ways we could offer our platform through Manalagi to uplift their work – many took up the offer in unexpected ways that has elevated the work of the project beyond even how I had imagined it.

Reciprocity in process

At these consultations we took with us packages that included Manalagi branded pens, t-shirts, caps, tote bags, water bottles, a USB thumb drive which had a copy of a draft questionnaire/survey instrument uploaded to it, which we had drafted across the summer and some mints, providing lunch and refreshments for all attendees. Although we were visiting communities outside the regions, we made sure that we took with us gifts to share and kai for everyone. Manaakitanga (kindness, generosity, hospitality) was at the centre of these visits. Both Phylesha and I were very cognisant that our communities are wary of research for many reasons, and we were doing what Professor Yvonne Underhill-Sem calls: resting on our connections. Not in a complacent, pejorative sense, rather, in an uplifting and empowering manner. It was our connections with different people across Aotearoa that was allowing our project and its work to be uplifted.

Our attempts to show fa'aaloalo (respect) and alofa (love), was a genuine attempt to make sure we demonstrated our gratitude in all that we did. We did this in respecting protocol, opening each session with a careful mihi and acknowledgement of all and the lands we were standing on. In addition to proper whakawhanaungatanga (establishing relationships, relating well to others), we also ensured that we took special gifts for the provider coordinators in each venue and attendees. Using our research costs budget to make sure we gave them an appropriate number of gifts as koha through the process was non-negotiable for the team. The issue of koha (gifts) in research is controversial for non-Indigenous, non-Pacific researchers, and praxis, but as a community-embedded researcher, if I could give all the resources to my community, I would happily do so. It is more than just about 'rewarding' or 'compensating' people for their time, it is about acknowledging that their presence in supporting the kaupapa (topic, matter for discussion) you are driving, is what makes you and your project possible. Without community we are nothing as Pacific researchers.

Manalagi simultaneously built this community effort in tandem with a wider, more visible digital presence. At the outset we were committed to ensuring that our communities would have access to our research and resources. We made them immediately available through the Manalagi Website that hosts an open-access repository. Because there was so little Pacific health research focused on Pacific Rainbow+ communities explicitly, we gathered a vast array of resources from art and performance worlds, opinion pieces, speeches, and audio-visual resources to complement the more academic texts we were finding and producing. As a team, we understood the need to create more scholarly resources for the next generation of Pacific Rainbow+

researchers to build upon and parse apart in filling the gaps we are leaving behind.

To make the repository and website a reality, I turned to other funding sources within the University, to fund research assistant positions for young Pacific students to be socialised into the project and research space. As a result, we were able to make use of our marketing collateral, which I sourced from a Pacific Rainbow+ graphic designer, Tapuaki Helu of Oddball Studios, to build a website, marketing materials that our research assistants (RAs) constructed, which included a focus on social media platforms for dissemination of research updates, creating the Manalagi branded gifts for communities for the consultation process, and helped us to generate momentum for the project before a single data gathering activity had taken place.

Inclusive collaborations and dissemination to serve community practitioners

My willingness to share the Manalagi platform has allowed for an interdisciplinary collaboration to take place that is now bringing work to regional economies, allowing community members' themselves to have their stories centred in creative ways, uplifting the entire kaupapa of Manalagi in the process. Thinking about research as a co-community and collective effort means allowing for non-conventional forms of dissemination to be considered, and better still, driven by community members themselves.

In Gisborne, following a wonderful and intimate talanoa, I was approached by a television producer and documentary filmmaker from Tairāwhiti TV who was engrossed by the kōrero we had engaged in. They asked me if I would consider working with them to develop a television series. Despite having no training in media and television, I said that we would be fully open to helping them develop a television series idea based on the research we were generating. Following the talanoa, tied to other mahi in my research programme, I was fortuitously asked by New Zealand On Air (NZOA) to speak to a member of their leadership team on ways we could better support Pacific representation across the screen sector. At this conversation, I raised the idea our community member had suggested at our talanoa. As a result, we were encouraged to pitch a proposal to one of NZOA's open funding rounds. Over the following months, I gave as much time as I could to drive the formation of a proposal with a collaborator with Tairāwhiti TV's Tee Wells. In September 2021 our Manalagi proposal was funded, and the research we are doing regarding the acknowledgement of the histories of Pacific Rainbow+ communities will now become a TV series, airing in 2026.

We are also currently working on an artistic exhibition and hoping to confirm the participation of a specific major arts and cultural institution to host an exhibition and Manalagi collection at the end of the project's part 2 life in 2027 at Te Papa Tongarewa. There are plans for a book publication to accompany the exhibition, allowing Pacific Rainbow+ community members themselves to not only participate in the research as sources of data, but actual generators of knowledge. All these ideas came from community members and have been generated by the platform Manalagi has created. This is where the potential for interdisciplinary collaboration matters in creating an inclusive research praxis.

Part of this inclusive research praxis is acknowledging the contributions of all members of our team irrespective of their prescribed role. Manalagi has been ably supported on this journey so far by RAs, each of the RAs that have worked on Manalagi have been included as co-authors on publications we have produced. This has allowed all our RAs to be given their first experiences with the peer-review and publishing process building their capacity as future research leaders as we have developed Manalagi. Furthermore, Allyssa Verner-Pula, who is Manalagi's main research assistant, is in many ways considered a vital, integral, and key member of our research team. Although not named as an investigator, Allyssa began working on the project two-thirds the way through her undergraduate degree and completed her master's degree at the end of the Manalagi Project. We as a research team value her input, opinions, and suggestions much like any other investigator and acknowledging her contributions and the contributions of all is a key community research praxis for the Manalagi Project. Allyssa, rather appropriately, provides her reflections on the process, to conclude this chapter.

Reflections of a research assistant on the Manalagi project consultation process

As a young Samoan queer woman from Manurewa, my queerness was never the aspect of my identity I made an effort to highlight. I often found it difficult to relate to my queer peers in Auckland; the queer space here largely caters to white interests, cultivating a culture of self-expression not always inclusive of one's ethnicity. However, my experience as the research assistant on the Manalagi community consultations proved quite the opposite. Among much needed talanoa about the issues facing our Pacific Rainbow+ communities in Aotearoa-New Zealand, the nature of these consultations was often predicated on celebration of self and community.

My experience with the Manalagi community consultations can be marked mostly by the fact that I gained a breadth of knowledge unable to be found within literature alone. As with the nature of talanoa, personal stories and conversations allow for nuances, complexities, and explanations to be laid out that cannot be fully encapsulated in text (Vaioleti, 2006). Pre-consultation process, I gathered a base of knowledge around the experience of Pacific and Rainbow+ communities separately, which showed how Pacific queer peoples are not often accounted for within discourse about Rainbow+ communities, and discourse within Pacific communities (Thomsen et al., 2021b). However, the Manalagi community consultations pointedly enhanced that understanding, allowing for conversations that spoke directly to the experience of Pacific queer communities in Aotearoa-New Zealand (Godfrey, 2021). These talanoa highlighted the burdens we face as Pacific queer people, but also were a site of empowerment and sharing.

These conversations highlighted a set of common issues that impact Pacific queer communities throughout the country. Many communities felt these conversations were happening at the beginning stages of their collective addressing of these issues.

While the existence of Pacific queer people in their communities had not been rejected, these talanoa were unprecedented opportunities to highlight the issues they faced. The Manalagi Project proved timely, as communities felt ready to tackle these issues, and take on the challenge of creating specific and much-needed solutions for their community. Within these communities, people were ready to share their experiences, including the issues they felt were prevalent for themselves and their peers. I felt that this offered the opportunity to build a foundation of knowledge around the history, presence, and stories of Pacific queer communities throughout the country. As a young queer, Pacific person, it was incredibly enlightening and heartening to hear these stories and anecdotes, particularly those shared by elders and pioneers within our community.

Having these conversations be community-led was incredibly important, as it highlighted the main issues existing within a certain region. These conversations also pointed to the fact that, despite commonalities throughout the country, there are also specific issues within specific communities. Quite naively, I did not initially think this would be such an important takeaway from the community consultation process. Currently, this diversity of these issues is not captured in its full essence, or even well known, which is ultimately a disservice to the communities facing them (Godfrey, 2021). I recall a young girl in Tokoroa, who shared her experiences having to travel outside of her region to receive gender affirming healthcare. Though, in Christchurch, issues of white supremacy and racial discrimination were highlighted the most. On a smaller scale, people in Wellington and Christchurch remarked to me how envious they were that I was able to experience certain Pacific queer-focused events in Auckland. This diversity in issues also highlights the different routes certain communities take to create solutions. By allowing communities to lead conversations about their wellbeing, you are also letting them create their own solutions. Perhaps it goes without saying, but it became apparent that community focused research must account for the fact that communities all have specific needs and aspirations. For me, I developed a better understanding of what communities should be given the tools to solve the issues that exist within their own communities. As a young researcher from Auckland, I could not possibly know the best way to engage with a community in Gisborne. If you, the researcher, are to dominate the space with conversation and ideas that do not reflect the current social landscape of the community you are visiting, you will not be able to understand the community effectively.

Letting the community lead the conversation gives them power and build trust and relationships between researcher and participant through actively listening, showing humility, and respect for their stories, among other things. However, it is also important to note that our communities have a history of rightful distrust in research and researchers (Hepi et al., 2007; Smith, 1999; Thomsen and Brown-Acton, 2021) and so this trust may not be built overnight.

During the pre-consultations, I was fearful that these communities would be sceptical about the research and its necessity. I know now that communities can see right through you. If you are coming into the research space, co-opting these relationships for the sake of personal gain, you will never be able to achieve research that can be beneficial. Any research methods and values employed must be done sincerely; if done so, communities will find you trustworthy enough to share those experiences with you. Having that trust was a responsibility I did not take lightly. I found myself becoming more and more protective over the stories being shared with me and I was consistently blown away by the magnitude of histories and personal accounts that ranged from stories of overcoming adversity to simple jokes about their experiences. As a young researcher, I did not account for how overwhelming it would be to hold such a responsibility, but I feel incredibly honoured to be handling such precious lived experiences in this research.

The process of community consultations can be gruelling and requires a level of adaptability when entering communities, you have not entered before. However, as a research assistant, I was not ready for how changing the experience would be. Towards the end of the community consultation process, I began to feel more comfortable in my queerness. Being able to see myself in the stories and presence of others in my communities throughout the country was emboldening and validating. I think this is also a feeling that exists beyond me. Through the Manalagi Project, we can create a visibility and validation for Pacific queer folk who have typically been disregarded or rendered invisible in conversations and spaces that consider the communities they are from. This, to me, has been an integral part of beginning to create change that will enhance the health and wellbeing of Pacific Rainbow+ communities.

Taualuga

We end this chapter not with a conclusion but a short taualuga or finale of sorts. In the Sāmoan context, a taualuga marks the end of a gathering and celebration of the lineages and connections that have been renewed at an event. The end of this chapter is the taualuga of the first gathering event of the Manalagi Project. In sharing our stories of carrying out the first few phases of the Manalagi Project, we bring together the narratives, the hopes, and aspirations of our communities as research representatives for them. Our sharing in this textbook is about honouring these connections, our own families, our own gafa or whakapapa, our own dreams, our alofa for all Pacific peoples and communities. All research, not just health research, should no longer be confined to just books, reports, and conventional forms of dissemination. But to effectively leverage the power of these non-conventional ways of disseminating research, you must understand the core principles of Pacific research which Manalagi embodies, about genuinely uplifting communities. The fact that we now have a TV Show and other community collaborations was not a pre-planned dissemination strategy, it came about because we were willing to offer a platform for community members to truly become co-creators while we went about developing the research. May our communities find joy in your work as a researcher, may their songs uplift you, may their dances fill your spirit with alofa, and may your work continue to be of service to all those you love and hold dear.

Ia manuia.

References

Crawley, L., Pulotu-Endemann, F. K., & Stanley-Findlay, R. T. U. (1995). *Strategic directions for the mental health services for Pacific Islands people.* Ministry of Health.

Durie, M. (1994). *Whaiora: Māori health development*. Oxford University Press.

English Standard Version Bible. (2001). ESV Online. https://esv.literalword.com/

Godfrey, D. (2021, April 27). New project looks at the challenges for Aotearoa's Pasifika Rainbow communities. *Radio New Zealand*. https://www.rnz.co.nz/international/pacific-news/441287/new-project-looks-at-the-challenges-for-aotearoa-s-pasifika-rainbow-communities

Health Research Council of New Zealand. (2014). *Pacific Health Guidelines 2014*. https://www.hrc.govt.nz/sites/default/files/2019-05/Resource%20Library%20PDF%20-%20Pacific%20Health%20Research%20Guidelines%202014_0.pdf

Hepi, M., Foote, J., Marino, M., Rogers, M., & Taimona, H. (2007). "Koe wai hoki koe?!", or "Who are you?!": Issues of trust in cross-cultural collaborative research. *Kōtuitui: New Zealand Journal of Social Sciences Online*, *2*(2), 37–53. https://doi.org/10.1080/1177083X.2007.9522423

Manuela, S., & Sibley, C. G. (2014). Why Do Pacific People with Multiple Ethnic Affiliations Have Poorer Subjective Wellbeing? Negative Ingroup Affect Mediates the Identity Tension Effect. *Social Indicators Research*, *115*(1), 319–336. https://doi.org/10.1007/s11205-012-0220-8

Ponton, V. (2018). Utilizing Pacific Methodologies as Inclusive Practice. *SAGE Open*, *8*(3), 215824401879296. https://doi.org/10.1177/2158244018792962

Prior, K. (2017, November 21). We're Here, We're Queer, We're Going Nowhere: FAFSWAG at The Basement in 2017. *Pantograph Punch*. https://www.pantograph-punch.com/posts/fafswag-at-the-basement

Queen's Birthday Honours 2019: The full list. (2019, June 3). *NZ Herald*. https://www.nzherald.co.nz/nz/queens-birthday-honours-2019-the-full-list/J5EDS75BOMRHS5ZGK2YYIOR5QM/

Ryan, D., Grey, C., & Mischewski, B. (2019). *Tofa Saili: A review of evidence about health equity for Pacific Peoples in New Zealand.* Pacific Perspectives Ltd. https://www.pacificperspectives.co.nz/publications/

Ryan, J. (2021, May 31). Yuki Kihara. *Sparkkle.* https://www.sparkkle.space/interviews/yuki-kihara

Smith, L. T. (1999). *Decolonizing methodologies: Research and indigenous peoples* (1st ed.). Zed Books.

Thaman, K. H. (2003). Decolonizing Pacific Studies: Indigenous Perspectives, Knowledge, and Wisdom in Higher Education. *The Contemporary Pacific, 15*(1), 1–17. https://doi.org/10.1353/cp.2003.0032

The Governor-General of New Zealand. (n.d.). *Phylesha Brown-Acton, of Auckland, MNZM, for services to the Pacific and LGBTQI+ communities.* Office of the Governor-General. https://gg.govt.nz/file/27805

The Coconet TV. (2014, October 28). *Tau'olunga Amanaki Prescott Faletau* [Video]. YouTube. https://www.youtube.com/watch?v=rpxyhTlI0SE

Thomsen, P. (2020b, May 30). We're part of New Zealand's Pacific story. *E-Tangata.* https://e-tangata.co.nz/reflections/were-part-of-new-zealands-pacific-story/

Thomsen, P. (2020a, October 1). *There are ghosts in this place: Growing up Sāmoan and queer in 1990s South Auckland.* Museum of New Zealand Te Papa Tongarewa. https://www.tepapa.govt.nz/discover-collections/read-watch-play/history/lgbtqi-histories-aotearoa-new-zealand/there-are-ghosts

Thomsen, P. (2022) Complex Criticalities: An Introduction to Pacific Rainbow+ Communities Health and Wellbeing in Aotearoa and the Pacific. BOOK TITLE (PP. X-X). PUBLISHER. DOI (*This is a cross-reference to Chapter 8 of this book)*

Thomsen, P., & Brown-Acton, P. (2021). Manalagi Talanoa A Community-Centred Approach to Research on the Health and Wellbeing of Pacific Rainbow LGBTIQA+ MVPFAFF Communities in Aotearoa New Zealand. *Pacific Health Dialog*, *21*(7), 465–471. https://doi.org/doi.org/10.26635/phd.2021.117

Thomsen, P., Leenen-Young, M., Naepi, S., Müller, K., Manuela, S., Sisifa, S., & Baice, T. (2021a). In our own words: Pacific Early Career Academics (PECA) and Pacific knowledges in higher education pedagogical praxis. *Higher Education Research & Development*, *40*(1), 49–62. https://doi.org/10.1080/07294360.2020.1852188

Thomsen, P., McLean-Orsborn, S., Ainea, H., & Verner-Pula, A. (2021b). Examining the State of Health Research on Pacific Rainbow Communities in New Zealand; Literature Review. *Pacific Health Dialog*, *21*(7), 449–457. https://doi.org/10.26635/phd.2021.111

Vaioleti, T. M. (2006). Talanoa Research Methodology: A Developing Position on Pacific Research. *Waikato Journal of Education*, *12*(1), 21–34. https://doi.org/10.15663/wje.v12i1.296

Loimata Suamalie and Tapasā Mo Aiga: Wayfinding sexual violence within a Samoan diaspora aiga

Fetaui Iosefo

Paul Muamai Vui Siope

Malaeulu Leatuavao Rebekah Rimoni

Fuimaono Puasina Salanoa

Nuualii Tupaimatuna

Luse Hellen Folau

Leah Sosofa

Leata Purea

Chapter summary

This chapter provides a case study around navigating healing of sexual abuse through the Tapasā Mo Aiga framework, developed within the Samoan diaspora context in Aotearoa-New Zealand. In centring a Samoan Indigenous Reference (SIR) point, the Tapasā Mo Aiga framework provides a real-life case study of how a Samoan family was able to, and continues to, heal sexual violence within their family history. Unfolded through wayfinding and critical auto-ethnography, the chapter is offered as an opportunity to explore the power of Indigenous healing as a way to overcome the trauma of sexual violence. Content warning: this chapter discusses instances of sexual violence such as rape and molestation.

Introduction

How can an entire family recover and heal as victims of sexual violence? Loimata Suamalie (meaning Sweet Tears, is a film (Marbrook, 2020) made about our family – that surprisingly and painstakingly discovers the impossible possible. Where we trans-language Sweet Tears via Tapasā Mo Aiga (TMA) a (family compass) (Iosefo, 2020) to reinterpret our salt filled tears into Sweet Tears, that become the Sweetest Tears. In this chapter we acknowledge the guttural difficulty of discussing sexual violence and the effects/affects and ethics of this within our aiga. We position ourselves within wayfinding and critical collective autoethnography as a means to decolonise western ideologies (Smith, 2021). The aim of this chapter is to share hope with other families who have been victims of sexual violence. We hope that families recognise that they are powerful agents of change and are able to create their own aiga tapasā to saili aiga manuia (navigate through the shame and secrecy to a place of peace).

We begin this journey consolidating Wayfinding, Vā, and Critical Collaborative autoethnography as our chosen methodology. We then traverse the lived experiences of four siblings Leah, Rebekah, Paul, and mother in and through and alongside TMA in relation to sexual violence.

Wayfinding Vā ethics and critical collaborative autoethnography

According to Hoturoa Barclay Kerr (2016) Wayfinding is a method that was and is used by our ancestral Pacific voyagers who navigated across the ocean without western instruments. Sua'ali'i-Sauni (2010) affirms that being Samoan is in our bones. Therefore, we do not need western instruments to navigate who we are as Samoans instead delve deeper into our bodies beyond the surface of our epidermis, into our bones because being Samoan is in our bones. Being Samoan is entrenched and enriched in our DNA. It is within our bones that our genealogical connections become our compass for who, how, and why we are who we are as Samoans.

His Highness Tui Atua Tupua Tamasese Taisi Efi (2009) implores that Samoans are not individuals. Our genealogical connections are relational. The density of our bones are interconnected and relationally connect aiga (family) with our atunu'u pele of Samoa. Anae (2016) confirms His Highness' relational genealogical claim and asserts that there is clear distinction between western and indigenous ethics namely vā tapuia, the sacred relationality. Critical autoethnography as wayfinding takes this notion further, insisting that wayfinding is not just a way of moving and inhabiting, but also a relational practice with the earth and sky, one that is dependent upon respectful and intimate knowledge of Wayfinding (Iosefo et al., 2020). Within this chapter we demonstrate how wayfinding, va', and critical collaborative autoethnography are used to disseminate the density of what is in our bones through a Samoan Indigenous Reference (SIR) (Efi & Sua'ali'i-Sauni, 2008). The dissemination is specifically in relation to a Samoan, Pasifika family, and their experiences of sexual violence.

McRobie (2013) discuss sexual violence within Pasifika families namely Samoan and Tonga. Sexual abuse, sexual violence is a violation to the values of Pasifika. As Anae (2016) and McRobie (2013) encourage that when working with Pasifika that professionals consider and understand the difference with western ideologies and Pasifika epistemologies and ontologies of the vā and sacredness of relationships. Furthermore, we front that these stories have undergone a rigorous ethical scrutiny with our aiga ethics. The aiga ethics komiti is once again based on SIR and places the aiga as the guardians of knowledge. It is a counter to the western notions of what is ethical and who gets to speak. This praxis has been part of our genealogical relational connection with our ancestors and has continued with our aiga in the diaspora. This has been noted in academia since 2016 (Iosefo, 2016, 2018a, 2018b, 2019, 2020, 2021; Iosefo et al., 2018; and Iosefo et al., 2020).

We preface the following quote as to one of the reasons why we as a family created the TMA.

> *'E fofo le alamea le alamea'. We grew up with this saying from our parents.*
> *alamea is a poisonous starfish in Samoa. If you stand on the starfish the spikes*
> *secrete a venomous fluid into your foot. The only way to get the poison out is*
> *to turn the starfish over and place your foot onto the spongy side. The starfish*
> *then soaks up the poison. This saying 'e fofo le alamea le alamea' within our aiga is metaphorically saying that the poison of life is inevitable; however, as a family we have the capacity to also be the antidote. So collectively we pick up the poisonous starfish and turn it over. Each of us holding onto each other as the poison returns to its home. Although this method suggests you can be healed within your family, we are not promoting that this is the only way to healing; one size does not fit all. Once the poison is sucked out of the wound it still needs to be treated. The voyage to healing is a collective approach. We understand it will be tempestuous and we will be shaken with the swells of life that smash against us and we will encounter water in many forms. However, we also know that we are not alone. Transformation takes place when we wayfind forward with critical autoethnography. Collectively we are wayfinders, duty bound to see beyond the horizon, imagine the impossible, and do everything we can to make it possible.* (Iosefo, 2020, p 50)

Tapasā Mo Aiga model

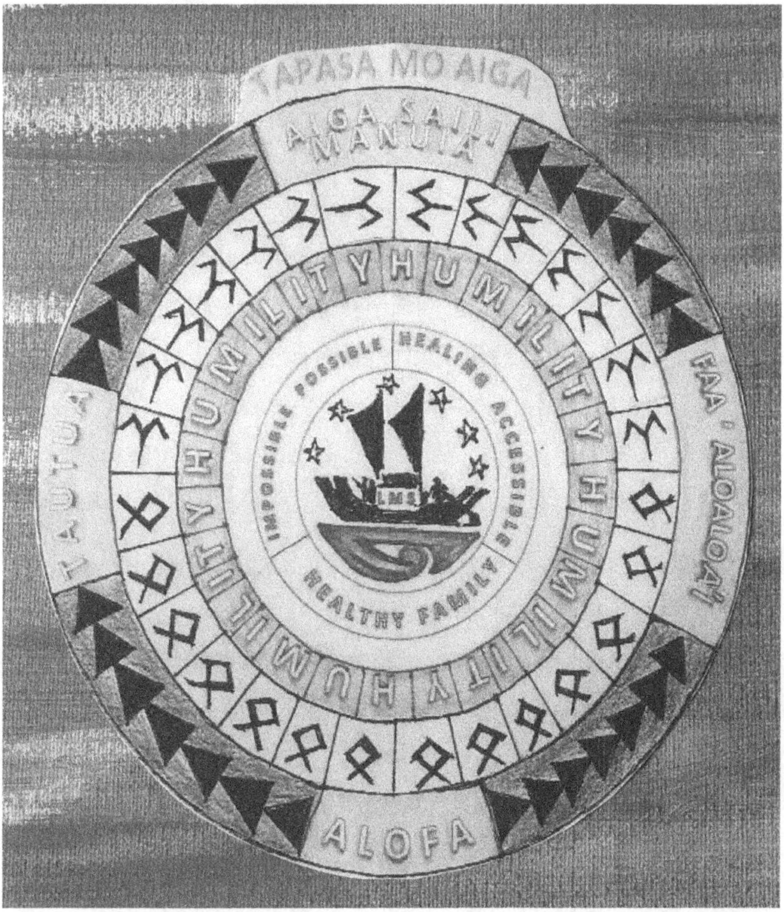

Figure Tapasā Mo Aiga: A family compass (Iosefo, 2020, p 49)

TMA is 'A Compass for Families.' This compass pays homage to the many Pasifika models that have made inroads for us to reclaim TMA, because TMA's musings and attempts to heal are extracted from the ancient wisdom of indigenous practitioners who have gone before us, and created space for our indigenous ways of knowing and being as the norm. Within TMA there are three purposes; four quadrants and seven sails. These will be further outlined and enhanced with the voices of the aiga.

Our purpose: The triadic intentions

Our sister Lilo (Fadi) was dying with cancer and she had asked us as her siblings and parents if we could help capture her life story on a film. The brevity of her life made it easy for us to prioritise and crystalise what we thought really mattered in terms of her fulfilling one of the things she had on her bucket list. But we had no idea, that filming Lilo's life story was going to unravel the sexual violence in our family.

With the pressure of death on Lilo's life and the juxtaposition of sexual violence in our family, the TMA evolved from a sympathetic intention to an empathetic purpose. The intention and purpose were organic as it was dynamic trying to respond to the reality of death and trauma. We were reluctant. Arguing in our subconscious until the intent became a solidified purpose. How do you let someone you love die with this horrific history? And if you quit, how do you live as an individual and as a family with this ugly memory? Would we allow death to creep up and hold us in the memory of sexual violence, or would we use death to bring healing to our memories of sexual violence? Our reflective and collective intention became a pulse at first in the reconstruction of our lives towards healing and wholeness in the following which was:

To make healing accessible

Each of us siblings were victims of sexual violence. Within the film, we discuss how accessing healing for sexual violence was difficult. To do any justice to Lilo's request to capture her life story on film, we had to make her wish, and her healing accessible, and in serving her and her dying wish, we accessed healing for ourselves and others.

To make the impossible possible

Between 40 and 57 years we had lived in the haunted spaces of our own memories. Would we be able to live through those haunted spaces when we would visit the places of our childhood? Admittedly, none of us felt we could have gone alone to visit any of our childhood homes to unravel the horror of sexual violence to find healing. But together could the impossible be possible? To allow the memory of sexual violence to stare at us in the visitation of these places was like suffering a second death. Could we escape that second death and how?

To make healthy structures for our families

We all knew at a certain point in the journey when the intentions became a purpose, we could not let the memories of sexual violence continue its control or limit anyone of us who was dying or living. We were to extract, analyse, reflect, talanoa, and evaluate the best we could find in our purpose to make our family (intergenerationally) healthier and safer.

Below is Leahs lived reality. Her lived experience emerges as a demonstration of the correlation of the three purposes of why and how the tapasā purposes was/is constructed.

Wayfinding, vā, purpose, and sexual violence

My journey for 53 years with sexual abuse has been a lonely journey. As a child I was sexually molested and was freed from that trauma when the offender sought me out and begged me for forgiveness in my late 20s. I believe children who are victims of sexual abuse and offenders who are children are all victims.

In my 30s I was again violated sexually and this time my world changed. I constantly felt sick, I was physically weak. I went from having my own style of dress into wearing my mum's clothes, I wore her thick hideous pale baggy pantyhose to cover my legs, long loose skirts, baggy cardigans. I am close to my father and my brothers, but I couldn't have them near me. Everyone at work noticed the physical change in my dress and appearance. I went to work to occupy my mind but when work was over for the day, I found myself struggling with thoughts of suicide. My body, mind and soul were slowly being destroyed, I numbed myself with copious amounts of illegal drugs. My GP sent me to Accident Compensation Corporation (ACC) Counselling, and it was there at Counselling where I talked about sexual abuse for the first time.

After one lot of sessions with ACC I requested a 2nd lot. When both blocks of counselling were completed, I told myself I was healed. Deep down inside I felt like I needed ongoing Counselling, but I felt I couldn't ask for more and it wasn't offered. I viewed Counselling as taking a dose of antibiotics where you come right once the bottle is finished. My GP prescribed antidepressants which I chose not to take as I had a concoction of illegal drugs that I felt were sufficient. Nobody told me how to access more help and I assumed in time

I would come right like I had in my 20s. When things got bad, I would go home to my parents and would seek my Dads advice in regard to my addiction with drugs, my failed relationships but never once did I speak to him or my mum about the sexual abuse.

As I embarked on this collective journey with my family, I truly believed that I had done all the work I needed to be healed from sexual abuse. I was 53, had quit drugs, had a meditational prayer life, had worked through my thoughts of suicide, attended healing workshops and over the years had found comfort in my parents' recliner where I often sought their wisdom and counselling. I felt all my hang ups I had in my 30s had been dealt with. It became evident very quickly in the beginning of our collective journey as a family that the remnants of sexual abuse were still embedded deep within me. After each visit into our past, after each talanoa I felt like hooks that I never knew were in me were being released from me physically and mentally. In retrospect had healing been accessible, and I had role models where I saw the impossible be possible happen (talanoa about sexual violence within our family) had healing been truly focussed on connecting our SIR to our diaspora identities within Aotearoa then maybe I would, we would not have suffered in silent shame.

Our principled quadrant: A family specific compass

We discovered the triadic intentions in our purpose needed non-negotiable indicators to give us some sense of location and direction while unravelling the memory of sexual violence. Central to our process was Lilo's request of us and presence of our Samoan parents. We had each explored many ways to healing but at this junction the elements demanded a different approach for us as family. We gravitated to integrate four indigenous Samoan values taught to us in our childhood and modelled for us by our parents. The following indigenous values were used to label four points on our Family compass:

Our True North 'Aiga Saili Manuia.'

'Aiga' means 'family.' 'Saili' means to 'seek, look, search,' while 'manuia' means, 'blessing, prosperity, benefit.' In other words: 'A Family in Search of a Blessing.' This term is also interpreted at a family in search of peace (Iosefo, 2020)

Our Eastern Vā 'Va' Faa'aloaloa'i'

Our Va' faa'aloaloa'i, means to tangibly care, honour, and respect your relationships with the best expression and means available.

Our Southern Vā 'Alofa'

Alofa means to love conceptually and concretely. Love encompasses the TMA unless there is love in the way we speak the way we hold ourselves then there is no TMA. Love holds us duty bound to custodians of SIR in love.

Our Western Vā 'Tautua'

which means to serve others. There are shades of meaning when it comes to the kinds of service. 'Tautua afu' to sweat in service; 'Tautua mata vela' to serve in the face of intense heat over a umu; 'Tautua toto' to serve by shedding your blood; 'Tautua oti' to serve by sacrificing your life.

Each of these points on the family compass locate where we as a collective or as an individual might be in terms of sexual violence, and where we or as an individual might be travelling in terms of healing. The labelled location and the anticipated point of travel towards healing still have an oceanic vā between points of sexual violence trauma that we had to carefully navigate. Like any compass the quadrants informs the recipients, but it does not give the details as to the environmental data, the cost for the journey or help with the baggage. How do you, or your family travel an oceanic gap from one point to the next? How do you read and relate to the internal and external environments on arrival? How do you cope with the changing seasons, and how do you carry this baggage of sexual violence successfully to find healing? The carriers of sexual violence baggage are not isolated from the physical victims of sexual violence; rather it effects/affects the family at large and eventually the greater society.

Below is Rebekah's lived experience as a sibling that was not sexually violated however, nonetheless she was still a victim:

Wayfinding the quadrants through my siblings

> *Sitting in silence and shame, I listened to Fadi [Lilo] calmly facilitate the sexual abuse she experienced as a child, then Fetaui also affirmed that she too had suffered similar traumatic sexual violence and expressed feeling resentment towards us older siblings for leaving home and not taking the perpetrators away. My anxiety levels heightened feeling horrendous; failure to protect my younger siblings, neglecting to confront the perpetrators. I continued to blame myself for being numb/dumb with unspoken and unresolved issues, suppressing horrific memories and living in denial. The guilt began to ravage the insides of me. I craved for my family to find peace and feel loved. I thought*

> *I had served my family and protected them. Yet hearing my sisters and brother share about sexual violence left me bereft. Through osmosis with hearing the talanoa of the sexual violence that had occurred with my siblings affected me I wept for days and still do. However, through the tapasā mo aiga process and on-going talanoa within our family, reassures me that collectively we are able to traverse through our past, present and future experiences together with unconditional love, by embracing forgiveness for self and others. The healing process is sacred and on-going to wholeness.*

Seven sails: Equitable space and process

As His Highness Tui Atua Tupua Tamasese Taisi Efi, (2005) suggests, we contemplate to unclutter the clutter. Intuitively, because of relevancy and currency we side stepped our western cluttered ways of healing to utilise the indigenous knowledge embedded linguistically in our Samoan language. Thus far within our TMA we have used three Samoan communication strategies and purposes to create the space to 'Talanoa' and four therapeutic principles to heal. Within this chapter we conclude with our seven sails. Please note that we have deliberately used Vā as the prefix for each of these terms/sails. This is deliberate so that we never forget the importance of relationality within all spaces of being Samoan, the Vā is in our bones. These sails below enable us to declutter western ideologies and traverse the oceanic gaps in the quadrant as diaspora Samoan Pasifika voyaging – from one point to the next – they are as follows:

1. Vā Soalaupule: Empowered an equitable dialogue

Vā soalaupule and the next two sails are best identified as communicative strategies to frame our conversation on sexual violence. 'Soalaupule' holds three words in one, 'soa' means to share, it subsumes a in the next word a partner 'lau' is your/s, and lastly 'pule' is authority. Ah Siu-Maliko (2015) calls it a consensual dialogue, while Lavatai (2018) develops it more fully as a method: A qualitive empirical inquiry and Kesi (2014) refers to it as a collaborative and consultative process. All of these specific interpretations and ruminations on 'soalaupule' created for us in our praxis an equitable space of equitable and equality to process our thoughts, needs, and wants for healing.

2. Vā Fealoaloa'i: Ensured healthy dignified boundaries

Va Fea'aloaloa'i helped us to understand the sacredness of spaces between people and things animate and inanimate within boundaries to be treated with dignity, honour, and respect.

3. Vā Saili Tōfā: Explore remedial/redemptive solutions

Saili Tōfā, is a commitment to wisely seek the best solution or outcome to enhance the wellbeing of the collective including the individuals. In our case there was a commitment to exploring solutions and outcomes that were remedial for our personal well-being and redemptive for our family.

On any point within the compass, the first three indigenous designed sails in the aforementioned enabled us to create a conducive environment to embark on the courageous conversation addressing sexual violence in our family.

4. Vā Faaleleiga: Establish reconciliation

The next four sails therapeutically facilitated our next steps in our journey towards healing. 'Faa'leleiga' means to make right what was wronged. Talking about the issues between ourselves was one huge achievement but the next steps was about making the choice to do something about it.

We found reconciliation existentially for us as victims was two-pronged necessitating a life time of many small and big choices, as well a life time commitment to stay reconciled with the past and the perpetrator. That is a hard sail to hoist individually, but with the cultural currency of the communication strategy and communal utility of the previous three sails already hoisted – we found the strength to hoist this new sail together.

5. Vā Feagaiga: Engage a covenant relationship

To maintain a reconciliation, we used the beautiful principle of 'Feagaiga' – a covenant relationship made up of a commitment of care, safety, and protection between us. Linguistically and culturally this concept in practice has a high currency rate in terms of its accessibility and reliability. A covenant relationship is an expression of love, if needed it prioritises the need of the other over their own need. During the journey and to date we have had to and continue to respond to each other as needed. Our indigenous understanding of 'feagaiga' enabled us to engage the memories of sexual violence, while allowing our relationships to grow in our care for each other as we became healthier and stronger survivor's.

6. Vā Taulaga Ofo: Exercise sacrificial giving

The word 'Tau' by itself has a variety of meanings 'tau' price, 'tau' pick, 'tau' fight, 'tau' weather, but in its linguistic usage as a 'taulaga' tau also means 'to arrive – tau mai' to connect with – tau atu and 'laga' means 'to bring up, to raise up, to expose and to address.' Taulaga subsumes all of these meanings and its usages in the context of relationships. While 'ofo' characterises the true nature of the offering – to be sacrificial means no demands on its expression to give, or any expectations in return.

In terms of making healing accessible, we all to some degree had to make a 'taulaga ofo' to our perpetrators, made possible, only in the spiritual realm of personal choice. To expect the perpetrators to pay for their wrongs would commodify the offence at our expense. But in the hoisting of this sail, we found a remedial way to heal and redemptive way to reform and rehabilitate the offender. The hoisting of this sail did not just involve the carrying of the traumatic baggage but the transformation of it to give ourselves and our offenders another possibility for ourselves to become.

7. Vā Faamagalo: Enabling and embrace forgiveness

Faamagalo means forgiveness. Within this one word we find five words with different shades of meaning when exegeted linguistically 'Faa'ma 'means to shame; 'Mā' means shame; 'Magalo' means to dilute what is bitter, caustic or sour in taste; 'Galo' means forgot or forget, and 'Faa'galo' means to forget. The word 'Ma' shame is centrally situated in the makeup of the word 'Faa'ma'galo' – forgiveness. To the left of 'Ma' shame is an accusative verb 'Faa'ma' – to shame, while on the right of 'Ma' is a wishing liberator in 'Galo' which means to forget. But linguistically, interesting is the combination of 'Ma-galo' which means the diluting and transforming of what is bitter, and sour in taste to a level of tolerability – but for us as a family make our 'Ma' shame – resolvable to a point where we can 'Faa'galo' forget where the 'Ma' shame held us – and in the 'Ma-galo' in the dilution – taste and remember where and how it freed us.

Wayfinding the seen/scene and unseen

There are multiple generations people who have been victims of sexual abuse. In the film Loimata, there is a scene where we are all in the lounge with our parents. This session is by far the hardest part for our parents. Our parents were never our sexual perpetrators and so for us siblings there was/is a sense of peace and security with our parents. However, despite having amazing relationships with our parents the topic of sexual abuse remained a space of shame and secrecy. Our parents journey shared in this piece is for the purposes of seeing elements of each of the sails in action. Below Paul shares as he wayfinds the scenario that was recorded and what followed.

Wayfinding the shame, silence, and hope for our Aiga

My siblings and I sat in the lounge with our parents. Four of us in our fifties, our baby sister in her forties, and Dad and Mum in their eighties. To start a seemingly impossible conversation with our Samoan parents I resorted to the indigenous best our parents had given to us as children – the principles of humility, love, service, respect, and truth telling. This is also known as soalaupule where ego is left outside and equity and equality are at the forefront. It is the chosen framed space that would help us navigate collectively forward.

Our faces were long and cold like sheets of creaseless tinfoil – hoping to breathe at least, and possibly heal, if allowed after all these years. Fadi started. 'Mum, do you remember when I told you about the sexual abuse?' No. Mum replied. 'Mum I told you'. Fadi insisted. 'I came to you and told you when it happened to me – and what happened to me'. No. I don't remember, Mum said.

Mum's reply punctured that creaseless tinfoil of hope and quickly wrinkled it into a lifeless ball of silver. How do we un-wrinkle a lost memory in Mums mind, and how do we mend a newly torn tear to our lifelong trauma?

Later that night. Fadi while fighting with cancer, was awoken by the presence of someone standing over her in the dark. Fadi sees Mums figure and hears Mums whimpering sobs while hovering over Fadi – saying, 'I remember. I remember. I'm sorry. I remember.' Fadi consoles Mum, and notices Mum is half naked. Fadi asks her about her dress then realises, Mum was depicting the way Fadi had told her when she was a girl. Repeating 'I'm sorry. I remember. I remember.'

The next morning in the lounge Mum tells us what happened. She said, 'before I slept I asked God in prayer to please help me remember what Fadi said, and then in my sleep everything came back' – 'moe manatunatu.' She wept saying, 'the reason why I could not remember was because I had prayed and asked God to help me forget what I was told.' She then turned and looked at us as if she had been transported back in time. She seemingly was reliving everything again. We saw our Mothers face of disgust, her irritable and abrupt demeanour and her voice filled with fury mixed with tears and bursts of compassion. She said – 'I wanted to kill. I wanted to finish it. To kill and finish it was easy for me to do. I just go and do it. But I thought about all of you. I would've gone to prison for murder. You all would have had no mother – your hard-working father – would've had no wife, and our whole family scattered. So, I prayed and asked God to help me to forget what I had heard. And I forgot until now. Now I want to kill. I wish I did kill. But I didn't and now I can't. I'm sorry my children. Please forgive me I am sorry.'

Fadi said, her healing in that moment was when Mum showed up half naked to prove she not only remembered when and what she was told, but how she looked when she told Mum.

When I heard Fadi's recount of Mothers empathic demonstration and saw and heard my eighty plus year old Mother's fury and passion stand up for me/us. The child in me holding that wrinkled tinfoil ball of hopelessness felt the impossible unravel in my Mother's words – we received a breathable bandage of love to heal the sexual trauma of my/our soul/s.

Continuum

This is not a conclusion but is a continuum as we understand that nothing is ever concluded.

The transparency, genuine love, acceptance, mutual respect, humility demonstrated with mum impacted us all. We all sat in awe of her vulnerability and truth telling without ego. She made this about us and not her. Mum reflected soalaupule. Her sharing deepened our understanding of vā fealoaloai and the role that vā saili tōfā has in healing. Mum being able to reconcile with Fadi (Lilo) mirrored the vā faaleleiga and she exposed the covenanted relationship that had been broken between mother and child. This scene that mum owned was her taulaga ofo for us as her children and for every generation to come. Finally, mum demonstrated what asking for forgiveness looks like vā faamagalo. Mum reflected TMA in its most sacrificial loving way has bonded us closer as a family and freed us in inexplicable ways.

The collective journey that our family continues with in regard to sexual abuse is made bearable simply because we are doing this journey together as a family. The Talanoa has and continues to be the most effective way. TMA is now our aiga praxis which all four generations are now implementing as a means of dealing with trauma. Healing as a family from sexual violence is possible. The three intentions which became a purpose is now our hope for others. To make healing accessible, to make the impossible possible and to make families healthier – by offering the TMA as another Pasifika mechanism for hope, help and healing. Forgiveness for sexual violence is essential to healing, but what we found helpful in our journey is the indigenous relevance and currency inherit in our languaging of relational values which wisely informed our communication and structural practice to heal, forgive and still be a united and healthy family. Whereas western epistemologies would of decimated and diluted the fullness that SIR frames for our aiga.

References

Ah Siu-Maliko, M. (2015). *Public Theology, Core Values and Domestic Violence in Samoan Society* [Doctoral thesis, The University of Otago]. OUR Archive. https://ourarchive.otago.ac.nz/handle/10523/5572

Anae, M. (2016). Teu le va: Samoan relational ethics. *Knowledge Cultures*, *4*(3), 117–130.

Barclay-Kerr, H. (2016). From Myth and Legend to Reality: Voyages of Rediscovery and Knowledge. In E. Emerald, R. E. Rinehart & A. Garcia (Eds.), *Global South Ethnographies* (1st ed., pp. 87–91). SensePublishers. https://doi.org/10.1007/978-94-6300-494-7_6

Efi, A. T. T. T. (2009). Bioethics and the Samoan indigenous reference. *International Social Science Journal*, *60*(195), 115–124. https://doi.org/10.1111/j.1468-2451.2009.01705.x

Efi, A. T. T. T., & Sua'ali'i-Sauni, T. (2008). *Su'esu'e manogi = In search of fragrance: Tui Atua Tupua Tamasese Ta'isi and the Samoan indigenous reference.* Centre for Samoan Studies, National University of Samoa.

Efi, T. A. T. T. T. (2005). Clutter in Indigenous Knowledge, Research and History: A Samoan Perspective. *Social Policy Journal of New Zealand*, *25*, 61–69.

Iosefo, F. (2016). Who is Eye? An Autoethnographic View on Higher Educational Spaces from a Pasifika Girl. In E. Emerald, R.E. Rinehart & A. Garcia (Eds.), *Global South Ethnographies: Minding the Senses* (1st ed., pp. 199–208). http://doi.org/10.1007/978-94-6300-494-7_16

Iosefo, F. (2018a). Scene, Seen, Unseen. In P. Stanley & G. Vass (Eds.), *Questions of Culture in Autoethnography* (1st ed., pp. 69–79). Routledge. https://doi-org/10.4324/9781315178738

Iosefo, F. (2018b). Transformer: More Than Meets the I/Eye. In S. Holman Jones & M. Pruyn (Eds.), *Creative Selves/Creative Cultures* (1st ed., pp. 183–195). Palgrave Macmillan, Cham.

Iosefo, F., Siope, L. E. T. F. V., Siope, F., & Iosefo, J. (2018). Way Finding Faasinomaga (Identity-I/Eye) in Higher Education. *Departures in Critical Qualitative Research*, *7*(4), 97–105. http://doi.org/10.1525/dcqr.2018.7.4.97

Iosefo, F. (2019). Settling the Soul through Va'(Relational) Ethics: An Ekphrastic Review of Hinekura Smith's "Whatuora: Theorizing 'New' Indigenous Methodology from 'Old' Indigenous Weaving Practice. *Art/Research International: A Transdisciplinary Journal, 4*(1), 420–424.

Iosefo, F., Harris, A., & Jones, S. H. (2020a). Wayfinding as Pasifika, indigenous and critical autoethnographic knowledge. In F. Iosefo, S. Holman Jones & A. Harris (Eds.), *Wayfinding and Critical Autoethnography* (1st ed., pp. 15–27). Routledge. http://doi.org/10.4324/9780429325410-3

Iosefo, F. (2020b). Wayfinding with aiga (family): Aiga saili manuia: Family in (re)search of peace. In F. Iosefo, S. Holman Jones & A. Harris (Eds.), *Wayfinding and Critical Autoethnography* (1st ed., pp. 38–52). Routledge.

Iosefo, F., Hawkins, H. S., & Fa'avae, D. T. M. (2021). Wayfinding the "Tapu" in Critical Autoethnography. In T. E. Adams, S. Holman Jones & C. Ellis (Eds.), *Handbook of Autoethnography* (2nd ed., pp. 483–492). Routledge.

Kesi, F. (2014). *Sailitofa: Samoan-born teachers' perspectives of ICT in Aoga Amata.* [Master's thesis, Auckland University of Technology]. Tuwhera. https://openrepository.aut.ac.nz/items/6c0b1984-7616-4112-81f5-23c70fdd21ae

Lavatai, S. F. (2018). *The Ifoga ritual in Samoa in anthropological and in biblical perspectives* [Doctoral thesis, Universität, Hamburg]. Missionshilfe Verlag, Hamburg.

Marbrook, A. (Director). (2020). *Loimata Suamalie (Sweetest tears)* [Film]. Anna Marbrook Productions.

Smith, L. T. (2021). *Decolonizing methodologies: Research and indigenous peoples* (3rd ed.). Zed Books.

Sua'ali'i-Sauni, T. (2010). "It's in your bones!": Samoan custom and discourses of certainty. *Yearbook of New Zealand Jurisprudence, 13*, 70–88.

Further reading

Agnew, F., Pulotu-Endemann, F.K., Robinson, G., Suaalii-Sauni, T., Warren, H., Wheeler, A., Erick, M., Hingano, T., & Schmidt-Sopoaga, H., (2004). *Pacific Models of Mental Health Service Delivery in New Zealand ("PMMHSD") Project*. Clinical Research and Resource Centre, Waitemata District Health Board Auckland and Health Research Council of New Zealand.

Amituanai-Toloa, M. (2006). Tapuia (Space Made Sacred) in Bridging Research and Relationships: Brown culture and commonsensical ethics. *AlterNative 3*(1), 4–17. https://doi.org/10.1177/117718010600300111

Daniell, B. (2021). *Pasifika sexual violence workforce submission on the National strategy for family violence and sexual violence presented to Joint Venture, Ministry of Justice on 30 June 2021*. TOAH-NNEST Te Ohaakii a Hine-National Network Ending Sexual Violence Together Pacific Steering Group.

Kingi V., & Jordan, J. (2009). *Responding to sexual violence: pathways to recovery*. Ministry of Women's Affairs.

McRobie, S. (2016). Working with Pacific survivors of sexual violence. Good practice guidelines for mainstream support services for survivors. In Wharewera-Mika, J., & McPhillips, K. (2016). TOAH-NNEST Good Practice responding to sexual violence in Aotearoa. Good practice guidelines responding to sexual violence. Te Ohaaki a Hine National Network Ending Sexual Violence Together. New Zealand. http://www.toahnnestgoodpractice.org and http://www.communityresearch.org.nz/wp-content/uploads/formidable/Good-Practice-Responding-to-Sexual-Violence-Crisis-Support-Services-2016-with-Reports.pdf

Notes

Complex criticalities

1. These projects include Counting Ourselves, Honour Project Aotearoa, Identify Survey and the Manalagi Project, see also Veale et al., 2019; Pihama et al., 2020; https://www.identifysur vey.nz/; https://www.manalagi.org/.
2. Although Le Vā has a published resources on their website that dates to 2014 of another of Phylesha Brown-Acton's speeches where she explains the origins of MVPFAFF+, in personal communications, Brown-Acton has commented on the importance of acknowledging that the term came from consultations and input from all Pacific advocates and delegates at this specific conference. She suggests that they must also be recognised, which is why it is important to reference the first time the speech was delivered.
3. Crenshaw's example demonstrated how US law does not see Black women as women, as the category woman was constructed with the White women archetype in mind; and does not see Black women as central to the Black antiracist struggle, because the archetype in that movement is Black men. This means that Black women were often erased from both narratives and struggle, allowing them to continue to experience multiple forms of discrimination from many aspects of society that does not see them as priority group with their own specific needs and concerns separated from the wider groups they are collapsed within.

Fonua Ola

1. Pacific peoples refer to the Indigenous and original inhabitants of island nations of Moana or the Pacific Ocean. Some of

them migrated to New Zealand over the years. These migrants and their descendants are also referred to as Pacific peoples.

2. Moana is one of the Indigenous names of what is now known as the Pacific Ocean. Māori, the Indigenous peoples of Aotearoa New Zealand, refer to Moana as 'Moana-Nui-a-Kiwa,' the Big Ocean of Kiwa, a legendary Māori navigator.

3. Address at Columbia University, New York, 2 December, 2020

4. In November 2021, the COP26 climate change summit of the United Nations was held in Glasgow, Scotland.

5. Co-hosted by the Health Promotion Forum of New Zealand (HPF) and the International Union for Health Promotion and Education (IUHPE) the theme of the 23rd IUHPE World Conference on Health Promotion Conference was 'Waiora: Promoting Planetary Health and Sustainable Development for All.'

6. The Sao Paulo Declaration was launched online by the Planetary Health Alliance and the United Nations Development on 6 October, 2021.

7. Fakapotopoto is a Tongan Indigenous leadership model, (See Tu'itahi, 2009)

Healthcare horizons

1. The New Zealand Health Survey is an important data collection tool for monitoring the health of the population. The information collected is an important source of supporting evidence for health and health service policy and strategy development.

   The survey comprises a set of core questions combined with a flexible programme of rotating topic areas/modules, for instance, the first module is on health service utilisation. The survey questionnaire is administered face-to-face to one adult and one child (if any) in each selected household. A parent or legal guardian is invited to complete the survey on behalf of children under the age of 15 years.

Index

Q

R

S

T

www.ingramcontent.com/pod-product-compliance
Lightning Source LLC
Chambersburg PA
CBHW060807150926
51501CB00044B/1109
* 9 7 8 1 9 1 8 0 2 6 2 7 6 *